Workbook for

McCurnin's Clinical Textbook for Veterinary Technicians and Nurses

Eleventh Edition

ELSEVIER

Elsevier
3251 Riverport Lane
St. Louis, Missouri 63043

Notice

Practitioners and researchers must always rely on their own experience and knowledge in evaluating
and using any information, methods, compounds or experiments described herein. Because of rapid
advances in the medical sciences, in particular, independent verification of diagnoses and drug dosages
should be made. To the fullest extent of the law, no responsibility is assumed by Elsevier, authors, editors
or contributors for any injury and/or damage to persons or property as a matter of products liability,
negligence or otherwise, or from any use or operation of any methods, products, instructions, or ideas
contained in the material herein.

Previous edition copyrighted 2022, 2018, 2014 and 2010.

Content Strategist: Melissa Rawe
Senior Content Development Specialist: Kristen Helm
Publishing Services Manager: Deepthi Unni
Senior Project Manager: Kamatchi Madhavan
Cover Designer: Gopal Venkatraman

Printed in India

Last digit is the print number: 9   8   7   6   5   4   3   2   1

 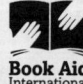

Working together
to grow libraries in
developing countries

www.elsevier.com • www.bookaid.org

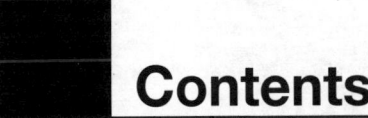

Contents

Contents

1 Introduction to Veterinary Nursing and Technology: Its Laws and Ethics

LEARNING OBJECTIVES

When you have completed this chapter, you will be able to:

1. Pronounce, define, and spell all the key terms in this chapter.
2. Describe the events from 1963 to 2019 that led to the development of modern veterinary technology in the United States and Canada.
3. Describe the educational and credentialing requirements established in most states and provinces for entry into the profession of veterinary technology.
4. Explain the structure, format, and scheduling of the Veterinary Technician National Examination (VTNE).
5. List the six features that characterize a profession.
6. Describe the five steps of the veterinary technician practice model.
7. Describe the scope of practice for veterinary technicians and list five duties performed only by veterinarians.
8. Describe areas of responsibility for veterinary technicians in clinical practice.
9. List the members of the veterinary health care team and describe their respective roles; include a list of the veterinary technician academies recognized by the National Association of Veterinary Technicians of America (NAVTA) in your definition of veterinary technician specialist.
10. Describe professional appearance, conduct, and communication.
11. Name the organizations represented by the acronyms AVMA, CVMA, CVTEA, NAVTA, AAVSB, and RVTTC and describe their roles in the education and credentialing of veterinary technicians.
12. Describe professional ethics.
13. Differentiate between statutes (laws) and regulations.
14. Describe the role of state boards in the credentialing of veterinary professionals.
15. List possible grounds for disciplinary action by state or provincial boards, list three levels of supervision defined in the NAVTA Model Rules and Regulations and describe how these levels affect the veterinary technician's scope of practice.
16. Describe steps and possible sanctions carried out during disciplinary action against a licensee.
17. Describe how laws related to labor, contracts, medical waste, controlled substances, and animals relate to the profession of veterinary technology.
18. Name and describe animal laws.

1. _____ carry out the orders of the veterinarian and perform all animal care duties except those that by law may only be performed by the veterinarian.

2. A(n) _____ may prognose, diagnose, and prescribe.

3. The _____ developed the Committee on Veterinary Technician Specialties (CVTS) to help guide and structure the development of specialties for veterinary technicians.

4. In the United States, the profession of veterinary technology, or nursing, is structured by _____ in each state.

5. The veterinary technician performs a patient _____, then prioritizes the patient's problems so that the most life-threatening issues are addressed first.

6. The veterinary technician _____ consists of five steps that are performed cyclically throughout a patient's hospitalization period.

7. The _____ is designed to evaluate the competency of entry-level veterinary technicians.

8. NAVTA has recognized 16 areas of _____ in veterinary technology.

9. Step three of the veterinary technician practice model includes establishing a series of nursing _____ to address the patient's care needs.

10. _____ are responsible for assisting the veterinary technician and the veterinarian by restraining animals, setting up equipment and supplies, cleaning and maintaining practice and laboratory facilities, and feeding and exercising patients.

11. Anything an employee develops while in the course of employment is covered under _____law.

EXERCISE 1.2 MATCHING #1: ACRONYMS RELATED TO ASSOCIATIONS, AGENCIES, AND COMMITTEES

Instructions: Match each acronym in column A with the corresponding description in column B by writing the appropriate letter in the space provided.

Column A

1. _____ AALAS
2. _____ CVMA
3. _____ AAVSB
4. _____ RVTTC
5. _____ ACC
6. _____ CALAS
7. _____ IACUC
8. _____ AVTE
9. _____ CVTEA
10. _____ US FWS
11. _____ AVMA

Column B

A. The committee that accredits veterinary technology programs in the United States under the auspices of the AVMA

B. A Canadian association that has established a certification program for laboratory animal technicians

C. The agency that coadministers the Endangered Species Act in the United States

D. An association dedicated to strengthening the registered veterinary technologist profession in Canada

E. An organization that accredits veterinary technology programs in Canada

F. A committee that works with research and educational institutions in the United States to help ensure compliance with and to enforce the Animal Welfare Act

G. A professional association in the United States that has established a certification program that certifies laboratory animal technicians

H. A group whose members are primarily instructors, staff, and managers of veterinary technology programs

I. The organization responsible for appointing members of the Veterinary Technician National Exam Committee (VTNE)

J. A committee that oversees the care and use of animals in education and research in Canada

K. The organization responsible for accrediting U.S. programs of veterinary technology

EXERCISE 1.3 MATCHING #2: ACRONYMS RELATED TO CERTIFICATIONS, LAWS, AND OTHER ENTITIES

Instructions: Match each acronym in column A with the corresponding description in column B by writing the appropriate letter in the space provided.

Column A

1. _____ RACE
2. _____ ALAT
3. _____ VTS
4. _____ RMLAT
5. _____ LATG
6. _____ AWA
7. _____ LAT
8. _____ VTNE
9. _____ HPA
10. _____ PES

Column B

A. The second highest level of certification for technicians caring for laboratory animals in the United States

B. A designation that a veterinary technician has the credentials to qualify as a specialist

C. The highest level of certification for technicians caring for laboratory animals in the United States

D. A program administered by the AAVSB to uphold quality standards of continuing education

E. An entity that works with the AAVSB to develop the Veterinary Technician National Exam

F. The U.S. law that requires minimum standards of care and treatment be provided for some warm-blooded animals bred for commercial sale, used in research and higher education, transported commercially, and exhibited to the public

G. A law designed to protect horses from the practice of "soring"

H. The first level of certification for technicians caring for laboratory animals

I. The highest level of certification for technicians caring for laboratory animals in Canada

J. A passing score on this test is required to practice in most states and provinces

EXERCISE 1.4 TRUE OR FALSE: COMPREHENSIVE

Instructions: Read the following statements and write "T" for true or "F" for false in the blanks provided. If the statement is false, correct the statement to make it true.

1. _____ Graduates of accredited Canadian Veterinary Technology programs are eligible for recognition in the United States.

2. _____ Most states and provinces require veterinary technicians to attend continuing education (CE) lectures and workshops to maintain licensure, certification, or registration.

3. _____ An additional 20 new questions are added to each VTNE, but these additional questions do not count toward the candidate's final score.

4. _____ Veterinary technicians are prohibited from entering drug prescriptions into the patient's record.

5. _____ According to the American Association of Veterinary State Boards (AAVSB) Veterinary Technology State Practice Act Model, a veterinary technician may provide a patient's chances of recovery to a client.

6. _____ Veterinary technicians often perform routine dental procedures.

7. _____ Routinely hospitalized patients, as well as emergency and critical care patients, should be evaluated using the same five-step systematic approach.

8. _____ Employment opportunities for veterinary technicians are expected to grow at a much faster rate than the average for all occupations.

9. _____ In order to call himself or herself a specialist, a veterinarian must be board-certified by a specialty organization.

10. _____ Because animals are often messy, uniforms are uncommon in small animal veterinary practices.

11. _____ The veterinary technician's professional apparel must include a watch with a second hand.

12. _____ The medical record is a legal document owned by the client but housed at the veterinary practice or supervising institution.

13. _____ Your e-mail address does not reflect on your level of professionalism.

14. _____ The Practice Act in most states includes a definition of the practice of veterinary medicine and veterinary technology, although in some states, the board has been left to define the practice of veterinary technology.

15. _____ The unlicensed practice of veterinary medicine is a criminal offense.

16. _____ Violations of laws or regulations may be punishable by fines or imprisonment.

17. _____ Someone convicted of crimes of moral turpitude may be denied a license to practice veterinary technology.

18. _____ Most jurisdictions require professional licensees, including veterinary technicians, to complete continuing education to renew their licenses.

19. _____ In virtually every state, a licensee may be prosecuted and disciplined for misconduct, even if the licensee's misconduct did not cause any harm to an animal.

20. _____ A veterinary technician may legally be the signatory on a document requiring the veterinarian's signature.

4

Chapter 1 **Introduction to Veterinary Nursing and Technology: Its Laws and Ethics**

21. ____ A licensee may be prosecuted and disciplined for misrepresentation, which may include telling a client that a certain treatment will cure a patient.

22. ____ A licensee may be prosecuted and disciplined for animal abuse, animal neglect, or animal cruelty.

23. ____ An unlicensed veterinarian may function as a veterinary technician.

24. ____ Any credentialed person who assists an uncredentialed person in performing tasks that the statute includes as the practice of the profession may be aiding an uncredentialed practice.

25. ____ Many states have continuing education requirements for veterinary technicians.

26. ____ If a licensee is found guilty of malpractice, the board can direct a monetary award to be paid to the animal's owner.

27. ____ The patient does not have to suffer any injury for the professional to be disciplined for malpractice.

28. ____ Veterinarians can be found negligent or guilty of malpractice because of a staff member's actions.

29. ____ Whenever a licensing board disciplines a veterinary technician for exceeding the technician's authorized scope of practice, the veterinarian responsible for supervising the technician may also be disciplined.

30. ____ When you are summoned to a disciplinary hearing by the board, the board must appoint an attorney to represent you.

31. ____ The Occupational Safety and Health Act confirms that all workers have a fundamental right to a safe workplace.

32. ____ Veterinarians are prohibited from using controlled substances in the practice of veterinary medicine.

33. ____ Private veterinary hospitals are inspected by the USDA under the Animal Welfare Act.

EXERCISE 1.5 MULTIPLE CHOICE: COMPREHENSIVE

Instructions: Circle the one correct answer to each of the following questions.

1. Which organization or agency accredits veterinary technology programs in the United States?
   a. State boards
   b. NAVTA
   c. AVMA
   d. AAHA

2. Which of the following is a recognized area of specialty for a veterinary technician?
   a. Veterinary otolaryngologist
   b. Veterinary psychologist
   c. Veterinary pulmonologist
   d. Veterinary behavior technician

3. Which organization or agency has established veterinary technician specialties?
   a. State boards
   b. NAVTA
   c. AVMA
   d. AAHA

4. What was the median annual wage veterinary technicians and technologists nationwide in 2021?
   a. $18,500
   b. $22,500
   c. $36,850
   d. $45,500

5. Approximately how many recommended and essential tasks are listed in the CVTEA handbook?
   a. 250
   b. 350
   c. 450
   d. 550

6. One of the most important duties of the veterinary technician in surgery is
   a. scrubbing the patient.
   b. washing the instruments and preparing surgical packs.
   c. placing the catheter.
   d. administering and monitoring anesthesia.

7. What is the format of the VTNE?
   a. Essay questions
   b. Multiple choice questions
   c. Short answer questions
   d. Short answer and multiple-choice questions

8. Where are the VTNEs administered?
   a. Veterinary technology schools
   b. Veterinary schools
   c. Board of Veterinary Medicine conference rooms
   d. Testing centers throughout North America

9. To whom does a veterinary technology student apply to take the VTNE?
   a. AAVSB
   b. AVMA
   c. State Board of Veterinary Medicine
   d. PES

10. Which of the following merits the highest priority in patient intervention?
    a. Chronic pain
    b. Acute pain
    c. Inadequate oxygenation
    d. Diarrhea

11. Which U.S. veterinary school awards the VMD degree rather than the DVM?
    a. University of Virginia
    b. University of Georgia
    c. Tufts University
    d. University of Pennsylvania

12. Which of the following types of organizations awards the designation of VTS (veterinary technician specialist)?
    a. An academy
    b. A college
    c. A board
    d. A society

13. Which government agency regulates the treatment of animals used in research facilities and teaching institutions?
    a. AVMA
    b. AWA (USDA)
    c. HSUS
    d. Board of Veterinary Medicine

14. How much additional training must graduate of AVMA- and CVMA-accredited programs complete in a registered facility before they are eligible for the Level 1 ALAT examination?
    a. 2 years
    b. 1 year
    c. 6 months
    d. 90 days

15. Which of these organizations wrote the veterinary technician code of ethics, the veterinary technician oath and the veterinary technician portion of the Model Practice Act?
    a. AVMA
    b. CVTEA
    c. NAVTA
    d. AALAS

16. When is National Veterinary Technician week?
    a. The first week in November
    b. The third week in October
    c. The second week in May
    d. The second week in February

17. Who has the ultimate decision-making authority over the care of an owned animal?
    a. The attending veterinarian
    b. The state
    c. The owner
    d. The veterinary technician

18. What is the overriding purpose of the Board of Veterinary Medicine?
    a. To protect the public
    b. To protect the animals
    c. To protect the veterinary profession
    d. To protect the veterinary and veterinary technology professions

19. Non-compete contracts are written to protect which of the following?
    a. The employer
    b. The employee
    c. The patient
    d. The client

20. Malpractice is also known as _____.
    a. unprofessional conduct
    b. negligence
    c. misrepresentation
    d. an illegal act

21. Conduct that increases the risk that negligence will occur, even if negligence has not yet actually occurred, is known as _____.
    a. malpractice
    b. unprofessional conduct
    c. incompetence
    d. practicing beyond the scope of veterinary medicine

22. What is considered the most severe penalty a board may impose?
    a. Revocation of a license
    b. Monetary fine
    c. Imprisonment
    d. Closing of the hospital

23. What is the term for the public censure of a licensee without suspension or probation?
   a. Ridicule
   b. Dunking
   c. Prohibition
   d. Reprimand

24. Which act establishes that USDA-registered facilities have IACUC (Institute of Animal Care and Use Committees)?
   a. Animal Welfare Act
   b. Occupational Safety Act
   c. Controlled Substance Act
   d. Medical Waste Tracking Act

25. The Horse Protection Act protects horses against which procedure?
   a. Slaughter
   b. Soring
   c. Castration without anesthesia
   d. Nerving

26. Which government agency co-enforces the Endangered Species Act?
   a. USDA
   b. DEA
   c. Commerce department
   d. FWS

EXERCISE 1.6 FILL-IN-THE-CHART: IDENTIFY LEVELS OF SUPERVISION

Use check marks to indicate which type of supervision is required in order for the licensed, registered, or certified veterinary technician to perform the following tasks.

Task	Immediate Supervision	Direct Supervision	Indirect Supervision
Euthanasia			
Intravenous catheterizations			
Dental procedures			
Inducing anesthesia			
Blood collection			
Radiography			
Applying a splint			
Handling biohazardous waste			
Dental extraction not requiring sectioning of the tooth			
Administering immunologic agents by parenteral routes			

EXERCISE 1.7 CASE STUDY: PROFESSIONAL ETHICS

1. You moved to a small town in a state that requires veterinary technicians to be licensed by the board. You secure a job in a two-veterinarian clinic; you are the only LVT in the practice and obtain a license. You spend the first week shadowing the veterinarians in the examination rooms with clients and assisting with canine and feline spays. The practices appear to provide quality medicine and surgery. The following week, you are left alone in the treatment area to collect samples, perform lab tests, and administer medications. You notice that an assistant is taking dogs and cats in and out of a room in the rear of the clinic, and when you walk in, you find someone you have not met performing castrations. When you ask the assistant about the situation, you are told that although he is not a veterinarian, he has worked at the practice for more than 25 years and has always performed neuters in the practice.

a. How should you respond to this situation?

_____

_____

_____

b. Should you say anything to the veterinarians? You are still in your probationary period.

_____

_____

_____

c. What are your legal and/or ethical responsibilities in this situation?

_____

_____

_____

_____

_____

2 Veterinary Practice Management

LEARNING OBJECTIVES

When you have completed this chapter, you will be able to:
1. Pronounce, spell, and define each of the key terms in this chapter.
2. List the terms used to describe various types of veterinary facilities.
3. List the roles and responsibilities of each member of the veterinary health care team.
4. Describe the basic flow of clients, patients, and employees through a typical veterinary hospital.
5. Outline the key elements of effectively working with clients, including the importance of communication skills, myths about communication skills, and how to diffuse the anger of difficult clients.
6. Describe the major job management functions needed to run a veterinary hospital efficiently.
7. Describe the primary components of excellent practice management.
8. List examples of stressors in the veterinary workplace and describe ways to ameliorate the effects of those stressors on veterinary personnel.
9. Describe the major areas in which veterinary practices employ internal and external marketing techniques.
10. List some of the major tasks associated with good financial management.
11. List reasons why management and financial analysis are important to the business of veterinary medicine.
12. Discuss the importance of efficient operations for practice revenue.
13. Discuss key areas in which computerization adds to the efficiency and productivity of veterinary practice.

EXERCISE 2.1 DEFINITIONS

Instructions: Define each term in your own words.

1. Hospital/Clinic: _____

_____

2. Outpatient Clinic: _____

_____

3. Strategic planning: _____

_____

4. Walk-in system: _____

_____

5. Appointment system: _____

_____

6. Mobile practice: _____

_____

7. Referral facility: _____

_____

8. AAHA: _____

_____

9. CVPM: _____

_____

10. Technician supervisor: _____

_____

11. PIMS: _____

_____

EXERCISE 2.2 MATCHING #1: KEY TERMS AND DEFINITIONS RELATED TO FINANCES

Instructions: Match each term in column A with its corresponding definition in column B by writing the appropriate letter in the space provided.

Column A

1. ____ Statement of cash flows
2. ____ Accounts receivable
3. ____ Key performance indictor
4. ____ Net income
5. ____ Revenue by category
6. ____ Budget

Column B

A. Money owed to the practice by the client for the sale of goods and services

B. A tool for managing the finances of a practice that includes estimated amounts for revenue and expenses

C. A metric used to analyze the types of services clients are choosing to receive

D. A statement reflecting the sources and uses of cash during a particular period

E. The amount of money left over after expenses are subtracted from revenue

F. A metric used by the practice to evaluate practice performance

EXERCISE 2.3 MATCHING #2: KEY TERMS AND DEFINITIONS RELATED TO VETERINARY FACILITIES

Instructions: Match each term in column A with its corresponding definition in column B by writing the appropriate letter in the space provided.

Column A

1. _____ Outpatient clinic
2. _____ Veterinary teaching hospital
3. _____ Haul-in facility
4. _____ Specialty facility
5. _____ Hospital/clinic
6. _____ Mobile practice
7. _____ Referral facility
8. _____ Emergency facility
9. _____ Center
10. _____ Mixed animal practice

Column B

A. A facility that treats both companion animals and livestock

B. A veterinary practice conducted from a vehicle with special medical or surgical facilities, or from a vehicle suitable for making house or farm calls

C. A facility in which consultative, clinical, and hospital services are rendered, and in which a large staff of basic and applied veterinary scientists perform significant research and teach professional veterinary students and house officers

D. A facility that is set up to allow large animals to be brought to the practice for examination or treatment

E. A facility in which the practice conducted typically or may include inpatient care as well as outpatient diagnostics and treatment

F. A facility in which veterinarians with a special interest in a specific species or area of veterinary medicine provide services

G. A word in the name of an animal care or veterinary facility that strongly implies an advanced depth or scope of practice

H. A facility with the primary function of receiving, treating, and monitoring emergency patients during its specified hours of operation

I. A facility in which the practice conducted may include short-term admission of patients, but where all patients are discharged at the end of the workday

J. A facility that provides services by board-certified veterinarian(s)/specialist(s)

EXERCISE 2.4 MATCHING #3: EMPLOYEE POSITIONS

Instructions: Match each job duty in column A with the title from column B of the veterinary personnel who would perform that duty (in a well-run practice) by writing the appropriate letter in the space provided. Each answer can be used more than once.

Column A

1. _____ Basic animal husbandry
2. _____ Performing surgery
3. _____ Updating client and patient information
4. _____ Animal restraint
5. _____ Making appointments
6. _____ Patient assessment
7. _____ Client education
8. _____ Completing medical record entries

Column B

A. Veterinarian
B. Veterinary technician/technologist
C. Veterinary assistant
D. Receptionist
E. Kennel attendant

EXERCISE 2.5 MATCHING #4: MARKETING

Instructions: Indicate whether each of the following activities would be considered internal marketing or external marketing by writing an "I" for internal or an "E" for external in the space provided.

1. _____Sending out vaccine reminders

2. _____Sponsoring a little league team

3. _____Personal appearance of staff

4. _____Sincere care for and concern about each client

5. _____Creating a Facebook page for the practice

6. _____Sending out newsletters

7. _____Placing an advertisement in the Yellow Pages

8. _____Full-service care

9. _____Practice app

10. _____A sign outside the practice

EXERCISE 2.6 TRUE OR FALSE: COMPREHENSIVE

Instructions: Read the following statements and write "T" for true or "F" for false in the blanks provided. If a statement is false, correct the statement to make it true.

1. _____For a veterinary practice to be successful, most of the staff will play some role related to management.

2. _____The types of staff positions needed in a practice will vary greatly depending on the size and type of the practice.

3. _____When it comes to naming veterinary facilities, the terms *hospital, clinic,* and *office* can be used interchangeably.

4. _____When it comes to delegating tasks, the best-run clinics assign tasks to the lowest paid person who can legally and competently complete the task.

5. _____In most well-run veterinary practices, job duties are performed by any staff member who is available to accomplish the task.

6. _____Pet owners who have owned pets previously usually have a good understanding of the care their pet needs.

7. _____A separate entrance and exit to the veterinary practice should be provided to make it easier for clients to enter and exit the practice.

8. _____To save time during an appointment, it is acceptable to have a client restrain his or her own pet.

9. _____If laboratory samples (e.g., blood, urine) need to be collected during an appointment, the patient should always be taken to the treatment area.

10. _____As long as clients wear the proper personal protective equipment, they can accompany their pet into the radiology suite.

11. _____Copies of all client communication documents that are sent home with the client should be kept in the medical record.

12. _____Pheromones, food enticements, and pharmacologic intervention are strategies to reduce stress for pets visiting a veterinary practice.

13. _____In a mixed-animal practice, the same examination rooms are used for large animal and small animal patients.

14. _____Many larger equine practices have a single room used for anesthetic induction and anesthetic recovery.

15. _____Job descriptions should be used for hiring new employees and for replacing existing employees.

16. _____If an applicant submits a résumé and cover letter to a practice, there is no need to have them also complete a job application.

17. _____When a practice hires a new staff member who has many years of experience from previous work at a different clinic, training is not necessary.

18. _____Stress can be caused by both positive and negative life events.

19. _____The terms *marketing* and *advertising* mean the same thing.

20. _____The main goal of external marketing is to attract new clients to the practice.

21. _____If a client does not respond to the first reminder they are sent, the practice should follow up by sending a second reminder and even a third reminder, if needed.

22. _____Digital marketing represents the most common form of advertising for veterinary practices and organizations.

23. _____Unlike in previous years, the majority of veterinary practices today are owned by corporate groups.

24. _____Pay-by-the-month wellness plans allow clients to pay a monthly amount that covers all treatment provided to their pets during the month the payment is received.

25. _____To ensure that clients pay their bills in full at the time of service, clinics should not offer payment options to clients.

26. _____If a pet is brought to the clinic with life-threatening injuries, the pet should be stabilized before a treatment plan/estimate is prepared.

27. _____Pet insurance works in a similar manner to human health insurance.

28. _____Ideally, physically counting the inventory in a veterinary practice should be done once a year.

29. _____Some veterinary practices have completely eliminated paper medical records and replaced them with electronic medical records.

Instructions: Circle the one correct answer to each of the following questions.

1. Increased competition, new technology, increasing numbers of malpractice threats, and shifting client expectations have
   a. caused many veterinary practices to go out of business.
   b. made effective management of a veterinary practice more complex.
   c. caused a significant drop in client compliance.
   d. caused many veterinary practices to hire more staff.

2. In a typical veterinary practice, the person who acts as the chief executive officer and delegates areas of responsibility is usually the
   a. financial manager.
   b. veterinarian-owner.
   c. hospital administrator.
   d. practice manager.

3. The individual typically responsible for all activities of the practice and running the hospital in conjunction with the practice's owner(s) is referred to as the
   a. office manager.
   b. practice manager.
   c. hospital administrator.
   d. associate veterinarian.

4. The best way to ensure that all of the major pieces of equipment in a veterinary practice are cleaned and maintained on a regular basis is to
   a. assign each member of the team a specific piece of equipment to clean and maintain.
   b. make sure that every member of the team takes part in equipment cleaning and maintenance during downtime.
   c. hire an outside vendor to clean and maintain the equipment, as most of it is very complex and expensive.
   d. assign one person in the practice to clean and maintain all of the equipment on a regular basis.

5. To minimize the amount of time clients have to wait in the reception area, there should be _____ examination rooms available for each veterinarian working on a particular day.
   a. one
   b. two
   c. three
   d. four

6. Placement of the laboratory and pharmacy in a central location is very important because
   a. they can be used in place of an examination room during busy periods.
   b. they are often used for examining and treating both outpatients and hospitalized patients.
   c. they are both important profit centers for the practice.
   d. this is where the material safety data sheets should be located.

7. Practices need to get the maximum use out of their storage area because
   a. this space is usually cluttered and disorganized.
   b. the practice must have enough inventory on hand to meet their clients' needs.
   c. this space typically generates very little income.
   d. it will reduce the chance that inventory becomes outdated.

8. It is more common to perform a necropsy when a large animal dies than when a small animal dies because
   a. there is a need to determine if the rest of the herd is threatened.
   b. large animals are a lot more expensive to replace than small animals.
   c. when a large animal dies, the owners are more likely to file a lawsuit against the practice.
   d. most small animal owners cannot afford to pay for a necropsy if their pet dies.

9. A client's judgment regarding the quality of medicine provided at a veterinary practice is generally based on
   a. the cost of the care provided.
   b. the amount of time the doctor spends with the patient.
   c. the health status of their pet.
   d. the level of client services.

10. One of the most common selection criteria used by clients when choosing a veterinary practice is
    a. the fees charged.
    b. the location.
    c. the number of staff.
    d. the hours of operation.

11. Complaints against veterinary practices are usually caused by
    a. long wait times in the examination room and/or reception area.
    b. the staff or DVM making a medical mistake.
    c. the fees charged.
    d. ineffective communication.

12. Forward booking is defined as
    a. booking a patient's next appointment before he or she leaves the practice.
    b. moving a confirmed appointment to a later date.
    c. completing scheduling for all appointments for set periods of time, typically two weeks to a month.
    d. setting all appointments at regular intervals, typically 20 to 30 minutes.

13. A document that is a visual representation of how authority and responsibility flow between the various areas of the practice or practice staff is called a(n)
    a. job description.
    b. business plan.
    c. organizational chart.
    d. employee manual.

14. It is best to base employee compensation on
    a. performance.
    b. seniority.
    c. experience.
    d. education.

15. One of the most important reasons for holding regular employee evaluations is to
    a. reprimand the employee for not following practice protocols.
    b. judge whether or not the employee's goals were met.
    c. determine if the employee deserves a raise.
    d. improve the employee's performance.

16. Which one of the following statements is the most accurate when it comes to describing marketing for a veterinary practice?
    a. Marketing is any effort the practice makes to increase sales and generate a profit.
    b. Marketing is any effort the practice makes to retain or obtain clients and make the practice more visible in the community.
    c. Marketing is advertising the services the practice offers using tools such as Yellow Book ads and a website.
    d. Marketing is any effort the practice makes to offer new and different products and services to existing and new clients.

17. The Occupational Safety and Health Administration
    a. does not have jurisdiction over practices with fewer than eight employees.
    b. requires annual hazard and chemical inspections.
    c. is primarily concerned with large-animal practices, particularly mobile practices.
    d. requires that all veterinary technicians and technologists receive continuing education on safety practices at least once every three years.

18. A veterinary practice's website should
    a. generate a return on investment.
    b. be developed by an outside professional.
    c. be updated frequently, on a regular basis.
    d. include a list of commonly phone-shopped fees.

19. One of the financial tasks that many practices will not do on their own is
    a. establish KPIs.
    b. determine profitability.
    c. calculate the practice's net worth.
    d. prepare a yearly tax return.

20. A financial report that lists a practice's assets and liabilities is called a(n)
    a. balance sheet.
    b. net worth statement.
    c. profit and loss statement.
    d. income statement.

21. A financial report used to evaluate the financial performance of a practice for a specified period of time is called a(n)
    a. profitability statement.
    b. cash flow statement.
    c. net revenue statement.
    d. income statement.

22. Which of the following is not typically a key performance indicator established by a practice?
    a. Average transaction charge
    b. Overtime hours
    c. Continuing education credits completed
    d. Revenue by category

23. One of the main reasons inventory management is so important in a veterinary practice is that
    a. inventory is a significant expense for a practice.
    b. inventory accounts for most of the revenue generated by a practice.
    c. extra inventory must be kept on hand to ensure the practice never runs out of anything.
    d. most items kept in inventory have a slim profit margin.

EXERCISE 2.8 CASE STUDY #1: VETERINARY PRACTICE MANAGEMENT

1. You are the head credentialed veterinary technician in a small animal private practice, and you are in charge of supervising all veterinary assistants. This role includes hiring, training, and disciplining the veterinary assistants that you supervise. The practice has only been open for one year, and business has grown steadily to the point where some members of the staff are becoming overwhelmed. Because of this, you speak to the hospital administrator about adding an additional veterinary assistant position. The hospital administrator is supportive of this idea and charges you with the task of creating a job description for the new veterinary assistant position. Create a short job description for a new veterinary assistant employee, making sure that you include all six components of a well-written job description.

_____

_____

_____

_____

_____

_____

_____

_____

_____

_____

_____

_____

_____

_____

_____

2. Now that you have a job description for the position, describe how you will attract applicants.

_____

_____

_____

_____

_____

3. You have invited several applicants for a face-to-face interview. What three things should you obtain from the applicants to give you more detailed information about the applicant's skills and experience?

    Item #1 _____

    Item #2 _____

    Item #3 _____

4. As you are preparing to interview the applicants, you make sure to review the types of questions that are illegal to ask during a job interview. Give two examples of questions that cannot be asked of an applicant during a job interview.

_____

_____

_____

_____

5. After going through the application and interview process, a decision was made to hire Lilly Rainsworth as the new veterinary assistant. What training must Lilly undergo as a new employee?

_____

_____

_____

_____

_____

_____

Cutie, a 12-year-old, female, spayed poodle mix was presented for a dental cleaning. A minimum patient database was acquired, and Cutie was prepared for the dental cleaning in a routine manner. The dental cleaning was performed, and during the course of the procedure, 15 teeth had to be extracted because of advanced periodontal disease. The client was not informed prior to the procedure because the possibility of extractions was discussed at the preop interview.

When the owner was notified of the number of teeth that were extracted, he became agitated and very angry, and said, "Great! Now she will never be able to eat normally! It is all your fault!"

1. What could you do to diffuse this client's anger in this situation?

_____

_____

_____

_____

_____

_____

3 Veterinary Medical Records

LEARNING OBJECTIVES

When you have completed this chapter, you will be able to:
1. Pronounce, define, and spell all key terms within this chapter.
2. Describe the key principles of the medical record's function.
3. List and describe the primary and secondary purposes of the medical record.
4. Explain the legal issues related to ownership of medical records, release of medical information, and maintenance of medical records.
5. Describe methods for formatting medical records and explain their respective advantages and disadvantages.
6. List and describe each problem-oriented veterinary medical record (POVMR) component.
7. Explain each portion of the veterinary technician SOAP note, the types of information included in each portion, and describe how each portion correlates to the steps in the veterinary technician practice model (presented in Chapter 1).
8. Describe the importance of cage cards, discharge instructions, discharge summary and medication administration/order record (MAOR) forms and why they are valuable in organizing the care of hospitalized veterinary patients.
9. Explain the advantages and disadvantages of electronic medical record keeping.
10. Compare and contrast the types of filing systems commonly used for paper medical records.
11. List and describe the types of forms and logs commonly used in veterinary practice.
12. Describe methods for collecting and storing medical information in ambulatory veterinary medical practices.
13. Locate your state's record keeping and retention requirements.

EXERCISE 3.1 FILL-IN-THE-BLANK: KEY TERMS AND DEFINITIONS

Instructions: Fill in each of the spaces provided with the missing key term or definition that completes the sentence. Acronyms may be used when appropriate.

1. A _____ should be maintained in such a manner that another veterinary professional could, by reading it, easily understand the case and proceed with proper care of the patient.

2. Interaction between veterinarians and their clients and patients is conducted under the_____, and medical records must be maintained for all patients with whom this relationship exists.

3. Through the use of the _____ veterinary medical record, an organized approach to clinical veterinary care is achieved, as information is grouped by problem and each problem is addressed separately.

4. The _____ veterinary medical record is a medical record format in which patient information is grouped by subject matter and clinical observations are entered as they become evident.

5. The _____ refers to the collective information that identifies an individual patient, such as the species, breed, gender, reproductive status, age, color, and distinctive markings.

6. Recorded information, such as a patient's date of birth, preventive medicine program, behavior, previous conditions, and known allergies, is included as part of the _____ in a comprehensive medical record.

7. A structured system of documenting patient evaluation and assessment in the progress notes is called the _____ format.

8. Patient information, such as presenting complaint, current medications, location and character of problems, treatment efforts, and recent changes in the environment, may be included as part of the _____ in a comprehensive medical record.

9. Major medical disorders experienced by a patient during its lifetime are included in the_____, which serves as an index to the patient's medical history.

10. Veterinary practices will often use the _____ to assist the veterinary health care team when working through current patient problems.

11. The ongoing daily management of hospitalized patients is documented in _____ so that therapeutic treatment and plans may be evaluated and adjusted accordingly.

12. Hypothermia, altered mentation, inappropriate elimination, and risk of infection are examples of _____, according to the veterinary nurse practice model.

13. To ensure that a hospitalized patient is given the treatments, diagnostic tests, and diet requested by the veterinarian, the _____, or ward treatment sheet, is used.

14. A _____ is a collection of all available information that would contribute to the diagnostic process of a patient when originally seen for a particular problem.

EXERCISE 3.2 MATCHING #1: TECHNICIAN SOAP NOTES

Instructions: Match each set of patient information with the appropriate component of technician SOAP notes by writing the appropriate letter in the space provided. Note that each answer can be used more than once.

Column A

1. _____ Temperature, weight, capillary refill time

2. _____ Awake, standing, wagging tail

3. _____ Limited daily exercise, cold compresses to injury

4. _____ Heart rate, respiratory rate, skin retraction time

5. _____ Cardiac insufficiency, hypotension, decreased perfusion

6. _____ Antibiotics prescribed, hypoallergenic diet, follow-up appointment

7. _____ Anxiety, panting, reduced mobility

8. _____ Lethargic, not eating well, lying in right lateral recumbency

Column B

A. Subjective

B. Objective

C. Assessment

D. Plan

EXERCISE 3.3 MATCHING #2: TECHNICIAN EVALUATIONS

Instructions: Match the clinical observations/assessments of a canine patient in column A with the appropriate physiologic need based on the Hierarchy of Patient's Physiologic Needs in column B.

Column A

1. _____ Bleeding gingiva, halitosis, difficulty chewing

2. _____ Body temperature of 94° F, acute abdominal pain, chemistry panel K + = 1.2 mmol/L

3. _____ Anxious, fearful, displays submissive urination

4. _____ Deep sores caused by licking and scratching at ears; owner won't use an Elizabethan collar as directed

5. _____ Restless at night, gets up slowly, pants heavily when exercised

6. _____ Dyspnea, blue mucous membranes, oxygen level 89% on pulse oximetry

7. _____ Delayed recovery of skin tenting, weak peripheral pulse, tacky mucous membranes

8. _____ Moaning frequently, reluctant to move, tail tucked between legs

9. _____ Urinating in the house, urinating more frequently, unable to hold urine overnight

Column B

A. Priority 1—Oxygenation

B. Priority 2—Critical Safety and/or Severe Pain

C. Priority 3—Hydration

D. Priority 4—Elimination

E. Priority 5—Nutrition

F. Priority 6—Noncritical Safety

G. Priority 7—Chronic Pain or Mild-Moderate Acute Pain

H. Priority 8—Activity

I. Priority 9—Utility

EXERCISE 3.4 TRUE OR FALSE: COMPREHENSIVE

Instructions: Read the following statements and write "T" for true or "F" for false in the blanks provided. If a statement is false, correct the statement to make it true.

1. _____ The medical record can be used as a legal document in a court of law and can be of critical importance in defending against malpractice suits.

2. _____ Completed consent and authorization forms provide veterinary practices with legal evidence of informed consent and can be signed by a pet owner of any age.

3. _____ Entries in written records may be corrected using correction fluid, provided the entry is signed and dated by the person who made the error, with a brief explanation of the correction.

4. _____ Only approved, standard abbreviations should be used in medical record keeping.

5. _____ Veterinary medical records are the property of the pet owner because the client purchased the veterinary services that generated the medical information.

6. _____ The owner of an animal should not be required to sign an authorization form to obtain a copy of his or her pet's record if it is only for himself or herself.

7. _____ If a veterinarian diagnoses a reportable disease, permission from the client to release the patient's record must be obtained prior to alerting local, state, and federal agencies.

8. _____ In general, the hard copy MAOR is preferred to the electronically generated one.

9. _____ The American Animal Hospital Association (AAHA) endorses the use of problem-oriented medical record keeping and insists on tis use for practices seeking AAHA certification.

10. _____ When recording physical examination results, abbreviations such as "BAR" and "WNL" should not be used because they may be interpreted differently by other veterinary health care providers.

21

11. ____The POVMR working problem list helps veterinarians and veterinary technicians think critically, identify and prioritize problems, and formulate an understanding of the patient's reactions to an illness.

12. ____Medication administration/order records should include the patient's full name, patient I.D. number and/or signalment, and any known allergies that the patient may have.

13. ____When documenting treatments on an MAOR, an "X" should be placed in the appropriate column at the time the medication is administered to the patient.

14. ____Medications given during surgical or anesthetic procedures should be entered on the MAOR along with all other medications that the patient receives.

15. ____When using the alphabetic system of medical record filing, a major disadvantage is that a client cross-reference list must be generated and maintained.

16. ____The American Animal Hospital Association requires that paper records for each patient be stored in standard letter-sized folders.

17. ____The primary medical record collection should include active records covering a three-year period (or other period established by the practice).

18. ____A recommended practice for purging files is to remove and shred all records that have been inactive for four years or more.

19. ____To ensure confidentiality and integrity, AAHA standards include the provision that the electronic medical record system automatically closes record notations after a user-specified period (maximum of 24 hours).

20. ____Consistency with paper records can be improved with use of exam forms, labels, or stamps.

21. ____A log is a hard-copy document noting specific procedures.

22. ____Two of the advantages of the numeric filing system are that fewer filing errors occur because numbers are easier to read and interpret than letters, and spelling is not a factor.

23. ____Practices must keep 12 different types of logs.

24. ____Voice recognition software can be used in the examination room, doctor's office, and/or operating room.

25. ____Although ambulatory practitioners may make handwritten notes on carbonized invoice sheets to be transcribed upon return to the office, many carry a mobile device such as a laptop or tablet to assist with record keeping.

EXERCISE 3.5 SHORT ANSWER: PROBLEM-ORIENTED VETERINARY MEDICAL RECORDS (POVMR)

Instructions: Provide a short answer to each of the following questions in the space provided.

1. In what way does the POVMR provide a more organized approach to clinical veterinary care than a SOVMR?

   _____

   _____

   _____

2. Although the POVMR includes SOAP notes that may be written by both veterinarians and veterinary technicians, the focus of their assessments is different. How does the focus of these assessments differ?

   _____

   _____

   _____

3. What are the four general components most commonly included in the POVMR?

   i. _____

   ii. _____

   iii. _____

   iv. _____

4. The working problem list is an important component of the POVMR that helps the veterinary health care teamwork through current problems. Explain the difference between the master problem list and the working problem list.

   _____

   _____

   _____

5. Why is it important that any entries in the discharge summary that indicate future care be documented accordingly, whether performed or not?

   _____

   _____

   _____

6. Ambulatory food animal and equine practitioners typically do not transport lengthy medical record files during their travels. Discuss different approaches they may use for record keeping.

_____

_____

_____

_____

_____

_____

_____

_____

7. The plan for patient care is an accumulation of interventions developed by the veterinary technician for each evaluation listed in the assessment portion of the SOAP.

a. What is the ultimate goal of developing a patient care plan?

_____

_____

_____

b. Give several examples of the general types of interventions that would be considered part of the care plan.

_____

_____

_____

8. POVMR discharge instructions provide pet owners with the information and resources to continue any prescribed homecare and monitoring of their pet. Summarize the information and procedures that should be included when discharging a hospitalized patient, so that a desirable outcome for both the patient and owner may be achieved.

_____

_____

_____

_____

_____

_____

_____

_____

4 Occupational Health and Safety in Veterinary Hospitals

LEARNING OBJECTIVES

When you have completed this chapter, you will be able to:

1. Pronounce, spell, and define all key terms in the chapter.
2. Do the following regarding safety in the veterinary hospital:
   - Explain the acronym OSHA and describe the role it plays in the development of safety programs in veterinary hospitals.
   - List the safety rights and responsibilities of veterinary hospital staff members.
   - List the safety rights and responsibilities of veterinary hospital owners and leaders.
3. List common workplace hazards in a veterinary facility, describe precautions that can be taken to reduce the risk of these hazards, and do the following:
   - Explain proper methods for lifting objects and animals.
   - List the hazards associated with the use of ethylene oxide, formalin, glutaraldehyde, anesthetic gases, and compressed gases.
   - Describe the requirements of the OSHA "right to know" law.
   - Explain the acronym SDS and describe the components of an SDS.
4. Do the following regarding medical and animal-related hazards:
   - List the hazards related to the capture and restraint of small and large animals.
   - Explain risks associated with excessive noise and methods taken to minimize these risks.
   - Describe hazards related to bathing and dipping animals and explain methods to minimize these risks.
   - Define the term *zoonotic disease* and list zoonotic and nonzoonotic diseases commonly encountered in veterinary practices.
5. Explain the importance of wearing goggles, gloves, and a surgical mask when performing dental procedures on animals.
6. List methods to minimize the risks associated with exposure to radiation, anesthetic gases, and medical waste.
7. List the equipment and supplies needed to protect veterinary personnel when handling hazardous pharmaceuticals, such as chemotherapeutic drugs, and describe methods for safely handling contaminated bedding and waste from oncology patients.

EXERCISE 4.1 MATCHING #1: KEY TERMS—INFECTIOUS AGENTS

Instructions: Match each term in column A with its corresponding definition in column B by writing the appropriate letter in the space provided.

Column A	Column B
1. _____ Giardia	A. A zoonotic viral disease that can affect any warm-blooded animal; spread by contact with saliva
2. _____ Lyme Disease	B. A condition of dogs caused by a highly infectious agent
3. _____ Panleukopenia	C. A tick-transmitted condition caused by *Borrelia burgdorferi*
4. _____ Parvoviral enteritis	D. A zoonosis that can cause hydrocephalus and mental retardation by affecting the human fetus
5. _____ Rabies	E. A protozoan; can be contracted by drinking contaminated water
6. _____ Ringworm	F. A skin condition caused by a mite of zoonotic concern
7. _____ Sarcoptic mange	G. A highly contagious viral disease that infects cats but not dogs
8. _____ Toxoplasmosis	H. A zoonotic skin condition caused by the agent *Microsporum* sp.

EXERCISE 4.2 MATCHING #2: KEY TERMS—ACRONYMS

Instructions: Match each acronym in column A with its corresponding description in column B by writing the appropriate letter in the space provided.

Column A

1. _____ CDs
2. _____ SDS
3. _____ OSHA
4. _____ PPE
5. _____ WAGs

Column B

A. Enforces federal laws that help to ensure a safe workplace for American workers

B. Risks associated with long-term exposure to these substances can be reduced by scavenging systems

C. Informational literature with additional precautions, instructions, and advice for handling specific chemical products in the workplace

D. Pharmaceutical agents used to treat cancer

E. Appropriate items that should be worn when working with hazardous materials

EXERCISE 4.3 MATCHING #3: KEY TERMS—CONDITIONS

Instructions: Match each condition in column A with the correct associated statement in column B by writing the appropriate letter in the space provided.

Column A

1. _____ Bone marrow disorders
2. _____ Cutaneous larval migrans
3. _____ Visceral larval migrans
4. _____ Diarrhea and cramping
5. _____ Toxoplasmosis

Column B

A. A zoonotic infection caused by the roundworm larvae resulting in a cyst-like growth; can result in blindness if the eye is involved.

B. A zoonotic infection caused by the hookworm parasite, characterized by red itchy lines on the skin that lengthen as the parasite moves from one part of the body to another subcutaneously.

C. A protozoal infestation that can have devastating effects on the development of a human fetus.

D. A potential risk of high-dose radiation exposure.

E. Characteristic of a zoonotic infection caused by the subclass of protozoal agents known as coccidia.

EXERCISE 4.4 MATCHING #4: CLASSIFICATION OF MEDICAL WASTE

Instructions: Match each item in column A with the appropriate classification in column B by writing "A" (for medical waste) or "B" (for normal trash) in the space provided.

Column A

1. _____ A needle used to draw blood for a heartworm test

2. _____ Waste from a patient infected with canine distemper virus

3. _____ Bloody gauze sponges used on a patient infected with brucellosis

4. _____ A bacterial culture plate used to culture *Pseudomonas* spp

5. _____ An IV catheter used to deliver a chemotherapy drug

6. _____ Tissues from a rabies suspect before receipt of test results

7. _____ Urine and feces from a patient that received a chemotherapy agent earlier in the day

8. _____ The uterus and ovaries of a patient that was spayed that day

9. _____ A scalpel blade used to remove a fatty tumor from a dog

10. _____ A blood tube used to draw blood for a thyroid hormone assay in a cat

Column B

A. Medical waste

B. Normal trash

EXERCISE 4.5 FILL-IN-THE-BLANK: COMPREHENSIVE

Instructions: Fill in each of the spaces provided with the missing word or words from the following list to complete the sentence.

Use the following key terms to fill in the blanks:

A. Ergonomic principles

B. Hazardous chemical

C. Ground-fault circuit interrupter

D. Hazardous materials plan

E. Hospital Safety Manual

F. "Right to know" law

1. Instructions on how the practice will maintain hazardous material documents and proper protective policies within the clinic should be detailed in the _____.

2. Enforced by OSHA, the _____ requires that the employee wear all appropriate PPE when handling hazardous chemicals.

3. Remember to follow sound _____ when positioning or restraining patients, especially when working with horses or food animals.

4. Safety-related policies adopted by a clinic should be found in the clinic's _____.

5. Drugs and medications are considered a type of _____.

6. When working around a wet area, any electrical appliances should be plugged into a _____.

EXERCISE 4.6 TRUE OR FALSE: COMPREHENSIVE

Instructions: Read the following statements and write "T" for true or "F" for false in the blanks provided. If a statement is false, correct the statement to make it true.

1. _____ An employee is required to admit an OSHA inspector regardless of whether the practice owner is present or not.

2. _____ It is appropriate to plug an autoclave into a surge suppressor to protect it from electrical fluctuations.

3. _____ Equipment with grounded plugs must never be used with adapters or with non-grounded extension cords.

4. _____ Flammable material should be stored a minimum of three feet from a water heater.

5. _____ Never attempt to fight a fire, regardless of its size, if you are unsure how to properly use the fire extinguisher.

6. _____ If you ever find yourself in a situation where someone demands money, drugs, or other material items while threatening your personal safety at work, do not withhold the things they demand.

7. _____ Whereas a clinic is required to provide safety equipment, it is the employee's decision whether or not to wear it.

8. _____ Water should be added to the concentrate when making a cleaning solution.

9. _____ Unless the SDS indicates otherwise, use a detergent when cleaning up a spill.

10. _____ Ethylene oxide, although a potential carcinogen, is an excellent cold sterilization solution.

11. _____ For optimal safety, an animal restrainer should focus her or his attention on the procedure being performed.

12. _____ Glutaraldehyde is a cold-sterilization solution used to sterilize instruments without the use of steam.

13. _____ The most common type of injury in the veterinary setting is animal-related.

14. _____ Noise from barking is irritating and frustrating but will not damage your hearing.

15. _____ The spray attachment on the tub should be used as an emergency eye flush because it offers more control.

16. _____ Ringworm is caused by a zoonotic parasite.

17. _____ Roundworm eggs in the soil can remain viable for long periods of time.

18. _____ Pregnant women should be advised to avoid contact with cats to prevent contracting toxoplasmosis.

19. _____ Whenever possible, store chemicals on shelves at or above eye level.

20. _____ It is possible to carry pathogens home to personal pets.

21. _____ Long-term exposure to low doses of radiation is considered relatively safe.

22. _____ Sunlight can cause false dosimetry badge readings.

23. _____ Portable x-ray units are considered less dangerous because of their limited power.

24. _____ It is permissible to dispose of used x-ray developing chemicals down the drain.

25. _____ You should wear your dosimetry badge at all times during your shift.

26. _____ The best method to reduce the amount of WAG exposure is to use a proper scavenging system.

27. _____ An absorption waste anesthetic gas scavenging canister should be checked for saturation by weighing it.

28. _____ Compressed gas cylinders can be stored anywhere in the clinic as long as they are empty.

29. _____ Used soda lime crystals should be disposed of as medical waste.

30. _____ Needles should be removed from syringes before depositing them in the sharps container to prevent overfilling.

31. _____ A biological safety cabinet should be used when preparing chemotherapy drugs.

32. _____ When raising safety concerns to your supervisor, it is best to leave the solutions to the supervisor.

33. _____ Employers are prohibited by law from removing an employee from a hazardous job based on pregnancy, potential pregnancy, or the effects of those hazards on the fetus.

34. _____ Fatigue is a factor in many workplace accidents.

35. _____ An appropriate area for eating and drinking in the veterinary practice is the reception room provided all patients are dismissed.

36. _____ A bite from a healthy animal poses no risk for rabies transmission.

EXERCISE 4.7 MULTIPLE CHOICE: COMPREHENSIVE

Instructions: Circle the one correct answer to each of the following questions.

1. Which is NOT a requirement of OSHA's "right to know" law?
   a. Employees must be informed of all chemicals to which they may be exposed.
   b. The employer must eliminate all hazards in the workplace.
   c. Employees must wear all PPE prescribed by the manufacturer.
   d. The employer must provide PPE at no cost to all employees.

2. If your clinic has more than 10 employees, you are entitled to all of the following except to
   a. see data that applies to your safety.
   b. be informed about the types of accidents that occurred in the clinic.
   c. be given information regarding other staff members.
   d. view a summary of work injuries/illnesses.

3. Which of the following is considered an acceptable method of providing clinic-specific training to employees?
   a. Staff meetings
   b. Continuing education courses
   c. On-the-job training
   d. All of the above

4. Flammable materials should always be stored at least _____ feet away from a furnace or other ignition source.
   a. 3
   b. 5
   c. 6
   d. 8

5. The _____ includes instructions for organizing and maintaining a clinic's "right to know" documents.
   a. OSHA poster
   b. Hazardous materials plan
   c. Safety data sheet
   d. Centers for Disease Control and Prevention website

6. The chemical formalin is primarily used for
   a. tissue preservation.
   b. disinfection.
   c. antisepsis.
   d. gas sterilization.

7. The most common type of injury in a veterinary clinic is
   a. strained/sprained back from improper lifting.
   b. carpal tunnel syndrome.
   c. slip and fall.
   d. animal-related.

8. The best way to protect yourself from animal-related injuries is to
   a. show you are not afraid.
   b. get training and practice.
   c. use force.
   d. try to outwit the animal.

9. A zoonotic disease that is associated with joint pain and fever is
   a. rabies.
   b. *Toxoplasmosis.*
   c. Lyme disease.
   d. *Giardiasis.*

10. _____ larva can migrate to virtually any organ and develop into visceral larval migrans.
    a. Roundworm
    b. Hookworm
    c. Protozoa
    d. Sarcoptic mange

11. *Toxoplasma* eggs sporulate and become infectious _____ after they are passed.
    a. immediately
    b. 2 to 4 hours
    c. 2 to 4 days
    d. 2 to 4 weeks

12. This parasite can cause cutaneous larval migrans in humans.
    a. Roundworm
    b. Hookworm
    c. Protozoa
    d. Sarcoptic mange

13. A zoonotic pathogen that can be acquired by drinking contaminated water is
    a. ringworm.
    b. roundworm.
    c. *Giardia.*
    d. *Toxoplasma.*

14. A pathogen found in the mouth of animals that can lead to cardiac and pulmonary problems in both humans and animals is
    a. *Pasteurella multocida.*
    b. *Escherichia coli.*
    c. *Toxoplasma gondii.*
    d. *Borrelia burgdorferi.*

15. When taking a diagnostic radiograph, the x-ray beam should be collimated to
    a. the size of the whole area of interest.
    b. the size of the cassette.
    c. an area larger than the size of the cassette.
    d. an area smaller than the size of the cassette.

16. When taking diagnostic radiographs, the dosimetry badge should be worn
    a. on your collar under the apron.
    b. on your collar outside the apron.
    c. on the waist tie outside the apron.
    d. on your belt under the apron.

17. According to OSHA, the level of halogenated anesthetic agents in the clinical air should not exceed
    a. 2 parts per million.
    b. 2 pounds per square inch.
    c. 2 cm of water.
    d. 2%.

18. The source of the majority of anesthetic gas in the room during a procedure is
    a. animal exhalation.
    b. leaks in the endotracheal tube.
    c. leaks in the machine.
    d. improper ventilation in the room.

19. Which type of scavenging system requires weighing and replacement of components?
    a. Passive exhaust
    b. Active removal
    c. Adsorption
    d. Accumulation

20. To prevent unnecessary exposure to WAGs when recovering a patient, you should do all of the following except
    a. keep the number of recovering animals in one room to a minimum.
    b. keep your face away from the animal's face.
    c. "flush" the system before extubation.
    d. extubate the animal as quickly as possible.

21. Which of the following materials is considered hazardous?
    a. IV catheter removed after a spay procedure
    b. Bandaging from a declaw procedure
    c. Scalpel blade used for a celiotomy
    d. Blood tubes from a dog infected with parvovirus

EXERCISE 4.8 CASE STUDY #1: FIRE AND EVACUATION

It is a busy Monday morning at the hospital where you work. The phones are ringing off the hook, the doctors are in rounds, appointments are about ready to start, and the other technicians are busy treating patients. Suddenly you smell smoke and notice it is coming from the laundry area. Apparently lint has clogged the outlet hose of the clothes dryer and caught on fire from the heat generated by the dryer. Smoke is billowing out into the room, and you can see flames through the glass door of the dryer. The fire does not appear to have spread or to involve the building, and at this point you do have a means of escape.

1. List the steps you should take to ensure everyone's safety. Keep the following in mind:
   ■ Your clinic does not have an automated fire alarm system.
   ■ You know where the fire extinguishers are located and have been trained on their use.

   _____

   _____

   _____

   _____

   _____

_____

_____

_____

_____

_____

_____

_____

_____

_____

EXERCISE 4.9 CASE STUDY #2: RRIGHTS AND RESPONSIBILITIES UNDER OSHA

Monday afternoon is just as busy as the morning was *(see Case Study #1)*. You have been asked to perform a variety of diagnostic tests, treat the hospitalized patients, and prepare several patients for release. In the process of taking thoracic radiographs on a patient, you notice that the lead glove on your left hand has a hole in it. The patient you are imaging is a wiggly little terrier that is very hard to hold. You decide to take off the lead gloves so you can hold it more easily. In the process of taking the radiographs, the patient bites you on the right forefinger, producing a painful, bleeding wound.

1. Considering your rights and responsibilities under the Occupational Safety and Health Act, what are you obligated to do as an employee of the practice under these circumstances?

_____

_____

_____

2. What is your employer required to do under the Occupational Safety and Health Act?

_____

_____

_____

5 Animal Behavior

LEARNING OBJECTIVES

When you have completed this chapter, you will be able to:

1. Pronounce, spell, and define all key terms in the chapter.
2. Explain why behavior problems can be life threatening to pets.
3. Summarize the veterinary technician's role in supporting behavioral health.
4. Describe how and when learning occurs in animals.
5. Understand the mechanisms and possible applications for:
   a. Classical conditioning and counterconditioning
   b. Desensitization
   c. Operant conditioning
   d. Applied behavior analysis
6. Recognize and protect against common problems with the use of punishment.
7. Understand the role of animal development in animal behavior.
8. Describe, identify, and respond to body language signals of canine, feline, equine, bovine, and small ruminant patients.
9. Understand and counsel clients and fellow-professionals in meeting the behavioral and social needs of animals in their care.
10. Recognize how to prevent and screen for the three most common unwanted behaviors in dogs and cats.
11. Recognize common behavior concerns in equine, bovine, and small ruminant patients.
12. Identify and immediately triage behavior emergencies in canine, feline, equine, and ruminant patients.
13. Describe how patients learn in the veterinary setting, and what technicians can do to influence the learning experience.
14. Define the fundamentals of Fear Free™ Veterinary Care for canine and feline patients.
    a. Determine a numeric FAS (Fear, Anxiety, and Stress) score.
    b. Apply Considerate Approach before and during patient interactions and handling.
    c. Use Touch Gradient to create a more relaxed and safer handling experience.
    d. Describe the use of Gentle Control to stabilize and restrain patients.
    e. Describe what information should be included in Emotional Medical Records

EXERCISE 5.1 MATCHING #1: TERMS AND DEFINITIONS

Instructions: Match each term in column A with its corresponding definition in column B by writing the appropriate letter in the space provided.

Column A

1. _____ Anthropomorphism
2. _____ Touch gradient
3. _____ Antecedent
4. _____ Aggression
5. _____ Buller steer syndrome
6. _____ Conspecific
7. _____ Repetitive behavior
8. _____ Trace conditioning
9. _____ Fear Free
10. _____ Considerate approach

Column B

A. Develops when one steer repeatedly stands and tolerates mounting by other steers

B. A form of communication that is a normal part of animal behavior

C. An animal that belongs to the same species as another

D. The attribution of human characteristics to non-human animals or objects

E. A method of touching animals in a systematic and sensitive way to decrease fear, anxiety, and stress during handling

F. Methodology governing the interaction between the patient and the veterinary care team that emphasizes control of the environment

G. Actions that have no discernable function and which may be a displacement behavior as a result of captivity

H. Stimulus that precedes an unwanted behavior

I. A type of conditioning that pairs touch with food to develop a strong response over multiple short trials

J. Training and certification program using methods to reduce anxiety during veterinary care interactions

EXERCISE 5.2 MATCHING #2: TYPES OF CONDITIONING

Instructions: Match each term in column A with its corresponding statement in column B by writing the appropriate letter in the space provided.

Column A

1. _____ Classical conditioning
2. _____ Counterconditioning
3. _____ Sensitization
4. _____ Habituation
5. _____ Operant conditioning
6. _____ Reinforcement
7. _____ Unconditioned response

Column B

A. Occurs when the animal develops a stronger response over time to the same stimulus

B. Occurs when a learner associates a previously meaningless stimulus with one that already evokes a response

C. Occurs when the learner's response to the same stimulus decreases in intensity over time

D. A form of learning where consequences drive future behavior

E. Used to replace the conditioned response with a different response

F. Anything that increases the future frequency, intensity, or duration of the behavior

G. A response that is intrinsic to the animal

EXERCISE 5.3 PICTURE QUIZ: DOG AND CAT BODY LANGUAGE

Instructions: Answer the questions about each photo.

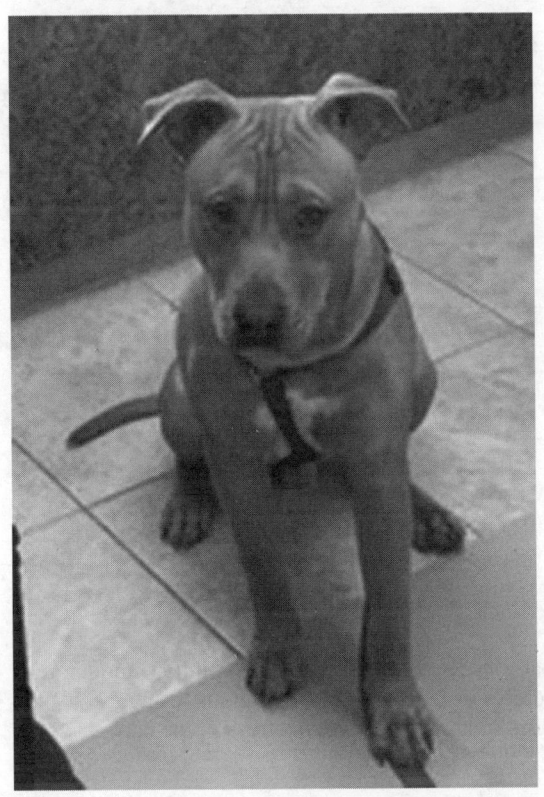

1. What stress level (relaxed, mildly, moderately, severely) does this dog's body language suggest? What factors indicate this level of stress in the dog?

_____

_____

_____

_____

_____

_____

_____

_____

_____

2. What stress level (relaxed, mildly, moderately, severely) does this dog's body language suggest? What factors indicate this level of stress in the dog?

_____

_____

_____

_____

_____

_____

_____

_____

3. What stress level (relaxed, mildly, moderately, severely) does this cat's body language suggest? What factors indicate this level of stress in the cat?

_____

_____

_____

_____

_____

4. What stress level (relaxed, mildly, moderately, severely) does this cat's body language suggest? What factors indicate this level of stress in the cat?

_____

_____

_____

_____

_____

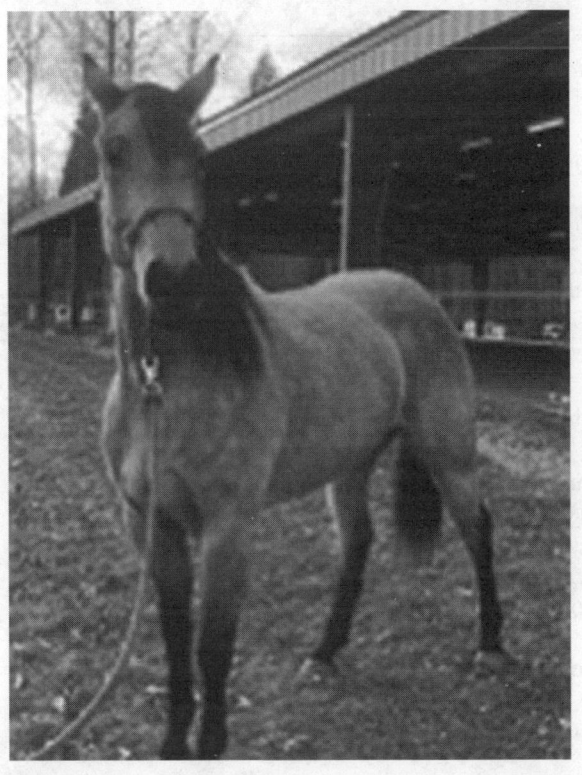

5. What stress level (relaxed, mildly, moderately, severely) does this horse's body language suggest? What factors indicate this level of stress in the horse?

_____

_____

_____

_____

_____

_____

_____

_____

_____

_____

6. What stress level (relaxed, mildly, moderately, severely) does this cow's body language suggest? What factors indicate this level of stress in the cow?

_____

_____

_____

_____

_____

_____

_____

Instructions: Read the following statements and write "T" for true or "F" for false in the blanks provided. If a statement is false, correct the statement to make it true.

1. ____ Questions about pet behavior should be included on any client history form.

2. ____ Client education about pet behavior problems is vital to preventing problems.

3. ____ A veterinary technician specialty in behavior does not currently exist.

4. ____ Keeping tactile contact with an animal can amplify the sensitivity of touch receptors (known as "wind-up").

5. ____ Punishment and negative reinforcement are the same thing.

6. ____ Some forms of aggressive behavior in dogs and cats may be preventable, particularly those related to play and related to common fears.

7. ____ The most common unwanted behaviors described by cat and dog owners who surrender their pets to shelters are unwanted elimination, destructive behavior, and aggression.

8. ____ Scratching and clawing are signs that a cat is experiencing distress.

9. ____ Only feline, canine, and equine animals require adequate clean spaces to reside, explore, and rest.

10. ____ Snorts and squeals are some vocalizations horses use to greet or call family, companions, or familiar humans.

11. ____ Used alone, medications rarely solve behavior problems.

12. ____ Research demonstrates most cats prefer fine-textured, unscented, clumping litter placed in an uncovered box with a large surface area.

13. ____ Placing a newborn ruminant's mouth on its mother's teat will almost certainly encourage it to stay latched on and stimulate nursing.

14. ____ By the juvenile period, most dogs will have resolved any fear periods.

15. ____ Kittens and puppies visiting the veterinary hospital around 7–8 weeks of age should be prosocial.

16. ____ Choke collars are a useful tool most reputable trainers employ in their work with canines.

17. ____ The best initial response to a dog exhibiting fear is to prevent its exposure to any of the things that cause the fear.

18. ____ A dog that injures itself during storms is considered a behavior emergency.

19. ____ All dog aggression is considered abnormal.

20. ____ Repetitive pawing behavior can be a desensitization behavior in horses.

21. ____ Bulls and cows both reach sexual maturity around 18 months of age.

22. ____ When feeling mildly stressed, dogs may lift a front paw or place paws on humans.

23. _____ Puppies and kittens use play fighting to gain coordination and learn social communication with conspecifics during youth.

24. _____ Management means controlling the animal's environment and experiences to avoid eliciting an unwanted behavior.

25. _____ Some of the most common tools used for positive reinforcement training in the veterinary hospital are food treats.

26. _____ It is critical to a foal's survival that it receives colostrum within several hours of birth.

27. _____ Increased heart rate, respiratory rate, blood pressure, temperature, blood glucose, and cortisol levels are immediate physiologic responses to stress.

28. _____ FAS scores range between 0 and 5, with 0 being completely relaxed and 5 often involving defensive aggression.

29. _____ Positive punishment is a fairly gentle approach to reprimanding an animal.

30. _____ A severely stressed dog may exhibit behaviors associated with learned helplessness.

31. _____ In general, negative punishment adds an element of pain or discomfort to a consequence for undesirable behavior.

32. _____ Urine marking is frequently a sign of kidney disease in dogs and cats.

33. _____ A frightened horse may injure its handler.

34. _____ Unfortunately, when horses feel threatened or fearful, they will rarely demonstrate this initially via subtle changes in body language.

35. _____ Cribbing is not seen in free-ranging horses.

36. _____ Equine aggression directed toward humans is unfortunately common and is often seen in free-ranging horses.

37. _____ Displays of aggression in small ruminants toward conspecifics or humans are usually due to fear or territorial behavior.

38. _____ Gregarious animals live in groups with others of their own species.

39. _____ Dairy bulls are notoriously aggressive toward humans.

40. _____ Historically, training techniques for horses have relied predominantly on negative reinforcement.

Instructions: Circle the one correct answer to each of the following questions.

1. Which of the following statements is not accurate?
   a. Fear and stress are adaptive.
   b. Fear and stress enhance memory consolidation.
   c. Fear and stress are more prevalent in cats than in dogs.
   d. Fear and stress decrease memory retrieval.

2. What is the term for carefully controlling a stimulus and gradually increasing its intensity?
   a. Counterconditioning
   b. Desensitization
   c. Negative reinforcement
   d. Classical conditioning

3. What type of conditioning focuses on voluntary behavior where the animal makes choices, and these choices lead to consequences?
   a. Operant conditioning
   b. Systematic desensitization
   c. Classical conditioning
   d. Habituation

4. In what type of conditioning does the learner's response to the same stimulus decrease in intensity over time?
   a. Classic conditioning
   b. Negative reinforcement
   c. Counterconditioning
   d. Habituation

5. Attempts at _____ can result in a potentially harmful sensitization response.
   a. Counterconditioning
   b. Operant conditioning
   c. Habituation
   d. Systematic desensitization

6. Giving a dog a food reward after each nail is trimmed is an example of which process?
   a. Operant conditioning
   b. Classical conditioning
   c. Flooding
   d. Systematic desensitization

7. Which of the following is classified as a tricyclic antidepressant (TCA)?
   a. Clomicalm
   b. Xanax
   c. Prozac
   d. Anipryl

8. When is the primary socialization period in puppies?
   a. 3 to 8 weeks of age
   b. 6 to 16 weeks of age
   c. 12 to 18 weeks of age
   d. 3 to 16 weeks of age

9. At what age does the socialization period start in kittens?
   a. 8 weeks
   b. 6 weeks
   c. 2 weeks
   d. 4 weeks

10. A dog in your clinic that is lip licking, yawning, and looking away from you is exhibiting behavior indicating that it is
    a. sleepy.
    b. anxious.
    c. aggressive.
    d. hungry.

11. _____ is/are the primary way our animal patients communicate with one another and with us.
    a. Vocalization
    b. Odiferous secretions
    c. Body language
    d. Aggression

12. A dog that is unable to accept food or accepts food only from its owner is showing signs that it may be
    a. full.
    b. severely stressed.
    c. aggressive.
    d. carsick.

13. If a kitten begins to bite you when playing, you should
    a. stop play immediately.
    b. give it a gentle swat on the backside.
    c. smack it on the face.
    d. throw a toy in another direction.

14. Which is not a component of the Happy Visit?
    a. Receiving treats in the parking lot
    b. Receiving treats in the lobby
    c. Receiving treats in the exam room
    d. Simulated medical care

15. What does the acronym ABC stand for in terms of behavior modification?
    a. Alert, Behavior, Consequence
    b. Alert, Behavior, Control
    c. Antecedent, Behavior, Consequence
    d. Ascertain, Behave, Control

16. Which drug is FDA-approved for the treatment of separation anxiety in dogs?
    a. Reconcile
    b. Valium
    c. Anipryl
    d. Ovaban

17. Which drug is FDA-approved for the treatment of canine cognitive dysfunction?
    a. Reconcile
    b. Valium
    c. Anipryl
    d. Ovaban

18. At what age does the primary period for socialization in the kitten occur?
    a. Weeks 2 to 7
    b. Weeks 4 to 16
    c. Weeks 8 to 10
    d. Weeks 12 to 18

19. A cat with its body hunched, ears flattened to its head, and pupils dilated is likely in which condition?
    a. Relaxed
    b. Mildly stressed
    c. Moderately stressed
    d. Severely stressed

20. A horse that moves slowly toward or away from an object or individual, or approaches after initial hesitation, is likely
    a. mildly stressed.
    b. moderately stressed.
    c. pleasantly curious.
    d. relaxed.

21. What tail position is seen in relaxed as well as moderately stressed cattle?
    a. Slowly swaying
    b. Wagging
    c. Inverted U-shape
    d. Tucked between legs

22. Stress in large animals leads to all but which of the following?
    a. Decreased quality of life
    b. More female offspring than male
    c. Lower levels of fitness
    d. Less income for agricultural businesses

23. Which of the following is a greeting call used by the horse?
    a. Snort
    b. Squeal
    c. Nicker
    d. Whinny

24. The vomeronasal organ is involved in which behavior in the horse?
    a. Aggression
    b. Olfaction
    c. Vision
    d. Touch

25. What does an out-of-context behavior mean?
    a. The animal may be stressed.
    b. The behavior occurs in a location that is not typical for the species.
    c. The animal's owner has offered an unusually attractive treat.
    d. The animal is ready to be weaned.

26. Nuzzling, licking, and close contact between a foal and its dam occur immediately after birth and continue for approximately what period of time?
    a. 24–36 hours
    b. 5–15 minutes
    c. 30–60 minutes
    d. 3–4 hours

27. Which of the following is not considered an urgent situation in large animal care?
    a. Self-harm
    b. Animal aggression toward humans
    c. Risk to human-animal bond
    d. Milking avoidance

28. Clicker or marker-based training is a technique used in which of the following?
    a. Habituation
    b. Operant conditioning
    c. Classical conditioning
    d. Counterconditioning

29. Today's management practices usually result in a foal being weaned at what age?
    a. 8 to 9 months
    b. 4 to 6 months
    c. 6 to 8 weeks
    d. 4 to 6 weeks

EXERCISE 5.6 CASE STUDY #1: HOUSETRAINING A PUPPY

Naomi Wasserman and her three children, ages 14, 8, and 6 years, have brought their 16-week-old male mixed-breed puppy, Baxter, to your veterinary clinic for his final booster vaccination. You ask how housebreaking is progressing, and Ms. Wasserman starts to cry. She tells you that she's thinking of getting rid of Baxter because he continues to poop and pee in the house. The family brought Baxter home from the shelter six weeks ago. During the day, Baxter roams the first floor of the house at will. Food and water are available in the kitchen at all times. The family lets Baxter out in the yard four times a day, including just before bedtime. When they find an accident in the house, they chastise Baxter by holding his face near the accident and yelling, "Bad dog!" At night, Baxter is closed up in the kitchen, where he has begun to chew the legs on the kitchen chairs.

1. What advice do you offer Ms. Wasserman for fixing this situation?

_____

_____

_____

_____

_____

_____

_____

_____

_____

_____

_____

_____

_____

_____

EXERCISE 5.7 CASE STUDY #2: CHOOSING A NEW PET

George Rodriguez and his partner have recently moved into an apartment and are considering adopting a pet. They come to the veterinary office to request help in deciding what kind of animal to get…or whether to get one at all. You congratulate them on taking this decision seriously and review the following questions from your practice's pet selection questionnaire with them. For each question and answer, what insight might you obtain and explore?

Example:
Question: *Have you had this animal/breed/etc. before? What was the outcome?*

Insight: *No history with this animal or breed points to the opportunity for education. Prior rehoming, surrender, or early-age euthanasia requires further investigation before recommendations.*

Question: Does everyone in the family want to adopt or purchase this animal?

Insight: _____

_____

Question: What kind of animal do you most want?

Insight: _____

_____

Question: How much time would you like to devote to grooming, exercise, and training?

Insight: _____

_____

_____

_____

_____

Question: What is the composition of your family? Adults, children, frequent visitors? High energy or low energy household?

Insight: _____

_____

_____

_____

_____

_____

Question: What is the family budget for pet care? Have you considered pet insurance or a pet care savings account? Are you familiar with the costs of training classes and any sports you might wish to try?

Insight: _____

_____

_____

_____

_____

Question: Are there any deal-breakers for you regarding a new pet?

Insight: _____

_____

_____

EXERCISE 5.8 CASE STUDY #3: THE VETERINARY NURSE'S ROLE IN SUPPORTING ANIMAL BEHAVIOR

You have agreed to meet with the college-bound daughter of a good friend. This young woman has expressed an interest in working with animals and would like to learn more about your job as a veterinary nurse. She has a particular interest in animal behavior but is under the impression that veterinary nurses are not involved in working with clients and patients on behavior issues.

1. What do you tell her about a veterinary nurse's role in supporting patient behavioral health?

    a. _____

    b. _____

    c. _____

    d. _____

    e. _____

6 Restraint and Handling of Animals

LEARNING OBJECTIVES

When you have completed this chapter, you will be able to:

1. Pronounce, spell, and define all the Key Terms in this chapter.
2. List three indications for animal restraint and describe methods for approaching dogs and cats before attempting restraint.
3. Do the following regarding canine and feline capture and restraint:
   - List the actions taken to diminish stress in dogs and cats during physical examinations and hospitalization.
   - List some of the equipment and the methods used in capturing and restraining both cooperative and uncooperative dogs and cats.
   - List the advantages and disadvantages of chemical restraint in dogs and cats.
   - Describe various positions for restraining cats and dogs, specifically for nail trimming and venipuncture of the cephalic vein.
4. Do the following regarding equine capture and restraint:
   - Explain the principles that affect equine perception and behavior.
   - Describe the physical abilities of horses and how these affect the ways in which horses are handled.
   - Describe methods for approaching and capturing adult and juvenile equine patients, including using restraint equipment, diversions, and pharmaceutical products, and identify special restraint techniques for horses and the circumstances in which they are used.
5. Do the following regarding capture and restraint of cattle:
   - Describe the principles that affect cattle behavior, and list principles used to move cattle in an effective and low-stress manner.
   - Explain the differences in housing between dairy and beef cattle and describe how these differences affect methods to handle and restrain them.
   - List the types of bulls known to be particularly dangerous to handle.
   - List the equipment used to restrain cattle in general and to restrain specific parts of their body. Also, describe the circumstances of their use.
6. Describe methods for observing and approaching swine of each gender and age group, and discuss methods used to capture and restrain adult and young pigs.
7. Do the following regarding small ruminant capture and restraint:
   - Describe the behavioral tendencies of small ruminants and explain how this influence the approach and capture of herds.
   - List the factors that affect levels of aggression in camelids and describe how aggression presents in these species.
   - Describe the approach, capture, and restraint of individual sheep, goats, and camelids.
   - List additional restraint techniques used in camelids but not in sheep or goats.
8. Describe restraint and handling techniques used with birds, small mammals, and reptiles.

EXERCISE 6.1 TERMS AND DEFINITIONS: ANIMAL RESTRAINT

Instructions: Define each term in your own words.

1. Rabies pole

   _____

   _____

2. Pig board

   _____

   _____

3. Chemical restraint

   _____

   _____

4. Diversionary restraint

   _____

   _____

5. Humane twitch

   _____

   _____

6. Manual twitch

   _____

   _____

7. Cat bag

   _____

   _____

8. Tail tie

   _____

   _____

9. Stocks

_____

_____

10. Emergency muzzle

_____

_____

11. Scruffing

_____

_____

EXERCISE 6.2 MATCHING #1: KEY TERMS AND DEFINITIONS

Instructions: Match each term in column A with its appropriate definition in column B by writing the appropriate letter in the space provided.

Column A

1. _____ FAS,

2. _____ Binocular vision

3. _____ Blind spot

4. _____ Freeze

5. _____ Defensive aggression

6. _____ Cow kick

7. _____ Fight-or-flight response

8. _____ Flight zone

9. _____ Point of balance

10. _____ Double barrel kick

11. _____ Near side

Column B

A. Vision in which both eyes are used synchronously to produce a single image

B. The name for the motion when a horse kicks straight back with both hind legs

C. A third term, in addition to fight or flight, used by some behaviorists to describe the tendency of some animals to become very still when they are nervous

D. Acronym for fear, anxiety, and stress; a numeric indicator of an animal's emotional wellbeing or lack thereof

E. An animal's personal space

F. Fear- and distress-induced defensive behavior in patients that may result in injury to handlers or the patients themselves

G. The name for the motion when a horse kicks out to the side with a back leg

H. The left side of a horse

I. Stimulation of the sympathetic nervous system in response to anxiety

J. The areas directly behind a horse, directly in front of its nose, and between its eyes

K. A specific location on an animal's anatomy from which the handler's step in either direction causes the animal to move in the opposite direction

Instructions: Match each species in column A with the technique used to restrain it in column B by writing the appropriate letter in the space provided.

Column A

1. _____ Raptors

2. _____ Hedgehogs

3. _____ Hamsters

4. _____ Lizards

5. _____ Small- to medium-size psittacine birds

6. _____ Mice

7. _____ Sugar gliders

8. _____ Nonvenomous smaller snake species

9. _____ Rabbits and chinchillas

10. _____ Gerbils

11. _____ Large psittacine birds

12. _____ Turtles

13. _____ Ferrets

Column B

A. Cover the head with a leather hood and restrain the body with jesses, leather gloves, and a towel.

B. Control the head with the thumb and index finger, being careful not to damage the large eyes. Most clinicians elect to use isoflurane immobilization.

C. Gently scruff the available skin along the neck and dorsum with the thumb and index finger and restrain the tail with the pinky finger.

D. Restrain the head and the torso with one hand and use the other hand to restrain the tibiotarsus of both legs.

E. Grasp the plastron and carapace with a sandwich-type grip with one hand and grasp the head behind the mandibles with the other hand.

F. Use a small hand towel. Inhalant isoflurane for immobilization is sometimes warranted after a small fasting period.

G. Carry like a football with the head in the crook of the arm and one arm supporting the chest and hindlimbs. It is important that the hind legs be under the control of the handler at all times.

H. Control the head at the base of the neck and wrap the animal's trunk with a towel, being careful not to restrict the thoracic wall. Maintain control of the head with one hand at all times. Slip the opposite hand and forearm under the animal's trunk to support the body and restrain the tail between the arm and body.

I. Gently scruff the dorsum of the neck, hold the body in a vertical position, and stabilize the hindlimbs with the other hand.

J. Restrain with leather gloves to avoid injury from the quills. Use of inhalant anesthesia may be needed.

K. Control the head with the thumb and middle finger, with an index finger on top of the head and the rest of hand gently encompassing the neck. Control the rest of the body with the other hand.

L. Gently cover the patient from the back with a towel and restrain the head and beak. Be careful to pay attention to respiratory rate and effort, and body temperature.

M. Control as with a hamster, being very careful not to grab the tail.

Instructions: Answer the questions about each photo.

1. Examine this technician's restraint technique of a dog. Why does she have her arms in these specific locations? What advantages do these positions afford?

   _____

   _____

   _____

   _____

   _____

   _____

   _____

   _____

   _____

   _____

   _____

   _____

   _____

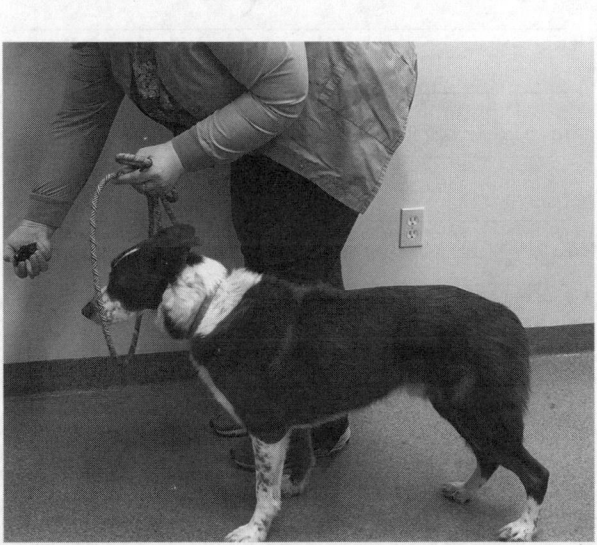

2. What is the handler attempting to do in this photo? What are the correct steps for this restraint?

   _____

   _____

   _____

   _____

   _____

   _____

   _____

   _____

3. What principles is this technician following when approaching this horse to minimize the risk of injury?

_____

_____

_____

_____

_____

_____

4. What principles is the technician following when working with this foal?

_____

_____

_____

_____

_____

_____

_____

_____

_____

_____

_____

_____

_____

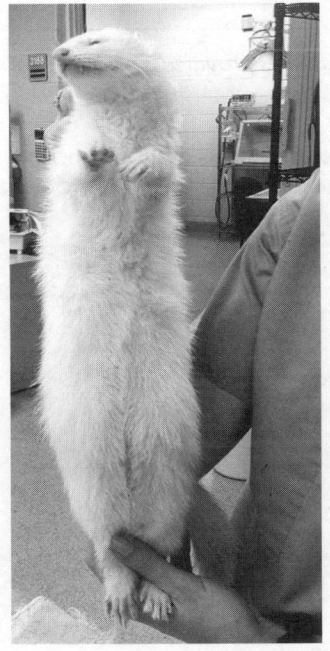

5. Describe the restraint of the animal in this photo.

_____

_____

_____

_____

_____

_____

_____

_____

_____

_____

_____

_____

_____

6. Describe the steps taken to administer oral medication to a bovine patient, as shown in this photo.

_____

_____

_____

_____

_____

_____

_____

_____

_____

_____

_____

_____

Instructions: Read the following statements and write "T" for true or "F" for false in the blanks provided. If a statement is false, correct the statement to make it true.

1. _____ Practice owners are responsible for any injuries incurred by veterinary personnel and clients during the performance of veterinary procedures.

2. _____ Only loose-knit blankets and towels should be used to restrain animals.

3. _____ Cats should be acclimated to the carrier prior to being loaded up for a visit to the veterinary clinic.

4. _____ In general, leather gloves offer the best protection when working with psittacines.

5. _____ An animal that freezes when you go to pick it up is no longer stressed.

6. _____ Cats tend to be more stressed on the examination table than in the carrier.

7. _____ A good practice is to allow animals to calm down in the waiting area prior to moving them to an examination and/or treatment area.

8. _____ A thick pheromone-infused towel may be a useful restraint device for working with cats.

9. _____ Kittens are generally harmless and are easily restrained in a veterinary clinic.

10. _____ It is better to ask for help in restraining an animal than to risk injury of either a patient or a veterinary team member.

11. _____ Because the patient often feels safest with its owner, clients should be encouraged to restrain their pets during examinations and procedures.

12. _____ Many dogs behave better with minimal restraint.

13. _____ Scruffing is the most commonly used method of restraining a cat.

14. _____ The veterinary technician should determine when chemical restraint is appropriate and which agents to use.

15. _____ Racehorses may become protective of their stalls and act aggressively when a stranger enters.

16. _____ Horses can kick with both front and hind legs.

17. _____ It is best to enter a stall quickly and grab a horse's halter before it has a chance to react.

18. _____ The best way to catch a foal is to stand between the mare and the foal.

19. _____ It is recommended that the lead rope be wrapped around the arm to help control the horse.

20. _____ It is counterproductive to attempt any procedures when the twitch is initially applied.

21. _____ The best way to restrain a foal is to place an arm around its chest and hind end and lift it off the ground.

22. _____ Dairy cattle tend to have shorter flight zones than beef cattle.

23. _____ The best way to move cattle is to herd them from behind.

24. _____ Cows do not have upper incisors.

25. _____ Herd animals such as cattle and horses are grazing, prey species.

26. _____ After the animal has been moved into a smaller pen, the first step of restraint for all small ruminant species is to control the head.

27. _____ If birds escape restraints, they may fly into windows and injure themselves.

28. _____ Birds do not have a diaphragm.

29. _____ Rabbits cannot breathe through their mouths.

30. _____ Hedgehogs are able to shoot their quills into enemies.

31. _____ Hedgehogs generate frothy sputum, which they lick onto their spines.

32. _____ Restricting the movement of an iguana's thorax will cause it to suffocate.

33. _____ Tongue depressors can be used as a protective barrier against a potential bite from a small to medium-sized turtle.

34. _____ The towel is the preferred method for restraining medium to large lizards.

EXERCISE 6.6 MULTIPLE CHOICE: COMPREHENSIVE

Instructions: Circle the one correct answer to each of the following questions.

1. Most of the aggressive behaviors seen in dogs and cats in the clinic are a result of which of the following?
   a. Dominance
   b. Fear
   c. Poor training
   d. Disease

2. When a fearful pet displays warnings as you approach its cage, the situation can be improved by doing which of the following?
   a. Backing up
   b. Feeding it
   c. Putting a snare around its neck
   d. Grabbing it with gloves

3. What can be sprayed onto towels, muzzles, and other equipment to make a dog feel more comfortable in the veterinary clinic?
   a. Citronella
   b. Doggieway
   c. Beef broth
   d. Dog-appeasing pheromone spray

4. The Air Muzzle may be especially useful with
   a. camelids.
   b. psittacines.
   c. brachycephalic dogs.
   d. turtles.

5. Care must be taken when scruffing ferrets with generalized alopecia because
   a. they can experience fur slip.
   b. they will emit a sticky froth to absorb odors from the environment.
   c. they will frequently have a brief grand mal seizure.
   d. they may experience skin bruising that will be quite noticeable after restraint.

6. The equine field of vision is almost
   a. 360 degrees.
   b. 180 degrees.
   c. 90 degrees.
   d. 60 degrees.

7. Most horses are traditionally and typically handled from which direction?
   a. Front
   b. Right side
   c. Left side
   d. Rear

8. What is the normal flight zone for a domestic horse in a field?
   a. 6 to 12 feet
   b. 10 to 30 feet
   c. 20 to 50 feet
   d. Domestic horses do not have a flight zone.

9. When capturing a yearling horse, the best initial move is to
   a. rapidly and firmly grasp the halter.
   b. establish eye contact.
   c. put a chain over its nose.
   d. squat down and scratch its withers.

10. Which is the best place to initially touch a horse?
    a. Withers
    b. Ears
    c. Muzzle
    d. Butt

11. Physical restraint of the adult equine begins with which piece of equipment?
    a. Stocks
    b. Head chute
    c. Lariat
    d. Halter

12. Which is not a part of a halter?
    a. Nose ring
    b. Noseband
    c. Throat latch
    d. Crown piece

13. What is the point of balance of a cow?
    a. Hip
    b. Head
    c. Shoulder
    d. Flank

14. The Rule of Twos means
    a. if a procedure takes more than 2 techs to perform, try a different plan.
    b. if a procedure requires more than 2 attempts, causes more than 2 seconds of intense struggling, or requires more than 2 arms on the animal to stabilize it, try a different plan.
    c. if a procedure takes more than 2 minutes and requires 2 techs, it's best to use chemical restraint if possible.
    d. it's best to have 2 of any herd animal when attempting to restrain and examine one of them.

15. Which action should not be performed as part of restraining a small ruminant?
    a. Grasping the horns of a mature goat
    b. Grabbing the wool or hair
    c. Working them in small groups
    d. Controlling the head

16. Lameness is a common disease of dairy cows and most commonly requires which treatment?
    a. Corrective shoes
    b. Casts
    c. Corrective trimming
    d. Surgery

17. Which of the following has the least herding instinct?
    a. Cattle
    b. Sheep
    c. Horses
    d. Pigs

18. Unlike ruminants, pigs have a genetic predisposition to which of the following?
    a. Anorexia nervosa
    b. Epilepsy
    c. Hyperthermia
    d. Laryngeal spasms

19. Which is the safest livestock animal to work with?
    a. Dairy cattle
    b. Swine
    c. Sheep
    d. Beef cattle

20. Ear protection is necessary when restraining which animal?
    a. Llamas
    b. Sheep
    c. Goats
    d. Pigs

21. The restraint methods of potbellied pet pigs should be similar to that used for
    a. adult farm pigs.
    b. piglets.
    c. dogs.
    d. sheep.

22. What is occurring when llamas and alpacas make a gurgling sound while being captured?
    a. Respiratory distress
    b. Getting ready to spit
    c. Diarrhea
    d. Colic

23. What are camelids doing when they "kush"?
    a. Spitting
    b. Rearing up
    c. Lying down
    d. Herding

24. The most challenging species of lizard to work with is the
    a. green iguana.
    b. gecko.
    c. bearded dragon.
    d. uromastyx.

25. What is the term for the rapid dilating and constricting of a parrot's pupils?
    a. Pinning
    b. Nystagmus
    c. Strabismus
    d. Miomydriasis

26. Being able to visualize a bird's keel while the bird is being restrained allows for the observation of
    a. body temperature.
    b. breathing.
    c. defecation.
    d. the beak.

27. With which animal are leather hoods often used as part of the restraint procedure?
    a. Macaw
    b. Ferret
    c. Alpaca
    d. Falcon

28. Which animal, if improperly restrained, can break its own back while still being held?
    a. Ferret
    b. Guinea pig
    c. Hawk
    d. Rabbit

29. Which rodent is normally most aggressive to handle?
    a. Guinea pig
    b. Ferret
    c. Hamster
    d. Mouse

30. In which animal is fur slip most likely to occur?
    a. Rabbit
    b. Gerbil
    c. Sugar glider
    d. Mouse

31. Snakes often threaten by doing which of the following?
    a. Hissing
    b. Growling
    c. Curling into a ball
    d. Spitting

32. Which of the following has a plastron?
    a. Iguana
    b. Macaw
    c. Box turtle
    d. Python

EXERCISE 6.7 CASE STUDY: RECAPTURING AN ESCAPED CAT

You are working with Troy, Mrs. Chang's newly acquired domestic short-haired cat. Troy is terrified and manages to escape into the lobby when Mrs. Chang reaches into his carrier to reassure him. What steps should be taken to capture Troy?

_____

_____

_____

_____

_____

_____

_____

_____

_____

_____

History and Physical Examination

LEARNING OBJECTIVES

When you have completed this chapter, you will be able to:
1. Pronounce, spell, and define all the key terms in this chapter.
2. Obtain an accurate and complete medical history in small animals by:
   - Explaining the role of the veterinary technician in obtaining the patient's medical history.
   - Listing questions commonly used to obtain a dog's or a cat's medical history.
   - Differentiating between an open-ended question and a leading question and why they are important.
   - Describing the type of information contained in each section of the patient's medical history for dogs and cats.
   - Explaining what a patient's signalment and mentation are and how they relate to patient assessment.
   - Listing the aspects of an animal's origin, background, and past medical history that may be relevant to a presenting complaint.
3. Describe the general procedures used to perform and document a physical examination in dogs and cats, including a subjective assessment of the patient in its surroundings and the measurement of temperature, pulse, and respiration.
4. Discuss methods for performing a comprehensive evaluation of each of the body systems in small animal species.
5. Obtain an accurate and complete medical history in large animals by:
   - Explaining the importance of determining owner/agent information.
   - Describing how the signalment and mentation of a large animal relates to patient assessment.
   - Discussing the individual history and chief complaint of the large animal.
   - Discussing the medication and treatment history.
   - Describing why the process of gathering historical information on herd health differs from taking an individual patient's history.
6. List and describe unique procedures used in the physical examination of horses and ruminants.

EXERCISE 7.1 FILL-IN-THE-BLANK: TERMS AND DEFINITIONS

Instructions: Fill in each of the spaces provided with the missing key term or definition that completes the sentence. Acronyms may be used when appropriate.

1. Significant true _____ may be present when heat-dissipating mechanisms cannot overcome excessive ambient temperatures or may occur secondary to certain drugs.

2. The acronym SOAP stands for _____.

3. A weak peripheral pulse may be caused by decreased cardiac output, also known as
_____.

4. Normally, it is not possible to palpate a dog's kidneys unless the dog is very thin or _____ is present.

5. An animal experiencing _____ will have poor perfusion and cardiac output, making this an emergency situation.

6. A lack of lung sounds in the ventral lung fields in the standing animal usually indicates_____.

7. The timing of the most recent heat cycle should be noted for all intact female dogs because _____, or purulent uterine infection, occurs most commonly two weeks to two months after a heat cycle.

8. Inspiratory crackles usually indicate _____, the presence of fluid within alveoli or interstitial spaces of the lungs.

9. The _____ lymph nodes, if palpable, will be in the subcutaneous space on the lateral aspect of the ventral thorax under the arm.

10. An inflammation of the colon, termed _____, may make obtaining a rectal temperature painful for the animal.

11. Obsessive self-grooming to the point of damaging the hair and skin is called _____.

12. _____ is the medical term for nostrils.

13. "Alert but slightly depressed" would be a subjective description of a patient's _____.

14. The _____ is the age, sex, breed, and species of a veterinary patient.

15. _____ is a congenital cardiac anomaly that results in rapid drop-off in diastolic pressure.

16. Simultaneous percussion and auscultation are used in a technique called abdominal _____, which is useful in detecting gas accumulations in the patient.

17. Decreased body temperature, or _____, usually results from impaired thermoregulation in any sick animal, especially cats.

18. "Has the urine strip been positive for sugar since your previous visit?" is an appropriate way to ask a client if she has noted _____ when performing home urine tests on the patient.

19. The absence or significant change in the quality of the pulse in the presence of an audible heartbeat is called a _____.

20. A congenital cardiac anomaly resulting in resistance to the flow of blood from the left ventricle into the aorta is known as _____.

21. Taking a rectal temperature can be made more difficult where the rectum or nearby anatomy is swollen or painful, as in cases of severe_____ or in the presence of a _____. _____.

22. _____ is an elevated body temperature usually caused by infection, inflammation, or neoplasia.

23. _____ may be auscultated during inspiration and/or expiration when air is moving through a narrowed airway.

24. A(n)_____ is one that potentially guides a client to a specific answer and can generate inaccurate historical information.

25. _____ discharge should be described in terms of amount (mild, moderate, severe) and appearance (waxy, black, hemorrhagic, purulent).

26. What you feel when palpating a pulse is called the _____ and represents the difference between systolic and diastolic arterial pressures.

EXERCISE 7.2 MATCHING #1: MEDICAL HISTORY

Instructions: Historical information can be divided into several sections. Match each statement in column A with the corresponding section of the medical history to which it belongs in column B by writing the appropriate letter in the space provided.

Column A

1. _____ I brought Winnie in today because she started vomiting about a week ago.

2. _____ Felix has no allergies to any medications as far as I am aware.

3. _____ Pepper was feeling well until last Tuesday.

4. _____ I am giving Spartacus hairball medicine twice a week.

5. _____ Bella is 3 years old and was spayed at 6 months of age.

6. _____ I don't see any change in the amount of water Max is drinking or the amount of urine in the box.

7. _____ Rocky was vomiting about once a day for a few days but is now vomiting a couple of times a day.

8. _____ Chloe got an infection 2 years ago from a cat bite and had a cold when she was a baby.

Column B

A. Signalment

B. Allergy history

C. Pertinent past medical history

D. Presenting complaint

E. Last normal

F. Progression

G. Systems review

H. Medications

EXERCISE 7.3 MATCHING #2: KEY TERMS

Instructions: Match each term in column A with its corresponding definition in column B by writing the appropriate letter in the space provided.

Column A

1. _____ Ataxia

2. _____ Anisocoria

3. _____ Pruritic

4. _____ Borborygmus

5. _____ Icterus

6. _____ Nictitating membrane

7. _____ Alopecia

8. _____ Ileus

9. _____ Costoabdominal breathing

10. _____ Excoriation

11. _____ Halitosis

12. _____ Stenotic Nares

Column B

A. A "third eyelid" that rests beneath the lower lid on the medial aspect of the orbit

B. Intestinal motility sound

C. Self-trauma caused by scratching in a pruritic animal

D. The use of thoracic and abdominal muscles to breathe

E. Foul odor to the breath

F. Uncoordinated muscle movements when walking

G. Complete absence of intestinal motility

H. Itchy

I. Hair loss

J. Yellow mucous membranes

K. Pupils of differing sizes

L. Narrow nostrils

Instructions: Read the following statements and write "T" for true or "F" for false in the blanks provided. If a statement is false, correct the statement to make it true.

1. _____ The medical record is a legal document.

2. _____ Congenital defects are more likely to be diagnosed in younger patients.

3. _____ There is no need to ask behavior-related questions when obtaining the history of a sick animal.

4. _____ Animals do not suffer from allergic reactions to medications.

5. _____ The equine insurance company and insurance agent should be noted in the medical record as they may be involved in the decision-making process for the affected animal.

6. _____ Mammary tumors are less common in dogs spayed before the first heat.

7. _____ Medical terminology should be avoided on the medical record.

8. _____ "You don't feed her table scraps, do you?" is an example of a leading question.

9. _____ The heart rate in a healthy animal should be twice the pulse rate.

10. _____ An animal in hypovolemic shock will have a strong pulse pressure.

11. _____ Gingivitis is a precursor to periodontal disease.

12. _____ The nictitating membrane is also known as the third eyelid.

13. _____ Normal tracheal airflow is turbulent, and the respiratory sounds should be loud and harsh.

14. _____ Hyperemia of the gingiva is usually caused by dehydration.

15. _____ The liver cannot be palpated in a healthy animal.

16. _____ The canine uterus cannot be palpated unless it is enlarged.

17. _____ The popliteal lymph nodes are medial to each thigh in the caudal ventral abdomen.

18. _____ All cranial nerves can be evaluated on a neurologic examination.

19. _____ The pupillary light reflex tests cranial nerves II and III.

20. _____ It is common for large animals to be attended by a person (or persons) other than the owner.

21. _____ It is acceptable to dip an animal thermometer in the horse's water bucket to provide lubrication before inserting it into the horse's rectum.

22. _____ A normal resting pulse rate in an adult horse is 16 to 26 beats per minute.

23. _____ Normal horses cannot breathe through the mouth.

24. _____ Murmurs are not uncommon in horses, although most equine murmurs are actually normal heart sounds.

25. ____ A horse's height is measured by hands, with one hand equal to six inches.

26. ____ When ruminants breathe through their mouths, it is usually considered a sign of distress or heat stress.

27. ____ Pings are normal findings when auscultating a ruminant's abdomen.

28. ____ In new patients, an effort should be made to secure medical records from previous veterinary care providers.

29. ____ SOAP stands for Subcutaneous, Ocular, Anal, Pathways

30. ____ Thermometers should be sanitized between uses.

31. ____ The terms heart rate and pulse rate mean the same thing.

EXERCISE 7.5 MULTIPLE CHOICE: COMPREHENSIVE

Instructions: Circle the one correct answer to each of the following questions.

1. Which term refers to sugar in the urine?
   a. Icterus
   b. Polyuria
   c. Glycosuria
   d. Hyperglycemia

2. What is seen in a polydipsic cat?
   a. Hypovolemia
   b. Increased drinking
   c. Ileus
   d. Increased urination

3. Which term refers to an elevated body temperature?
   a. Ileus
   b. Hypothermia
   c. Hypertension
   d. Hyperthermia

4. A cat with a body temperature of 97° F is exhibiting which of the following?
   a. Hyperthermia
   b. Hypothermia
   c. Stridor
   d. Hypovolemia

5. Which condition may cause a cat to resist having a rectal thermometer placed?
   a. Ileus
   b. Polydipsia
   c. Colitis
   d. Icterus

6. Which may be a sign of upper airway disease?
   a. Ileus
   b. Ataxia
   c. Pyometra
   d. Stertor

7. The aural temperature is taken from which site?
   a. Rectum
   b. Ear
   c. Mouth
   d. Vagina

8. From which vessel is the pulse generally taken in a dog or cat?
   a. Jugular vein
   b. Carotid artery
   c. Femoral artery
   d. Cephalic vein

9. A pulse deficit occurs in which situation?
   a. When the heart rate is less than the pulse rate
   b. When each audible heartbeat is not accompanied by a pulse wave
   c. Whenever the pulse slows down
   d. Whenever the pulse is weaker than normal

10. Which is caused by a cardiovascular problem?
    a. Glycosuria
    b. Stertor
    c. Colitis
    d. Shock

11. Which can cause a weak peripheral pulse?
    a. Hypovolemia
    b. Stertor
    c. Hypothermia
    d. Ileus

12. The rolling of the lower eyelid in toward the eye is known as
    a. ectropion.
    b. entropion.
    c. hypyon.
    d. miosis.

13. Which of the following will cause an eyeball to feel firm on palpation?
    a. Mucocele
    b. Ophthalmitis
    c. Glaucoma
    d. Retinitis

14. What is the medical term for pupils of different sizes?
    a. Heterotopic
    b. Cataract
    c. Mydriasis
    d. Anisocoria

15. Petechiation inside the pinna may be a sign of which disorder?
    a. Thrombocytopenia
    b. Otitis externa
    c. Hematoma
    d. Otitis media

16. Stenotic nares are commonly seen in
    a. aortic stenosis.
    b. brachycephalic breeds of dogs.
    c. dolichocephalic breeds .
    d. Arabian horses.

17. Which device is used for auscultation?
    a. Otoscope
    b. Ophthalmoscope
    c. X-ray machine
    d. Stethoscope

18. Which term refers to increased fluid in the thoracic cavity?
    a. Pleural effusion
    b. Colitis
    c. Pyometra
    d. Ascites

19. Capillary refill time is used to assess which condition?
    a. Anemia
    b. Dehydration
    c. Perfusion
    d. Heart rate

20. What does a respiratory sinus arrhythmia indicate in a dog?
    a. Normal cardiac function
    b. Cardiomyopathy
    c. Congestive heart failure
    d. Shock

21. What causes the jugular veins to be distended all the way up the neck?
    a. Hypotension
    b. Increased central venous pressure
    c. Dehydration
    d. Anemia

22. Which is a sign of a bacterial skin infection?
    a. A nodule
    b. Broken hairs
    c. Pustules
    d. A mass

23. What is seen in an animal that is described as obtunded?
    a. Hyperactivity
    b. Head tilt and circling
    c. Weakness in the rear end
    d. No interest in surroundings

24. Nystagmus often suggests that a lesion is located where in the patient?
    a. Vestibulocochlear nerve (cranial nerve VIII)
    b. Optic nerve (cranial nerve II)
    c. Sciatic nerve
    d. Nasal passage

25. Which of the following might be observed when examining a patient's eyes?
    a. Ataxia
    b. Stertor
    c. Excoriation
    d. Anasocoria

26. Black walnut shavings may cause which problem in horses?
    a. Colic
    b. Laminitis
    c. Thrush
    d. Asthma

27. What is the normal rectal temperature for an adult horse?
    a. 98° F to 99° F
    b. 99° F to 101.5° F
    c. 100.5° F to 103° F
    d. 102° F to 104.5° F

28. From which vessel is the pulse most commonly felt in the horse?
    a. Femoral artery
    b. Carotid artery
    c. Facial artery
    d. Jugular vein

29. Which term refers to the absence of intestinal sounds and may be noted in the horse?
    a. Borborygmus
    b. Icterus
    c. Ileus
    d. Colitis

30. What is the normal eructation rate in a normal cow?
    a. 6 per hour
    b. 12 per hour
    c. 18 per hour
    d. 24 per hour

EXERCISE 7.6 FILL-IN-THE-CHART: REGURGITATION AND VOMITING

Instructions: Asking specific questions to determine whether the dog is truly vomiting or displaying regurgitation is critical to obtaining an accurate history.

Fill in the chart with the following key:

R—Rarely to never

O—Often

N—Never

S—Sometimes

A—Always

Historical Differentiation Between Regurgitation and Vomiting

	Regurgitation	Vomiting
Bile		
Digested food		
Active abdominal retch		
Hypersalivation		
Gagging		
Odynophagia		

EXERCISE 7.7 FILL-IN-THE-CHART: REFLEX RESPONSES

Instructions: A neurologic examination of the limbs involves an assessment of postural reactions, reflexes, and sensation. Fill in the chart below with the description of each of the grades of reflex responses.

Grading of Reflex Responses

Grade	Description
0	
1	
2	
3	
4	

Instructions: A cranial nerve examination is an essential part of every complete neurologic examination. Fill in the chart below with the missing answers.

Test Response

Nerve	Test	Normal	Abnormal
I. Olfactory	Volatile substance	Blink	No response
II. Optic	Menace Pupillary light reflex	Direct, consensual responses present	
III. Oculomotor	Pupillary light reflex Observe the eye following an object	Direct, consensual responses present Normal eye movement	
IV. Trochlear	Observe		Muscle atrophy
	Palpate temporalis		No blink
	Corneal reflex		No blink
	Palpebral reflex		
V. Trigeminal	Observe the ability to chew	Normal jaw movement	
	Palpate masseter muscle	Normal muscle tone	
	Pupillary light reflex		No direct or consensual response present
VI. Abducens	Observe	Normal eye position	
VII. Facial	Observe		
	Corneal reflex	Eye blink	
	Palpebral reflex		No blink
	Menace	Eye blink	
VIII. Acoustic	Hand clap	Startle response	
	Move head horizontally, vertically	Normal nystagmus	
IX. Glossopharyngeal	Gag reflex	Swallow	No response
X. Vagus	Gag reflex	Swallow	
	Oculocardiac reflex	Bradycardia	
	Laryngeal reflex	Cough	
XI. Accessory	Palpate neck muscles	Normal muscle tone	
XII. Hypoglossal	Tongue stretch		No response

EXERCISE 7.9 CASE STUDY: HISTORY AND PHYSICAL EXAMINATION FINDINGS

A 16-year-old, spayed female Burmese cat named Coco presents with vomiting of 4 days' duration. Coco's vaccinations are current, and she is strictly an indoor cat. This is Coco's first visit to your hospital. The doctor has asked you to take a history, perform an initial physical examination, and give her the results so that a decision can be made regarding next steps. You ask all the standard questions required at your clinic, including each of the following.

1. Briefly explain why each question is important.

   a. What brings you to the practice today?

   _____

   _____

   b. Can you describe the vomitus?

   _____

   _____

   c. Are there other animals in the house?

   _____

   _____

   d. What, when, and how often do you feed her?

   _____

   _____

   e. What prior medical problems has she experienced?

   _____

   _____

   f. When was she last normal?

   _____

   _____

   g. Is the problem getting better, worse, or remaining the same?

   _____

   _____

   h. Has there been a change in her appetite or water consumption?

   _____

   _____

Coco is quiet and depressed but purrs as you begin your physical examination. The pertinent physical findings are:

- Body temperature of 97.5° F
- Heart rate of 260 beats per minute
- Poor pulse quality
- Pale, dry mucous membranes
- Normal respiratory effort
- No abnormal lung sounds noted
- Prolonged capillary refill time
- Body condition score of 4/9
- Prolonged response to the "skin pinch" test
- Cool extremities
- Severe halitosis
- Poor dentition
- Vomit stains under chin and sternum
- Oral ulcerations along the gingiva

2. Which of these physical findings suggests poor perfusion? Why?

_____

_____

_____

3. Which physical findings suggest dehydration?

_____

_____

_____

4. Is this an emergency case that needs immediate attention? Why or why not?

_____

_____

_____

5. The owner inquires about her halitosis and tells you that it was noticed several months ago. What other physical examination findings listed previously are possibly linked to the halitosis?

_____

_____

_____

8 Preventive Health Programs

LEARNING OBJECTIVES

When you have completed this chapter, you will be able to:
1. Pronounce, define, and spell all of the key terms in this chapter.
2. Compare and contrast the issues and information discussed during wellness visits at various life stages of a dog or a cat (puppy/kitten, adult, and senior/geriatric), and discuss the importance of grooming.
3. Do the following regarding immunity in cats and dogs:
    - Differentiate between active and passive immunity and discuss why it is necessary to administer a series of vaccinations to young puppies and kittens.
    - Differentiate between noninfectious and infectious types of vaccines and explain the purpose of adjuvants.
    - Describe the storage, handling, reconstitution, and dosing of animal vaccines.
    - List the recommended administration locations for various canine and feline vaccinations.
    - Distinguish between core and noncore vaccines and explain what is meant by duration of immunity.
    - Identify the core and noncore vaccines that are used for dogs and cats.
    - Describe potential adverse vaccine events and how to deal with various adverse events should they occur.
4. Explain the importance of discussing potential canine and feline parasitic infections with owners and describe general preventive measures that can be taken.
5. Describe a routine preventive health program for horses, including physical examination, vaccinations, parasitic infection prevention, dental and hoof care, and nutrition.
6. Describe vaccines and other preventive measures that can be used during various life stages of pigs, cattle, sheep, and goats.

EXERCISE 8.1 TERMS AND DEFINITIONS: PREVENTATIVE HEALTH PROGRAMS

Instructions: Define each term in your own words.

1. Active immunity

_____

_____

2. Biosecurity

_____

_____

3. Anaphylaxis

_____

_____

4. Toxoid

_____

_____

5. Adjuvant

_____

_____

6. Passive immunity

_____

_____

7. Congenital

_____

_____

8. Fomite

_____

_____

9. Colostrum

_____

_____

10. Antitoxin

_____

_____

EXERCISE 8.2 MATCHING: ABBREVIATIONS RELATED TO PREVENTIVE HEALTH PROGRAMS FOR DOGS AND CATS

Instructions: Match each term in column A with its corresponding definition in column B by writing the appropriate letter in the space provided.

Column A

1. _____ T_4
2. _____ FVRCP
3. _____ FeLV
4. _____ FHV-1
5. _____ FCV
6. _____ FPV
7. _____ FIV
8. _____ CPiV
9. _____ CAV-2
10. _____ CPV-2
11. _____ DA_2PP

Column B

A. Highly contagious virus in dogs that produces vomiting, diarrhea, leukopenia, and fever

B. Combination vaccine for cats, including herpesvirus, calicivirus, and panleukopenia

C. Lentivirus that causes immunosuppression in cats

D. Retrovirus that causes immunosuppression, anemia, and lymphoma in cats

E. Upper respiratory disease in cats that causes oral ulcerations

F. Combination vaccine for dogs, including distemper, parvovirus, adenovirus type 2, and parainfluenza

G. Serum hormone that may be high in senior cats and low in senior dogs

H. Herpesvirus that causes sneezing, ocular, and nasal discharge and fever

I. Paramyxovirus that is one of the causes of kennel cough in dogs; main clinical sign is a nonproductive, self-limiting cough

J. Parvovirus in cats that causes leukopenia fever, lethargy, anorexia, dehydration, vomiting, and diarrhea

K. One of the causes of canine infectious tracheobronchitis; the modified live vaccine gives cross-immunity for infectious canine hepatitis

EXERCISE 8.3 FILL-IN-THE-BLANK: COMPREHENSIVE

Instructions: Fill in each of the spaces provided with the missing word or words that complete the sentence.

1. Preventive health programs are especially important in situations where animals are housed _____ .

2. Puppies and kittens are vaccinated every 3 to 4 weeks until they are 16 weeks old to stimulate a(n) _____ immune response once _____ immunity declines.

3. Vaccines should be injected within _____ of reconstitution.

4. Vaccines recommended for all animals to protect against highly contagious pathogens are called _____ vaccines.

5. _____ vaccines are recommended for animals at high risk to develop disease.

6. _____ of _____ is the length of time an animal is considered to be immune from developing disease after exposure to a pathogen.

7. Kittens that are infected with feline panleukopenia can develop _____ in utero or shortly after birth.

8. The trivalent vaccine for equine encephalomyelitis protects against _____, _____, and _____ viruses.

9. Heavy parasite loads in horses lead to decreased _____ and _____ performance plus weight loss and colic.

10. The American Association of Feline Practitioners (AAFP) has identified six life stages in cats: Kitten (0-6 months), Junior (_____), Adult (_____), Mature (_____), Senior (_____), and Geriatric.

11. To minimize the risk that disease will spread, _____ pigs should be worked with before _____ pigs.

12. Swine operations do not routinely deworm because pigs are not housed _____.

13. A virus that causes reproductive failure, respiratory disease, and chronic infections in pigs is called porcine _____ and _____ syndrome virus.

14. Beef calves are weaned at about _____ months of age by removing the calf from the dam, whereas dairy calves are raised away from their dams, so weaning is a(n) _____ adjustment and not as stressful.

15. Cattle vaccinated against brucellosis are identified with a(n) _____ ear tag and tattoo in the _____ ear.

16. Cattle vaccines are administered in the _____ region to preserve _____ quality.

17. Deficiency of _____ causes white muscle disease in lambs.

18. To dehorn goats at a young age, the horn bud is destroyed by a(n) _____ instrument.

EXERCISE 8.4 TRUE OR FALSE: COMPREHENSIVE

Instructions: Read the following statements and write "T" for true or "F" for false in the blanks provided. If a statement is false, correct the statement to make it true.

1. ____ Neutering eliminates intermale aggression, separation anxiety, enlargement of the prostate, and testicular cancer.

2. ____ Serum thyroxine levels are frequently measured in senior pets to rule out hyperthyroidism in dogs and hypothyroidism in cats.

3. ____ Culling of small ruminants with chronic severe parasitism is recommended because such animals have low parasite resistance.

4. ____ Active immunity can only be stimulated by an antigen injected in the form of a vaccine.

5. ____ Foals that fail to ingest colostrum at birth are vaccinated with core vaccines within 24 hours of birth.

6. ____ The AAHA-AVMA Canine and Feline Preventive Health Guidelines recommend that adult dogs and cats be examined biannually, with some animals requiring more frequent visits.

7. ____ Noninfectious vaccines are more likely to cause hypersensitivity reactions than infectious vaccines.

8. ____ Administering an intranasal vaccine subcutaneously or intramuscularly may cause serious side effects.

9. ____ Sites for canine vaccination are not standardized, but the rabies vaccination is frequently administered in the left hind leg and the DA$_2$PP in the left front leg, in keeping with feline recommendations.

10. ____ Cats will test positive on the antibody-based FIV screening test after vaccination.

11. ____ Minor side effects to vaccines include lethargy, soreness at injection site, and decreased appetite.

12. ____ Conditions that may be delayed adverse reactions to vaccination include immune-mediated thrombocytopenia, immune-mediated hemolytic anemia, and thyroiditis.

13. ____ The AAHA Senior Care Guidelines for Dogs and Cats define as seniors animals that are in the last 5% of their predicted life span.

14. ____ All dogs and cats should receive the same designated vaccine dose, per manufacturer recommendations, regardless of the age or size of the animal.

15. ____ Thrush occurs on the sole of the horse foot as a result of a moist environment and dirt accumulation allowing bacterial growth.

16. ____ Preventive medicine is important in livestock species to maintain herd productivity.

17. ____ Kids and lambs born to unvaccinated does and ewes are vaccinated at 6 and 10 weeks of age.

18. ____ The barber pole worm causes anemia in sheep by attaching to their abomasums, and this parasitism is a major issue in small ruminants.

19. ____ Horses are wormed for bots and tapeworms in the spring with either moxidectin or ivermectin, with praziquantel.

20. ____ Core vaccination in cattle protects them from leptospirosis, campylobacteriosis, rotavirus, and coronavirus.

EXERCISE 8.5 MULTIPLE CHOICE: COMPREHENSIVE

Instructions: Circle the one correct answer for each of the following questions.

1. Spaying before the second heat cycle in cats and dogs decreases
   a. aggression.
   b. vaccine-induced sarcoma.
   c. lymphoma.
   d. mammary carcinoma.

2. Older dogs may require more frequent nail trims because of decreased exercise associated with
   a. kidney disease.
   b. cognitive dysfunction.
   c. degenerative joint disease.
   d. hyperthyroidism.

3. Passive immunity in puppies and kittens primarily occurs
   a. when antibodies pass to the offspring in utero via the placenta.
   b. by vaccination within 24 hours of birth.
   c. by ingestion of colostrum within 24 hours of birth.
   d. with intravenous infusion of antibody-rich plasma at birth.

4. To maximize the chance of successful treatment in the event that a vaccine-induced sarcoma develops, it is now recommended that feline vaccines be administered
   a. distal to the shoulder or hip.
   b. proximal to the shoulder or hip.
   c. in the intrascapular region.
   d. intranasally.

5. Core vaccines for the cat are
   a. feline leukemia, panleukopenia, calicivirus, and rabies.
   b. feline leukemia, feline immunodeficiency virus, panleukopenia, and rabies.
   c. feline viral rhinotracheitis, calicivirus, panleukopenia, and rabies.
   d. feline viral rhinotracheitis, *Chlamydophila felis*, panleukopenia, and rabies.

6. Core vaccines in the dog protect against
   a. parvovirus, adenovirus-2, leptospirosis, and rabies.
   b. distemper, parvovirus, *bordetella*, and rabies.
   c. distemper, parvovirus, leptospirosis, and rabies.
   d. parvovirus, distemper, adenovirus-2, and rabies.

7. Many of the core feline combination and canine combination vaccines are administered every
   a. year.
   b. 2 years.
   c. 3 years.
   d. 5 years.

8. Cats should test negative before vaccination against
   a. feline immunodeficiency virus.
   b. feline panleukopenia.
   c. *Chlamydophila felis.*
   d. calicivirus.

9. Which noncore feline vaccination is recommended for multi-cat households with a past history of bacterial upper respiratory infections?
   a. Feline leukemia
   b. Feline immunodeficiency virus
   c. *Chlamydophila felis*
   d. *Giardia*

10. A disease process in dogs that manifests as a dry, honking cough and that is transmitted dog to dog through respiratory secretions is caused by
    a. canine distemper virus.
    b. canine coronavirus.
    c. *Bordetella bronchiseptica.*
    d. canine parvovirus.

11. Veterinary assistance should be sought if, following vaccination, the animal exhibits
    a. mild fever and decreased appetite.
    b. soreness at the injection site.
    c. sneezing after an intranasal vaccine.
    d. facial swelling and difficulty breathing.

12. For most core vaccines, the recommended length of time between initial and booster vaccines during the initial vaccine series in dogs, cats, and horses is generally
    a. 2 weeks.
    b. 4 weeks.
    c. 6 weeks.
    d. 8 weeks.

13. Foals born to unvaccinated mares are routinely vaccinated at
    a. 1 to 2 months.
    b. 3 to 4 months.
    c. 5 to 6 months.
    d. 7 to 8 months.

14. Head tossing, excessive chewing of the bit, and bucking in the horse can be signs of
    a. tick infestation.
    b. internal parasitism.
    c. nutritional deficiency.
    d. dental issues.

15. Young horses and horses with dental issues should have dental exams
    a. every 6 months.
    b. once a year.
    c. every 2 years.
    d. every 3 years.

16. Which animal is not considered a natural reservoir of rhabdovirus?
    a. Skunk
    b. Coyote
    c. Rattlesnake
    d. Raccoon

17. To maintain proper balance and avoid problems with lameness in the horse, hooves should be trimmed
    a. every 2 to 4 weeks.
    b. every 4 to 6 weeks.
    c. every 6 to 8 weeks.
    d. every 8 to 10 weeks.

18. Thrush is treated by frequent cleaning of the sole of the foot and application of
    a. copper- or iodine-based solutions.
    b. moxidectin or ivermectin.
    c. praziquantel.
    d. fenbendazole or oxibendazole.

19. Anemia is prevented in piglets with supplementation of
    a. selenium.
    b. magnesium.
    c. iron.
    d. calcium.

20. Piglet tails are docked to prevent
    a. chewing by other piglets.
    b. fecal contamination.
    c. maggot infestation.
    d. increased price of meat.

21. Before entering the breeding herd, pigs are vaccinated for
    a. parvovirus, erysipelas, and leptospirosis.
    b. parvovirus, brucellosis, and pseudorabies.
    c. leptospirosis, pseudorabies, and brucellosis.
    d. brucellosis, pseudorabies, and erysipelas.

22. To prevent disease transmission, newly acquired pigs are not introduced to the rest of the herd for
    a. 10 days.
    b. 14 days.
    c. 21 days.
    d. 30 days.

23. Passive immunity blocks active immune response in calves that are vaccinated when younger than
    a. 3 months of age.
    b. 4 months of age.
    c. 5 months of age.
    d. 6 months of age.

24. Bovine leukosis virus in cattle may cause
    a. cancer.
    b. reproductive failure.
    c. respiratory disease.
    d. corkscrew hooves.

25. Dairy cows are vaccinated against mastitis caused by
    a. *Clostridium perfringens.*
    b. *Escherichia coli.*
    c. *Streptococcus equi.*
    d. *Campylobacter fetus.*

26. Dairy cows should have their hooves trimmed
    a. every 3 months.
    b. every 6 months.
    c. at least once a year.
    d. every 2 years.

27. During the first few weeks of life, either tail docking or castration in sheep can be performed by
    a. using a hot metal instrument to burn tissue off.
    b. applying a tight elastic band around the tail or to the scrotum.
    c. surgical removal.
    d. using an emasculatome.

28. Diarrhea in sheep and goats is caused by single-celled parasites called
    a. *Leptospira pomona.*
    b. *Clostridium perfringens type C and D.*
    c. *Haemonchus contortus.*
    d. *Coccidia.*

29. Sheep and goats can be rapidly screened for anemia by checking the
    a. conjunctiva.
    b. red blood cell count.
    c. mouth.
    d. capillary refill time.

30. Core vaccination in sheep and goats protects against
    a. rabies.
    b. *Haemonchus contortus.*
    c. *Clostridium perfringens* and *Clostridium tetani.*
    d. contagious ecthyma.

Instructions: Find the words that are identified by the clues given below. The words may be located horizontally, vertically, or diagonally, and may be reversed.

```
S R S C O T P I R A I X O N I L I A L S N
A T E I P E B R U C E L L O S I S I C I U
A Z R V L O Z L C I M R E A R R L O E T Q
L M N A E I E R R G T C I S E R K O L I N
M E S E N F H S A A Y E S R R X R O S L S
N S K R U G E J O H N E S D I S E A S E A
I S I S I L L S O R U S R T B U N J I Y O
S O E L A N F E R R P R S P R T S B O M T
U R A N U S B N S O N F T D H T A T D O E
R E C A E T E O I M H T Z R I R P I T L Z
I M R S I S O I R E T C A B O L Y P M A C
V O V I I I I B B H N X A D N C Y E E H L
E U E O U E S S E A R I U M R M M E R P O
L T F U V T T I S R R E U H O R I S Y E S
I H S U H U U S U U S L A Q O T N D S C T
N E L S I S O R I P S O T P E L O A I N R
T N S T T U Y A O R M V B V S H T P P E I
S I T I V I T C N U J N O C O T A R E K D
E Q U I N E H E R P E S V I R U S S L E I
W E I R X V L A U S R P I I A E I A A N U
R O L R A R P S U P R R L G A I S A S R M
```

Strangles
Potomac Horse Fever
Johnes Disease
Purpura Hemorrhagica
Rabies
Encephalomyelitis
Sore Mouth

Campylobacteriosis
Brucellosis
Leptospirosis
Clostridium
West Nile Virus
Erysipelas

Equine Herpes Virus
Pseudorabies
Equine Influenza
Botulism
Anthrax
Keratoconjunctivitis

EXERCISE 8.7 CASE STUDY: FELINE PREVENTIVE HEALTH

Lily, a calico, female, domestic shorthair cat of unknown age presents for a check-up and vaccinations. According to the client, Ms. Rose, she found Lily wandering the neighborhood and decided to bring her into her home. As the veterinary technician, you take Ms. Rose and Lily back to an examination room and obtain the following information about Lily.

Weight and Vital Signs: Weight: 4 lbs; Heart Rate: 180 bpm; Respiratory Rate: 32 bpm; Temperature: 101.8° F.

Recent History: Lily has been in the neighborhood for about 4 weeks, since the neighbor on the corner moved away. Ms. Rose believes the neighbor who moved left Lily behind. Ms. Rose has been feeding Lily for the last 2 weeks, and she appears to eat well but not gain weight. She has no information as to urinations or bowel movements as Lily is outside. She has decided to bring her inside with her two indoor cats, Petunia and Violet. She is concerned about Lily's introduction into the home and wants to make sure her other cats are not exposed to any diseases. She is also concerned that Lily may not acclimate to being an indoor-only cat since she has lived outdoors for a while.

Physical Examination Findings: Lily's adult canine teeth are erupted, indicating she is 6 months old. Lily is thin and black specks are noticed in her hair coat. The rest of her physical examination findings are unremarkable. A spay scar cannot be palpated on the ventral midline. It expected that she may not be spayed.

Instructions: Answer the following questions based on the case with regard to the best preventive health program for Lily and Ms. Rose, considering the home and the environmental situation.

1. Because Lily has been an outdoor cat with no known vaccination history, what are the first diagnostic tests Lily should receive based on current recommendations?

   _____

   _____

   _____

2a. How could you explain the black specks in Lily's hair coat? What external parasite might they indicate?

   _____

   _____

   _____

2b. What is a commonly recommended treatment protocol that could be used for Lily to treat this parasite, including both eggs and adults?

   _____

   _____

   _____

   _____

   _____

3a. Assuming the diagnostics in #1 are negative, discuss the core vaccinations Lily should receive, including the site of injection for each.

_____

_____

_____

_____

3b. How often should each vaccine be boostered, assuming Lily will be living exclusively indoors?

_____

_____

_____

_____

_____

4a. Describe potential adverse effects to the vaccines that you will have Ms. Rose monitor for.

_____

_____

_____

4b. What are some serious adverse effects that warrant immediate notification of the veterinary practice if they occur?

_____

_____

_____

5. If Lily exhibits any of the more serious side effects, what steps might the veterinarian take to minimize the likelihood of these effects in the future?

_____

_____

_____

_____

_____

6a. If Lily develops a lump at the site of a vaccine injection, what are some possible reasons for this?

_____

_____

_____

_____

_____

6b. What might be done by the attending veterinarian to differentiate these causes?

_____

_____

_____

_____

_____

_____

_____

7. Discuss a surgical procedure that would keep Lily from having an unwanted pregnancy, and describe the other health benefits this procedure provides.

_____

_____

_____

_____

_____

_____

_____

_____

8a. If after surgery, Lily will not stay indoors, discuss the noncore vaccines she should receive, including the recommended injection site for each.

_____

_____

_____

_____

_____

8b. How often should each vaccine be boostered?

_____

_____

_____

8c. If Lily continues to go outside, how does that affect the vaccines given to Violet and Petunia?

_____

_____

_____

_____

_____

9 Animal Nutrition

LEARNING OBJECTIVES

When you have completed this chapter, you will be able to:
1. Pronounce, spell, and define the key terms in this chapter.
2. Compare and contrast the concepts of energy units, energy partitioning, metabolizable energy measurement, Atwater factors, energy density, and measurements of energy expenditure.
3. List the macronutrients and micronutrients found in pet feeds. Do the following regarding nutrients:
   - List the building block molecules that make up proteins, fats, and carbohydrates.
   - Discuss the requirements for protein, fat, carbohydrates, fiber, vitamins, and minerals in the diet of dogs and cats.
   - List the energy-producing and non–energy-producing components of food.
   - Differentiate between microminerals and macrominerals and give examples of each.
4. Explain the rationale for and steps of the nutritional assessment of small animals.
   - Calculate the RER for a cat and dog.
   - Determine the body condition score of a cat and dog.
5. Describe the unique feline physiology and the impact on nutrition.
   Explain various aspects regarding commercial pet food, including the following:
   a. Explain how pet food manufacturing is regulated in the United States and identify the government agencies and organizations involved in the regulation of pet food.
   b. Describe which marketing language bears little nutritional significance and explain how veterinary therapeutic diets may be used appropriately and inappropriately.
   c. List the components of pet food labels and explain how the information provided in each component should be interpreted.
6. Explain the myths that are associated with small animal nutrition.
7. Describe feeding protocols for healthy dogs and cats at each stage of life, including pregnant and lactating females.
8. Describe the rationale and indications for assisted feeding in cats and dogs.
9. Regarding the nutrition of horses:
   - Explain the importance of grass and hay in the equine diet.
   - Describe how pregnancy and lactation alter a mare's nutritional requirements.
   - List steps taken to provide appropriate nutrition to foals and young, growing horses.
   - Describe general guidelines for feeding sick horses.
10. Describe the rationale and method for performing an assessment of nutrition status in large animals.
    - List the variables affecting energy requirements of livestock.
    - Describe how nutrient excesses and deficiencies lead to toxicity in large animals.
    - Describe how the nutritional requirements of each of these species are affected by the animal's stage of life and by its energy expenditure (maintenance, growth, lactation, etc.).
    - List advantages and disadvantages of pasture feeding livestock.
11. Discuss the requirements for protein, fat, carbohydrates, fiber, vitamins, and minerals in the diet of birds, small mammals, and reptiles.

Across

2. Unit of energy
6. Any fat or oil or related compound that is insoluble in water but soluble in nonpolar solvents
7. The building blocks of fat (2 words)
9. Energy available to the animal after energy from feces, urine, and combustible gases has been subtracted from gross energy. Used to express the energy content of foods and commercial diets
10. Substances that provide nourishment for growth and maintenance of life
11. The number of calories provided in foods

Down

1. Evaluated periodically to assess weight gain or loss (3 words)
3. The name of a type of nutritional support that should be started withing 3 days of the onset of anorexia in stable, ill patients (2 words)
4. Assigned energy values of the macronutrients (2 words)
5. Description of the taste, texture, aroma, and other characteristics of pet food
8. The building blocks of proteins (2 words)

EXERCISE 9.2 MATCHING #1: KEY TERMS

Instructions: Match each key term in column A with its corresponding definition in column B by writing the appropriate letter in the space provided.

Column A

1. _____ Calorie
2. _____ Nutrient
3. _____ Energy density
4. _____ Amino acids
5. _____ Forage
6. _____ Palatability
7. _____ Modified Atwater factors
8. _____ Assisted feeding
9. _____ Resting energy requirement
10. _____ Essential fatty acid
11. _____ Metabolizable energy
12. _____ Body condition score
13. _____ Lipid
14. _____ Kilojoule
15. _____ Concentrates
16. _____ Digestible energy
17. _____ Digestion

Column B

A. Something essential that a plant or animal obtains from the environment for growth and maintenance of life

B. The small molecules that are the building blocks of proteins

C. Molecules that provide and store energy, make up cell membrane structure, and act as signaling agents and hormones

D. A component of cell membranes found in animal fats

E. A measure of energy defined as the energy needed to move a 1 kilogram weight 1 meter by 1 newton

F. The energy needed to increase the temperature of 1 gram (g) of water from 14.5° C to 15.5° C

G. Result of subtracting the energy lost in urine and gases produced by the body from the digestible energy (DE) of a food or diet

H. Used to determine the digestibility of commercial pet foods

I. The kcal per unit of a food ingredient or pet food

J. A widely used estimate of how many calories an animal needs to maintain its weight in a controlled environment

K. Grass, legumes, and hays

L. A method used regularly to assess the weight gain or weight loss of an animal

M. A measure of how well overall an animal likes a food

N. Providing nutritional support to a sick, injured, or hospitalized pet

O. Grains or high-starch compounds

P. Subtraction of the energy lost in the feces from the consumed GE

Q. The process of protein, carbohydrate, and fat breakdown into absorbable nutrients

EXERCISE 9.3 MATCHING #2: ENERGY PARTITIONING

Instructions: Match each abbreviation in column A with its corresponding description in column B by writing the appropriate letter in the space provided.

Column A

1. _____ kcal
2. _____ BV
3. _____ ME
4. _____ RER
5. _____ DE
6. _____ GE
7. _____ NE
8. _____ BCS
9. _____ DER

Column B

A. An estimate that establishes the baseline energy needs of an animal

B. Total potential energy of a foodstuff

C. Digestible energy—energy lost in urine and gas

D. Percentage of true absorbed protein that is available for productive body functions

E. Metabolizable energy minus the energy used in digesting and absorbing food

F. The standard measurement for energy that is also referred to as "calories" to an animal owner

G. An assessment to assist in monitoring adequacies of daily food intake

H. Calculated by multiplying RER by standard factors related to energy needs

I. A food's gross energy minus the energy which is non-absorbable and lost in the feces

EXERCISE 9.4 MATCHING #3: PET FOOD LABELS

Instructions: A client presents a bag of food to you with the following information. Help the client understand this information by matching each piece of information with the section of the food label that it is listed in from column B by writing the appropriate letter in the space provided.

Column A

1. _____ Purina Dog Chow
2. _____ Crude protein 42% (minimum)
3. _____ Chicken, brewers rice, corn gluten meal
4. _____ Adult maintenance
5. _____ Feed 1–1½ cups per 5–10 lb. dog.
6. _____ Picture of the product

Column B

A. Product vignette

B. Guaranteed analysis

C. Feeding directions

D. Ingredient statement

E. Principal display panel

F. Statement of nutritional adequacy

EXERCISE 9.5 TRUE OR FALSE: COMPREHENSIVE

Instructions: Read the following statements and write "T" for true or "F" for false in the blanks provided. If a statement is false, correct the statement to make it true.

1. _____ Nutrients are most commonly listed in kilogram (kg) units on a pet food label.

2. _____ Although pet owners should be advised to be cautious with vitamin supplements, mineral supplementation is generally considered safe.

3. _____ Cats have a minimum requirement for 25% carbohydrates in their diet, while dogs require 55% carbohydrates in their diet.

4. _____ The ad-lib feeding method is typically recommended to the owners of healthy, normal cats and dogs.

5. _____ Essential fatty acids, including linoleic acid, are required in the diets of dogs and cats.

6. ____ The USDA enforces regulations on chemical and/or microbiologic contamination in pet food.

7. ____ Guinea pigs require vitamin C in their diets.

8. ____ Vitamin requirements in the diet vary among different species of animals.

9. ____ The expressions "as-fed," "dry matter," and "metabolizable energy" refer to measurements of a nutrient in a diet and are interchangeable with each other.

10. ____ Dietary taurine is essential in cats and clinical disease results if insufficient amounts are present.

11. ____ The main problems with offering raw foods to pets are the expense and the lack of digestibility.

12. ____ Naturally derived antioxidants are difficult to use as the sole source of preservatives in commercial pet foods.

13. ____ Energy needs for pregnant dogs are highest during the 6th to 8th week of gestation.

14. ____ Spayed or neutered animals often have higher energy needs than intact animals.

15. ____ In general, cats have higher protein requirements than dogs.

16. ____ A cat or dog weighing 10–19% more than optimum for its breed is considered obese.

17. ____ Constipation is a common finding in mature dogs and cats.

18. ____ A sick, hospitalized patient should not be fed, in order to allow the GI tract to rest.

19. ____ The most serious and potentially life-threatening complication of parenteral nutrition in equine patients is overfeeding.

20. ____ Force feeding or syringe feeding is the best method for providing assisted enteral nutrition.

21. ____ Complete feeds for horses are typically a mixture of 60% roughage to 20% concentrate.

22. ____ Hypoglycemia is a frequent finding in the normal neonatal foal.

23. ____ In large animals, physiological response indicative of anorexia manifests as endogenous protein catabolism.

24. ____ A cow at peak lactation may need an average of 15 gallons of water a day.

25. ____ Protein requirements for camelids are similar to those for horses.

26. ____ The most commonly used type of NPN for sheep and goats is uric acid.

27. ____ All-seed foods are suitable as the main component of the diets of most species of birds.

28. ____ One of the most common disorders seen in reptiles is metabolic bone disease.

29. ____ Ferrets should not be fasted for longer than 3 hours.

30. ____ Combining different types of proteins has no effect on the biologic value.

31. ____ Ruminants have the ability to break down fiber content to be used as energy, and this allows them to utilize feed that other animals cannot use.

32. ____ Horses should not have access to salt, as an overdose can lead to toxicity.

33. ____ Muscle condition scoring is an evaluation independent from body fat content assessed by body condition score.

85

Instructions: Circle the one correct answer to each of the following questions.

1. All of the following components are legally required on a pet food label except
   a. ingredient statement.
   b. guaranteed analysis.
   c. freshness date.
   d. feeding directions.

2. The nutrients that supply energy to an animal include
   a. vitamins, carbohydrates, and fats.
   b. fats, protein, and minerals.
   c. protein, carbohydrates, and fats.
   d. carbohydrates, vitamins, and minerals.

3. Each of the following is a major function of proteins except
   a. serving as a primary component of many body tissues.
   b. maintaining an oncotic force in blood vessels.
   c. serving as a source of soluble fiber.
   d. transporting molecules in the blood.

4. Which of the following statements is false regarding fat in the diet?
   a. Fat is the source of essential fatty acids.
   b. Fat provides 4 kcal of energy per gram.
   c. Fat enhances palatability.
   d. Fat is necessary for the absorption of some vitamins.

5. Which of the following is not a disease typically associated with inadequacies in the hand-fed diets of large animals?
   a. Osteodystrophia fibrosa
   b. Lactic acid indigestion
   c. Azoturia
   d. Foot rot

6. Which of the following items is optional in a guaranteed analysis on a pet food label?
   a. Crude protein
   b. Moisture
   c. Calcium
   d. Crude fiber

7. Fiber is often a component of dog or cat foods and
   a. is an essential nutrient.
   b. comes from protein found in animal tissues.
   c. is broken down by the body into glucose.
   d. resists digestion in the gastrointestinal tract.

8. Which of the following is not considered a risk factor finding to address during a nutritional assessment of a small animal?
   a. Poor hair or skin coat
   b. Inadequate housing
   c. Treats accounting for 5% of total calories
   d. Abnormal body condition score

9. Anemia may be caused by a deficiency of
   a. fat.
   b. carbohydrate.
   c. protein.
   d. calcium.

10. Dogs and cats have minimum dietary requirements for all of the following nutrients except
    a. protein.
    b. fat.
    c. carbohydrate.
    d. vitamins and minerals.

11. The essential nutrients required in the diet of cats include all of the following except
    a. taurine.
    b. arachidonic acid.
    c. vitamin C.
    d. arginine.

12. Raw meat diet recipes
    a. contain adequate levels of calcium and phosphorus to support growth.
    b. are safe for people to handle and for animals to eat.
    c. rarely cause GI upset, as the ingredients do not contain preservatives.
    d. may include bones, which can obstruct or perforate the GI tract.

13. Consider this scenario: An outbreak of *Salmonella* has been traced to a facility that manufactures several brands of dog food. These contaminated products will be recalled through a mandate by the
    a. AAFCO.
    b. USDA.
    c. FDA.
    d. FTC.

14. AAFCO, an important organization in the pet food industry,
    a. is a government agency that ensures the safety of all pet food ingredients and products.
    b. publishes the Nutrient Requirements of Dogs and Cats with guidelines for formulating dog and cat foods.
    c. establishes protocols for animal feeding tests with various pet food products.
    d. performs feeding tests on dogs and cats using a variety of products in a laboratory setting.

15. A diet deficient in protein will result in
    a. dull, dry hair coat.
    b. reduced fecal production.
    c. weight gain.
    d. increased activity level.

16. Which nutrient is specifically involved in normal neural, retinal, and auditory development in kittens and puppies?
    a. Magnesium
    b. High biologic-value protein
    c. Omega-3 fatty acids
    d. Soluble fiber

17. During the growth phase, a puppy's daily energy requirement is approximately
    a. the same as its mother's during gestation.
    b. three times its resting energy requirement.
    c. 50% more than it is estimated to be at expected adult weight.
    d. double kcal of its weight in grams.

18. The owner of a 5-month-old, intact male Labrador wants to know how much to feed his dog per day. The most appropriate recommendation is
    a. feed the dog ad libitum until he reaches 12 months of age.
    b. calculate the RER for this dog, and feed that amount per day.
    c. use the feeding instructions on the dog food bag, and monitor BCS frequently.
    d. feed the dog 4 cups of food.

19. Skylar is a sedentary, 5-year-old, spayed female mixed-breed dog at her ideal weight of 25 kg. Her calculated RER (kcal/day) would be
    a. 534.
    b. 662.
    c. 783.
    d. 897.

20. Griffin, a 3-kg, active, 7-month-old, male, domestic shorthaired feline, would require approximately how much energy supplied by the diet (kcal/day)?
    a. 160 to 320 kcal/day
    b. 320 to 480 kcal/day
    c. 480 to 640 kcal/day
    d. 640 to 800 kcal/day

21. Predisposing factors for obesity in pets include all of the following except
    a. high fat content in the diet.
    b. overfeeding.
    c. high fiber content in the diet.
    d. sedentary lifestyle.

22. The deficiency of which nutrient in the diet of pregnant cows can contribute to the development of white muscle disease in their calves?
    a. Calcium
    b. Selenium
    c. Linoleic acid
    d. Vitamin D

23. Fiber in a feline diet
    a. is an essential nutrient required by the species.
    b. is useful for thin animals to improve weight gain.
    c. can improve GI function and prevent hairballs.
    d. reduces fecal quantity.

24. Which should be available to a rabbit ad libitum?
    a. Dry cat kibble
    b. A salt lick
    c. Ground corn pellets
    d. Grass or hay

25. Which feeding tube should be considered in an animal with anesthesia risks?
    a. Jejunostomy
    b. Gastrotomy
    c. Nasoesophageal
    d. Esophagostomy

26. Which pet rodent typically has the highest dietary protein requirements?
    a. Rats
    b. Gerbils
    c. Hamsters
    d. Mice

27. Which factor is not considered a cause of metabolic bone disease in reptiles?
    a. Insufficient vitamin D3
    b. Excessive phosphorous
    c. Excessive sodium
    d. Insufficient calcium

28. To measure the body condition score of an animal, you will
    a. put the animal on a scale and record its weight in kilograms.
    b. measure the circumference of the animal's chest, just behind the elbow.
    c. use calipers to measure the thickness of a skin fold.
    d. feel along the rib cage and check for a waist and abdominal tuck.

29. Which nutrient is considered the most important for sustaining life?
    a. Essential fatty acids
    b. Energy
    c. Protein
    d. Water

30. An appropriate weight loss diet for a canine should include
    a. a minimum of 25% crude protein (DMB) and a maximum of 55% carbohydrates (DMB) and 9% fat (DMB).
    b. approximately 12-20% crude protein (DMB), 55% carbohydrates (DMB), and 5% fat (DMB).
    c. a maximum of 25% crude protein (DMB), 50% carbohydrate (DMB), and 25% fat (DMB).
    d. a minimum of 25% crude protein (DMB) and a maximum of 40% carbohydrate (DMB) and 9% fat (DMB).

31. What is the primary energy source used in livestock rations?
    a. Proteins
    b. Fat
    c. Carbohydrates
    d. Minerals

32. Sheep are more susceptible to toxicity from this mineral than are other species.
    a. Zinc
    b. Copper
    c. Iron
    d. Magnesium

33. Which nutrient is the most important in a horse's diet?
    a. Roughage
    b. Carbohydrates
    c. Protein
    d. Water

EXERCISE 9.7 FILL-IN-THE-BLANK: COMPREHENSIVE

Instructions: Fill in each of the spaces with the missing word or words that complete the sentence.

1. Macronutrients consist of _____, _____, and _____ and are used by the body to produce _____.

2. _____ is an important nutrient that contributes to 50% to 70% of an animal's body weight. Deficiencies of this nutrient lead to a state of _____ in the body.

3. Cats have a _____ need for protein than dogs have.

4. The protein in poor- to moderate-quality ruminant feed is typically _____ through rumen metabolism.

5. Essential fatty acids are required in the diets of animals that cannot synthesize them. _____ and _____ are fatty acids essential to both dogs and cats.

6. Diets high in insoluble fiber are inappropriate for dogs and cats with _____ energy requirements, such as puppies and kittens.

7. In terms of nutrition, iron and zinc are considered _____, while calcium and sodium are considered _____.

8. Vitamins are divided into two major categories: _____ and _____.

9. When large animal feed is measured, as opposed to being weighed, the risk of overfeeding or underfeeding is _____.

10. _____ is/are a category of dietary supplements that may delay or prevent oxidative processes in the body and in food.

11. Cats have a special need for four amino acids _____, _____, arginine, and cysteine.

12. Food allergies are typically caused by immune reactions to _____ in the diet.

13. The only current certification in nutrition for veterinarians in the United States is conferred by the _____.

14. A nutrient that has a lower digestibility will need to be fed in _____ amounts.

15. It's recommended that growing horses should be weighed _____ times a week.

EXERCISE 9.8 CASE STUDY #1: WEIGHT LOSS

Spunky, a 4-year-old, spayed, female mixed-breed dog, presents to your clinic. Her owners are concerned about her weight gain over the last four months. In obtaining a history, you learn that there are four people in the house: owners Jen and Brian, a toddler, and a new baby. Jen and Brian have taken to leaving all-purpose dog food out all day, because they realized they had each forgotten to feed Spunky on several occasions since the birth of the baby. Spunky's exercise is limited to spending time in the fenced yard, rather than the walks she used to enjoy. Spunky spends much of her time indoors and is quick to eat food the toddler has dropped. On physical examination, Spunky weighs 55 lbs. with a BCS of 4/5. Her ideal weight is 45 lbs. All other examination findings were unremarkable. CBC, chemistry, and thyroid hormone levels were also unremarkable.

1. Is Spunky's weight excessive? Why or why not?

_____

_____

_____

2. What does Spunky's body condition score indicate about the fat percentage of her body?

_____

_____

_____

3. Risk factors for obesity include being spayed or neutered, excessive caloric intake, decreased physical activity, genetic susceptibility, age, type of food, and feeding method. Address each of these risk factors, based on the information you obtained in Spunky's history.

_____

_____

_____

_____

_____

_____

_____

4. When you mention that Spunky would benefit from weight loss, Jen, her owner, says, "Okay, we'll just put out half of the food we usually give her." Is this plan advisable? Why or why not?

_____

_____

_____

_____

5. Based on your knowledge of the nutrients required in an energy-restricted diet, what values (in percentages; use ppm for L-carnitine) will you look for in the dog food you suggest for Spunky's weight loss plan?

Maximum dietary fat (DMB) _____

Range of dietary fiber (DMB) _____

Minimum crude dietary protein (DMB) _____

Maximum dietary carbohydrate (DMB) _____

Recommended level dietary L-carnitine (DM) _____

6. Other than feeding an energy-restricted diet, what else might her owners do that would help Spunky lose weight?

_____

_____

_____

_____

7. Why is it important to address obesity in pets?

_____

_____

EXERCISE 9.9 CASE STUDY #2: HOSPITALIZED PATIENT

Sulu, an 8-year-old, neutered, male, domestic shorthair cat, presents to your clinic with a 3-day history of anorexia and acute vomiting. Physical examination revealed a string foreign body under his tongue, a painful abdomen, approximately 7% dehydration, and a current body weight of 5 kg. Abdominal radiography supports the presence of an intestinal foreign body. Sulu is stabilized with intravenous fluids and taken to surgery for removal of the foreign body. The plan is to provide some nutritional support to Sulu, as he has been anorexic for 72 hours.

1. What routes could be used to provide nutrition to this patient?

_____

_____

_____

2. It was decided at the time of surgery to place a 5-French jejunostomy tube (J-tube). Discuss some of the factors to be considered when choosing a tube for parenteral nutrition.

_____

_____

_____

3. Calculate the RER for Sulu at his current body weight of 5 kg (11 lbs.).

_____ kcal/day

4. Ensuring that Sulu receives adequate nutrition is critically important. What are the ways malnutrition impacts the following body organs and systems?

Gastrointestinal tract: _____

_____

_____

_____

Kidneys: _____

_____

_____

_____

Immunity: _____

_____

_____

Pulmonary: _____

_____

_____

_____

Cardiovascular: _____

_____

_____

Metabolic: _____

_____

_____

10 Animal Reproduction

LEARNING OBJECTIVES

When you have completed this chapter, you will be able to:

1. Pronounce, define, and spell each of the key terms in this chapter.
2. Locate the anatomic parts of the reproductive system, including endocrine organs in the cranium.
3. Describe hormonal changes that occur during the estrous cycle and pregnancy.
4. Compare and contrast the processes of oogenesis and spermatogenesis.
5. Explain the process of fertilization and embryo development, including the anatomic locations of these events.
6. Compare and contrast canine, feline, and equine estrous cycles, gestation, and parturition and describe the collection process and interpretation of canine vaginal cells and state the importance of vaginal cytologic examination in breeding dogs.
7. Compare and contrast the bovine, ovine, caprine, and camelid estrous cycles, gestation, and parturition.
8. Identify and put in order the important aspects of a breeding soundness examination in a male and a female animal.

Across

2 The term used to describe parturition in the camelid species.
4 The estrous cycle of the mare is divided into the _____ phase and the luteal phase.
7 The tail of the spermatid is referred to as a _____.
8 The term used to describe the life stage at which a given species is capable of reproduction.
10 When semen is frozen in liquid nitrogen for preservation, it is said to be _____.
11 The term for the delivery of fetuses in the canine species.
13 The word used to describe a system that utilizes actual physical contact of the stallion and the mare to help determine the presence of physiologic estrus in the mares that do not exhibit signs of heat.
15 The term for the male of the canine species.
16 This word, when used as an adjective, relates to the "kind" of cycle.

Down

1 The name of the thick tunic that covers the ovary in the mare. (2 words)
3 The term for the oviductal entry into the uterus.
6 The placentation type of the bitch indicating a narrow band of attachment of the chorioallantoic membrane to the endometrium.
5 The term used for male species if one or both testes have not descended into the scrotum.
8 The equine species is a seasonally _____ animal, thereby influenced greatly by increasing amounts of light in the spring of the year.
9 The breeding _____ examination is performed on all male species before they are used for breeding.
14 The term for the female of the canine species.
12 The noun that describes the period of time the female is in "heat" or sexually receptive.

EXERCISE 10.2 TERMS AND DEFINITIONS

Instructions: Define each term in your own words.

1. Ovulation: _____

_____

2. Oviduct: _____

_____

3. Fertilization: _____

_____

4. Prolactin: _____

_____

5. Puberty (in the female): _____

_____

6. Anestrus: _____

_____

7. Mare: _____

_____

8. Stallion: _____

_____

9. Foaling: _____

_____

10. Gelding: _____

_____

11. Ovariectomized mare: _____

_____

12. Foal heat: _____

_____

13. Queening: _____

_____

14. Ewe:_____

_____

15. Wether:_____

_____

16. Allantois:_____

_____

17. Meiosis:_____

_____

18. Doe:_____

_____

19. Buck:_____

_____

20. Kids:_____

_____

21. Heifer:_____

_____

22. Queen:_____

_____

23. Bull:_____

_____

24. Steer:_____

_____

25. Calf:_____

_____

26. Cria:_____

_____

Instructions: Match each definition in column A with its corresponding term in column B by writing the appropriate letter in the space provided.

Column A

1. _____ The study of reproduction in animals

2. _____ Cells that cover the ovum upon being released from the follicle

3. _____ Successive fertilization of ova by two or more fathers during the same heat

4. _____ A second conception while a female is pregnant

5. _____ The type of placenta found in the human and rodent

6. _____ Physical and biochemical cell membrane changes of the sperm, allowing for fertilization

7. _____ The type of placenta present in the horse, swine, and ruminants

8. _____ The term for uterine lining where the placenta attaches

9. _____ The term for a bitch if the uterus and gonads have been removed

10. _____ The hormone that influences early development of the follicle and estrogen production in the canine species

11. _____ A rapid rise in luteinizing hormone at the start of estrus

12. _____ The passage of blood from the uterine lining through capillary walls into the uterine cavity

13. _____ Difficult birth

14. _____ To cause regress

15. _____ The term for a young mare that usually implies she is between and two years of age

16. _____ The term used for a newborn equine

17. _____ A secretion of the hypothalamus that stimulates the secretion of follicle-stimulating hormone

Column B

A. Capacitation

B. LH surge

C. Filly

D. Cumulus

E. Dystocia

F. Spayed

G. Superfecundation

H. GnRH

I. Theriogenology

J. Hemochorial

K. Diapedesis

L. Endometrium

M. Superfetation

N. Foal

O. FSH

P. Lyse

Q. Epitheliochorial

Instructions: Match each definition in column A with its corresponding term in column B by writing the appropriate letter in the space provided.

Column A

1. _____ The stage in the canine estrous cycle when the bitch stops accepting the male

2. _____ The gland that is affected by the use of artificial lighting to induce early estrus in the mare

3. _____ A thick covering on the ovary preventing ovulation anywhere except at the ovulation fossa

4. _____ The hormone produced by endometrial cups formed from embryonic cells which invade the uterine lining

5. _____ A substance commonly used to induce parturition

6. _____ The structure expected to rupture during stage II of parturition in the equine and bovine

7. _____ Used for correcting abnormalities of the vulva

8. _____ The term used for the neutered male of the porcine species

9. _____ Increases during estrus and decreases after ovulation in the feline

10. _____ The type of placentation noted in the feline

11. _____ The term used for the delivery of fetuses in the sheep

12. _____ The process of feeding a higher level of nutrition to a ewe with a low-body condition score prior to breeding to increase the number of oocytes

13. _____ The term used for the birthing process in the goat

14. _____ The term used for the birthing process in the bovine

15. _____ The device that utilizes a dye packet to detect mounting when breeding cows

16. _____ The chemical signal released by the zygote once it reaches the uterus

17. _____ The classification of the placenta in which the contact points are evenly distributed over most of it

18. _____ The first secretion of a cow's udder, which is important for calves to consume by means of nursing

19. _____ An example of a polyestrous species

20. _____ The device typically used to count sperm for determining concentration levels

Column B

A. Zonary

B. Camelids

C. Chorioallantois membrane

D. Heat detector patches

E. Pineal

F. Diffuse

G. Equine chorionic gonadotropin

H. Flushing

I. Hemocytometer

J. Barrow

K. Kidding

L. Lambing

M. Diestrus

N. Estrogen

O. Calving

P. Colostrum

Q. Tunica albuginea

R. Caslick's surgery

S. Oxytocin

T. Early conception factor

EXERCISE 10.5 ORDERING: BREEDING SOUNDNESS EXAMINATION IN THE MALE

Instructions: Place the eight parts of the breeding soundness examination in the proper order (from first to last) by placing the appropriate letter in the space provided.

Column A

1. _____
2. _____
3. _____
4. _____
5. _____
6. _____
7. _____
8. _____

Column B

A. Examination of sperm motility

B. A detailed examination of the external and internal genitalia

C. Other tests as necessary

D. Identification of the patient (ideally through a microchip, tattoo, or brand)

E. Examination of sperm morphology

F. A thorough history focusing on the reproductive system

G. Determination of a sperm count

H. Semen collection

EXERCISE 10.6 TRUE OR FALSE: COMPREHENSIVE

Instructions: Read the following statements and write "T" for true or "F" for false in the blanks provided. If a statement is false, correct the statement to make it true.

1. _____ Although the follicle matures as ovulation approaches, the ovum within only matures following ovulation.

2. _____ When an oocyte is released from an ovarian follicle, it is covered with cumulus cells.

3. _____ Regression of the corpus luteum is accompanied by a rapid drop in progesterone.

4. _____ Superfetation is a normal occurrence.

5. _____ When animals are bred naturally, semen deposited at the beginning of a heat will still be capable of fertilizing the oocyte after ovulation.

6. _____ The general body temperature is higher than that of the testes.

7. _____ The production of sperm is cyclical.

8. _____ Capacitation is a process by which an ovum is made ready for fertilization.

9. _____ The castrated male canine is referred to as a neutered male.

10. _____ The canine estrous cycle does not include the stage of anestrus.

11. _____ During canine estrus, the bitch may play with the male in the beginning of "courtship" to establish a friendly behavioral relationship.

12. _____ The ova in the bitch can be fertilized at the time of ovulation.

13. _____ Parturition in the bitch occurs during the diestrus period of the estrous cycle.

14. _____ Parturition takes place in the bitch within approximately 24 hours after the CL is no longer functional.

15. _____ Progesterone and luteinizing hormone levels can be used to predict when a bitch should be bred.

16. _____ Once thawed, frozen semen has a short life span.

17. _____ Frozen semen can be potentially stored for thousands of years in liquid nitrogen.

18. _____ When using fresh semen, canine insemination should be performed 2 to 3 times to ensure fertilization takes place.

19. _____ Vaginal cytology is used for predicting insemination time in the bitch after progesterone assay concentrations have reached greater than 10 ng/mL.

20. _____ Radiography is used to determine the number of pups in utero, their size, and their position.

21. _____ The drop in body temperature that occurs in the canine before stage II of whelping is related to a decrease in estrogen.

22. _____ It is normal to see a blackish-green vaginal discharge during whelping.

23. _____ Parturition in queens that lasts for over 9 hours typically results in fetal death.

24. _____ The queen is a seasonally polyestrous animal.

25. _____ Relaxin is produced in the queen by the fetoplacental unit.

26. _____ The queen is an induced ovulator.

27. _____ The queen is one of many animals commonly seen in a veterinary office that is capable of assisting itself with dystocia.

28. _____ Increased vocalization during estrus in the queen is a normal occurrence.

29. _____ Vulvar discharge in the queen should occur during the estrus stage of the heat cycle.

30. _____ Prostaglandin $F_2\alpha$ has the ability to induce abortion in the queen and in the bitch.

31. _____ Fertilization in the queen occurs in the oviducts, and the fertilized eggs then migrate to the uterine horns where they implant.

32. _____ Ultrasonographic imaging starting at approximately day 15 postbreeding is an excellent resource for diagnosing pregnancy in the queen.

33. _____ By days 12 to 15 in feline gestation, the amniotic vesicles coalesce and are no longer individually discernible by abdominal palpation of the uterus.

34. _____ The uterine size will take weeks to reduce to a normal size after stage III parturition has occurred in the queen.

35. _____ Dystocia is a common occurrence in the queen.

36. _____ A newborn foal is not referred to as a yearling until after 12 months of age.

37. _____ Although a mare may be called spayed, her uterus is rarely removed.

38. _____ Foals obtain IgG transplacentally.

39. _____ Fillies younger than three years have an increased abortion rate of up to 50%.

40. _____ Although twin ovulations occur about 18% of the time, the live birth of equine twins is rare.

40. _____ It is not uncommon for mares to show signs of heat without being in physiologic estrus.

42. _____ The foal needs to be mature and at 330 days or more of gestation for parturition.

43. _____ Mares will always exhibit signs of heat during physiologic estrus.

44. _____ It may be necessary to use tranquilization when examining the reproductive tract of a mare.

45. _____ A mare in heat exhibits the flehmen response when she is approached by a stallion.

46. _____ The equine ovum requires no additional time for maturation once released, allowing fertilization to occur immediately if the sperm are present.

47. _____ The CL is fully functional within approximately 5 days postovulation in the equine.

48. _____ At 30 days postovulation, progesterone concentration in the equine begins to decrease.

49. _____ Foals born on December 31st are considered 1 year old the next day.

50. _____ Artificial lighting is not of significance when it pertains to the estrus cycle in mares.

51. _____ Examination of the anatomical conformation of the vulva in the mare is a very important part of a reproductive tract evaluation.

52. _____ The use of progestogens can lengthen the period from follicular development to ovulation in the mare.

53. _____ The cervix and vaginal wall should be easily visible once the vaginal speculum has entered the vagina during examination of the mare.

54. _____ A "deep" intrauterine insemination technique is the usual method for performing artificial insemination in the mare.

55. _____ Equine chorionic gonadotropin is also known as pregnant mare serum gonadotropin.

56. _____ The United States has more horses than any other country in the world.

57. _____ The most accurate method of diagnosing pregnancy in the equine is palpation of the reproductive tract via rectal examination.

58. _____ The age of puberty in bovines depends on breed and level of nutrition.

59. _____ The desired age at first calving in the bovine is 4 years.

60. _____ The cow is a seasonally polyestrous animal.

61. _____ A sign of estrus in the cow may include the presence of clear stringy vaginal discharge.

62. _____ The approximate estrous cycle length of a cow is 21 days.

63. _____ The cow has an average of 75 to 120 uterine caruncles, which are irreplaceable once damaged or destroyed.

64. _____ Pregnancy in the cow is primarily determined with the use of ultrasonographic examination.

65. _____ Sheep are seasonally polyestrous animals.

66. _____ Lambs and doelings bred in the fall of their first year generally have earlier and higher lifetime production levels than those first bred as yearlings.

67. _____ Abortion rates in sheep and goats are generally low.

68. _____ The flushing of ewes with a body condition score above 2.5 is highly recommended.

69. _____ Both sheep and goats respond to male pheromones, which can shorten anestrus by a week or more.

70. _____ The semen deposited during breeding by the ram at the beginning of a ewe's heat cycle will still have the capability to fertilize oocytes during ovulation.

71. _____ Use of intravaginal controlled internal drug release (CIDR) inserts that release estrogen allows estrus synchronization in ewes.

72. _____ The estrus cycle in sheep is 36 hours.

73. _____ The gestation period in sheep is typically 145–152 days.

74. _____ Pregnancy determination may be performed via ultrasonographic rectal examination in the ewe at 25 days into gestation.

75. _____ Infectious causes of abortion in sheep and goats include leptospirosis, toxoplasmosis, and *Chlamydophila abortus.*

76. _____ Camelid females in heat will adopt a position of sternal recumbency and allow breeding shortly after a male is introduced.

77. _____ Camelid species are induced ovulators.

78. _____ Pregnancies in camelids occur predominately in the left horn.

79. _____ The size of the testes or the scrotum is important information to obtain during the breeding soundness examination of a male animal.

80. _____ The horse is the only domestic species in which the penis is cleansed prior to the collection of semen.

81. _____ The sperm of most species move rapidly forward in a straight line.

82. _____ The head of a sperm cell is characterized as rounded, not flat.

83. _____ During a breeding soundness examination, the motility of sperm is assessed before the morphologic examination is performed.

84. _____ Uterine cultures are more easily obtained on smaller animals.

85. _____ The uterine lumen is sterile in all species.

86. _____ The mare and cow are the only species in which endometrial biopsies may be obtained through the vaginal lumen.

87. _____ Cultures of the reproductive tract of the bitch should be obtained by the use of a conventional culture swab.

Instructions: Circle the one correct answer to each of the following questions.

1. Prior to placentation, which of the following comprise the maternal and fetal layers?
   a. Endothelium
   b. Mesoderm
   c. Epithelium
   d. All of the above

2. Antibody protection of the newborn at birth is solely dependent upon which of the following?
   a. A diffuse placenta
   b. The chorionic epithelium remaining in contact with the maternal component
   c. Maternal layers remaining intact
   d. Colostrum consumption after birth

3. Within the testes, developing sperm cells are surrounded by
   a. Sertoli cells.
   b. a layer of mucous.
   c. interstitial cells.
   d. primordial germ cells.

4. The hormone that acts on Sertoli cells to increase primordial sperm cell division and release more sperm cells is
   a. testosterone.
   b. FSH.
   c. GnRH.
   d. LH.

5. After sperm cells are released, they attain motility and the ability to fertilize in the
   a. seminiferous tubules.
   b. epididymis.
   c. tunica albuginea.
   d. female reproductive tract.

6. The length of time required from the initiation of sperm development until formation of a mature sperm cell is approximately
   a. 27 days.
   b. 33 days.
   c. 55 days.
   d. 62 days.

7. The age at which puberty is reached in the bitch is approximately
   a. 4 to 6 months.
   b. 7 to 12 months.
   c. 6 to 24 months.
   d. 24 to 42 months.

8. Once mature, ova in the bitch remain fertilizable for
   a. 12 hours.
   b. 36 hours.
   c. 24 hours.
   d. 3 days.

9. Which of the following choices represents the proper order of the canine estrous cycle?
   a. Proestrus, estrus, diestrus, anestrus
   b. Estrus, diestrus, proestrus, and anestrus
   c. Estrus, proestrus, anestrus, and diestrus
   d. Anestrus, estrus, proestrus, and diestrus

10. The approximate length of the canine estrous cycle is
    a. 2 months.
    b. 4 months.
    c. 6 months.
    d. 8 months.

11. The proestrus and estrus stages of the bitch will each last approximately
    a. 3 days.
    b. 5 days.
    c. 7 days.
    d. 9 days.

12. In most canine breeds, anestrus will last approximately
    a. 2 months.
    b. 4 months.
    c. 6 months.
    d. 8 months.

13. The release of ova from the ovaries in the bitch will occur approximately _____ days following the LH spike.
    a. 1
    d. 2
    c. 4
    d. 5

14. Once released and mature, the ova of the bitch will remain fertilizable for
    a. 3 days.
    b. 6 days.
    c. 9 days.
    d. 12 days.

15. During the natural breeding process of the canine species, the male and female will be "locked together" for up to _____ minutes.
    a. 15
    b. 30
    c. 45
    d. 50

16. The period of least reproductive activity in the bitch will occur during
    a. estrus.
    b. proestrus.
    c. diestrus.
    d. anestrus.

17. The BSE in males is designed to assess
    a. semen quality.
    b. attitude.
    c. disposition.
    d. All of the above

18. Because of its short life span, once frozen semen has thawed, fertilization should occur within
    a. 6 hours.
    b. 8 hours.
    c. 12 hours.
    d. 15 hours.

19. Examination for pregnancy in the bitch by palpation is possible in most bitches between _____ and _____ days of gestation.
    a. 12, 25
    b. 15, 38
    c. 21, 30
    d. 30, 36

20. In the bitch, the length of gestation from the point of fertilization is approximately
    a. 48 days.
    b. 60 days.
    c. 72 days.
    d. 84 days.

21. A drop in body temperature to 99° F in a near-term pregnant bitch signals that whelping is imminent. This change generally occurs about _____ hours before stage II.
    a. 8
    b. 12
    c. 24
    d. 48

22. Which animal can assist itself in dystocia?
    a. llama
    b. mare
    c. bitch
    d. queen

23. The approximate weight at which the queen will reach puberty is
    a. 3 to 4 pounds.
    b. 5 to 6 pounds.
    c. 6.5 to 7 pounds.
    d. 7.5 to 8 pounds.

24. Estrous in the queen can last
    a. 2 to 19 days.
    b. 20 to 30 days.
    c. 31 to 35 days.
    d. 40 to 45 days.

25. If no ovulation occurs after breeding or if there is no breeding, the queen will return to estrus in
    a. 1-2 days.
    b. 3-14 days.
    c. 15-21 days.
    d. 22-28 days.

26. Less than _____ of all queens will ovulate with a single mating.
    a. 15%
    b. 25%
    c. 35%
    d. 50%

27. The average duration of pregnancy in the queen following breeding is
    a. 55 days.
    b. 63 days.
    c. 75 days.
    d. 82 days.

28. What stage of parturition in the queen is characterized by lactational secretion, increased fetal movements, and relaxation around the perineal area?
    a. Stage I
    b. Stage II
    c. Stage III

29. What is the age at puberty of the porcine species?
    a. 6–7 months
    b. 12–14 months
    c. 4–6 months
    d. 18–24 months

30. The speed of movement of sperm is reflected in
    a. the size of the individual sperm cells.
    b. the quantity of sperm cells.
    c. the rotation of the sperm cells.
    d. the age of the sperm sample.

31. The approximate age range at which the estrous cycle is initiated in the filly is
    a. 6 to 12 months.
    b. 12 to 24 months.
    c. 24 to 48 months.
    d. 48 to 60 months.

32. The peak of estrous activity in the equine species occurs near which of the following dates?
    a. June 21st
    b. August 21st
    c. December 21st
    d. May 21st

33. The average length of heat in the mare is
    a. 5 days.
    b. 6 days.
    c. 7 days.
    d. 9 days.

34. The average length of the estrous cycle in the equine is
    a. 16 days.
    b. 21 days.
    c. 24 days.
    d. 36 days.

35. Which behavior is not related to estrus in the equine?
    a. Frequent urination
    b. Raised tail
    c. Frequent opening and closing of the vulva exposing the clitoris
    d. Increased tendency to kick

36. The best time to breed a horse is
    a. the first day of estrus.
    b. 1–2 days after ovulation.
    c. the last days of estrus before ovulation.
    d. the first day of diestrus.

37. Sperm of the equine species usually have a high fertilizing life span of
    a. 12 hours.
    b. 24 hours.
    c. 48 hours.
    d. 72 hours.

38. Postovulation insemination performed in the equine species is highly successful when performed within
    a. 6 hours.
    b. 8 hours.
    c. 12 hours.
    d. 16 hours.

39. The breeding season for the equine species in North America is approximately
    a. January 1st to June 1st.
    b. February 1st to July 15th.
    c. July 1st to December 1st.
    d. October 1st to March 1st.

40. Spermatogenesis is completed within the testicles, but sperm are not completely mature until they pass through the
    a. vesicular glands.
    b. bulbourethral gland.
    c. prostate.
    d. epididymis.

41. The desired age for first calving in the cow is approximately
    a. 2 years of age.
    b. 3 years of age.
    c. 4 years of age.
    d. 7 years of age.

42. Pregnancy must occur at which of the following ages in order for a first calving to occur at the desired time?
    a. 10 months
    b. 15 months
    c. 20 months
    d. 24 months

43. The estrous cycle length of the cow is approximately
    a. 18 days.
    b. 21 days.
    c. 24 days.
    d. 32 days.

44. Ovulation in the cow will occur about _____ hours after the end of standing heat.
    a. 4 to 6
    b. 6 to 8
    c. 8 to 12
    d. 12 to 16

45. The gestation length of the cow is approximately
    a. 256 to 259 days.
    b. 265 to 269 days.
    c. 279 to 283 days.
    d. 341 to 345 days.

46. The length of the estrous cycle in the ewe is approximately
    a. 10 days.
    b. 13 days.
    c. 18 days.
    d. 19 days.

47. The estrous cycle length in the goat is
    a. 21 days.
    b. 28 days.
    c. 32 days.
    d. 34 days.

48. The estrus stage of the goat estrous cycle lasts approximately
    a. 1 to 2 days.
    b. 3 to 4 days.
    c. 5 to 6 days.
    d. 7 to 10 days.

49. The female camelid will reach puberty at the approximate age of
    a. 6 to 10 months.
    b. 10 to 12 months.
    c. 12 to 18 months.
    d. 18 to 24 months.

50. The average length of estrus in a camelid is between
    a. 1 and 4 days.
    b. 1 and 7 days.
    c. 2 and 8 days.
    d. 3 and 15 days.

51. The gestation period of the camelid is
    a. 290 to 310 days.
    b. 310 to 330 days.
    c. 340 to 350 days.
    d. 360 to 380 days.

52. In the camelid, ovulation and fertility will return postpartum at approximately
    a. 4 days.
    b. 9 days.
    c. 12 days.
    d. 20 days.

EXERCISE 10.8 FILL-IN-THE-BLANK: COMPREHENSIVE

Instructions: Fill in each of the spaces provided with the missing word or words that complete the sentence.

1. After ovulation, the empty follicular sac fills with clotted blood, forming a _____.

2. _____ is important in the regulation of seasonal and diurnal rhythms, including the seasonal breeding cycles of long- and short-day breeders, such as cats, sheep, goats, and horse.

3. When sperm are mixed with accessory sex gland fluid, the result is called _____.

4. Sexual receptiveness in the female is brought about by the ratio of the hormone _____

   to the hormone _____.

5. The _____ gland is particularly important to reproduction. Both it and the hypothalamus are part of the _____ system, which is the part of the brain that regulates _____ and _____ functions.

6. During estrus, the uterine feels turgid and tightly coiled when palpated. This is due to increasing levels of _____.

7. The ectoderm of the zygote will develop into hair, skin, and the _____ system.

8. In the male, testosterone is produced by the _____ cells of the testes.

9. During embryonic development, the testicles are covered by a capsule of connective tissue known as the _____.

10. The external location of the testes maintains their temperature _____ °C cooler than the body core.

11. _____ from the pituitary stimulates testosterone production. As testosterone increases, it inhibits secretion of _____ from the hypothalamus.

12. In the male, the changes in blood flow that initiate an erection are mediated by the _____ branch of the autonomic nervous system. In contrast, ejaculation is mediated by the branch of the autonomic nervous system.

13. The female canine that has had the _____ removed is referred to as an ovariectomized bitch.

14. The canine estrous cycle consists of _____, _____, _____, and anestrus.

15. The beginning of proestrus in the bitch is indicated by the commencement of a from the vulva.

16. During proestrus in the bitch, the endometrium becomes highly _____ and engorged with blood.

17. _____ is the microscopic evaluation of cells from the vagina.

18. Radiographic diagnosis of pregnancy in the feline is possible from _____ day to term; it is most useful for fetal counts at around day _____.

19. Uterine involution following whelping or in the nonpregnant bitch is not complete until approximately 120 days following _____.

20. During estrus, increased vocalization is the norm in the queen. In addition, she may display _____, in which she arches her spine and raises her hips.

21. The foal may also be called a _____following separation from its mother or reaching 6 to 12 months of age.

22. When a nearly mature follicle is present, ovulation can be induced in the equine by the administration of _____ or _____.

23. The findings on genital palpation of a mare in heat include a decrease in _____ tone, relaxation of the _____, and an increase in size of the follicles present.

24. Secondary CLs maintain the _____ in the mare until day 120 and then are no longer required.

25. Equine chorionic gonadotropin is produced by the _____ cups.

26. Foal heat occurs within 18 days following _____.

27. The cow has year-round estrous cycles with minimal seasonal influence. Therefore, it is considered to be _____.

28. Ovicaprine estrous cycles have four stages: proestrus, estrus, _____, and _____.

29. The _____ reflex is a neuroendocrine mechanism whereby the dilation of the cervical lumen stimulates the release of _____, which further dilates the cervix.

30. Cows are usually in sternal or _____ recumbency at the time of delivery.

31. Rams that have been _____ are frequently used as part of an artificial breeding program.

32. The rate of embryonic loss in camelids is 10% to 50%, which is _____ than in most domestic species.

33. Mating of camelids occurs in a recumbent position called _____.

34. The placenta of the camelid should be passed within 6 hours; if retained, the patient should be treated with _____.

35. Although spermatogenesis is completed in the testicles, the spermatozoa must pass through the _____ for maturation to occur.

36. Scrotal circumference is measured when performing a breeding soundness examination of _____.

37. The _____ gland is the only accessory sex gland present in the dog.

38. Any vaginal examination or diagnostic technique in the mare should be preceded by a thorough cleansing of the _____ area.

39. The _____ is the portion of the uterus most involved with pregnancy maintenance.

EXERCISE 10.9 CASE STUDY: PARTURITION

Ms. Allen, a longtime client, calls your hospital asking for advice. She has several feral cats living under her porch. Although she has worked with a local humane organization to have all of the cats trapped, neutered, and released, a new female (who she named Emily) showed up a few weeks ago.

Emily is tame enough that Ms. Allen was able to coax her into the garage and was even able to handle her a little bit. Emily seems very healthy but appears to be pregnant. Ms. Allen is calling today to make an appointment to bring her in for a checkup, pregnancy check, and any other care she might need, and would like some information concerning what to expect when the kittens are born (assuming Emily is pregnant, as Ms. Allen suspects).

1. Answer her question by describing the series of events that takes place during parturition in the queen, starting from stage I to birth of the kittens, as well as the likelihood of dystocia in the queen. (For the purposes of this exercise, you may use clinical terminology.)

_____

_____

_____

_____

_____

_____

_____

_____

Hematology and Cytology

LEARNING OBJECTIVES

When you have completed this chapter, you will be able to:

1. Pronounce, define, and spell all key terms in this chapter.
2. Describe proper collection techniques, handling of blood samples, and components of a complete blood count (CBC).
3. Describe the advantages, disadvantages, and capabilities of automated hematology analyzers.
4. Do the following regarding blood counts:
   - Compare and contrast procedures used to determine red blood cell (RBC) mass (packed cell volume [PCV], hematocrit [HCT], hemoglobin, and RBC count) and discuss the causes and significance of abnormal values.
   - Describe methods used to calculate RBC indices and red cell distribution width (RDW) and discuss the causes and significance of abnormal values.
   - Describe methods used to determine plasma protein concentration and discuss the causes and significance of abnormal values.
   - Describe methods used to determine the white blood cell (WBC) count and the platelet count.
5. Do the following regarding blood smears:
   - Describe the technique used to prepare a stained blood smear, list factors that influence smear quality, and discuss the evaluation process.
   - Describe normal and abnormal morphology of RBCs, WBCs, and platelets in each species as they appear on a blood smear.
   - Discuss the causes and significance of RBC, WBC, and platelet abnormalities commonly observed on a blood smear.
   - Describe the procedure used to perform a differential WBC count and calculate absolute values.
6. Do the following regarding coagulation testing:
   - Explain normal primary and secondary hemostasis, including intrinsic, extrinsic, and common pathways.
   - Discuss bleeding time, activated clotting time (ACT), activated partial thromboplastin time (APTT), and prothrombin time (PT), and the uses and significance of each.
   - Discuss tests used to evaluate fibrinolysis, including fibrin(ogen) degradation products (FDPs), D-dimer tests, and fibrinogen tests.
7. Do the following regarding cytology:
   - Explain uses for and limitations of cytology.
   - Describe procedures used to evaluate the cytology of solid tissue masses, enlarged organs, thoracic and abdominal effusions, and synovial fluid.
   - Discuss procedures used to submit cytology samples to a reference laboratory.
   - Describe collection and preparation of otic cytology samples and identify common findings on normal and abnormal otic cytology preparations.

Across

2 A test that gives information about the numbers and types of circulating cells.
4 Stacking of red blood cells.
7 Vacuolization, Döhle bodies, and cytoplasmic basophilia in neutrophils. (2 words)
10 Nonnucleated fragments of cytoplasm released from megakaryocytes.
11 A nucleated red blood cell.
13 Falsely decreased in patients with red blood cell agglutination.
17 Percentage of RBCs in a specific volume of blood. (3 words)
18 Large in some poodles, very small in goats, and oval in camels. (3 words)
21 Variation in cell size.
23 A test that evaluates the intrinsic pathway of the coagulation cascade.
24 The term "leukopenia" means decreased numbers of these. (3 words)
25 The most abundant granulocyte in rabbits.
26 In most species, this is approximately equal to the PCV divided by 3.

Down

1 Becomes a macrophage in the tissues.
3 Used to evaluate exfoliated tissue cells.
5 MCV, MCHC, and MCH. (4 words)
6 This change in RBC distribution occurs in patients with immune-mediated hemolytic anemia (IHA).
8 Normally very few in circulation, but may be the most abundant leukocyte in some species of turtles.
9 The predominant circulating white blood cell in cattle, sheep, and goats.
12 Evaluated by the PT and ACT.
14 May contain Döhle bodies.
15 Counted to differentiate regenerative from nonregenerative anemia.
16 A red blood cell that has lost a portion of its membrane.
19 In cats, this cell contains numerous small, rod-shaped granules.
20 An increased number of circulating bands. (2 words)
22 An immature neutrophil.

EXERCISE 11.2 MATCHING #1: ABBREVIATIONS RELATED TO HEMATOLOGY AND COAGULATION

Instructions: Match each abbreviation related to hematology and coagulation in column A with its corresponding description in column B by writing the appropriate letter in the space provided.

Column A

1. _____ MCV
2. _____ MCHC
3. _____ FDP
4. _____ PT
5. _____ MCH
6. _____ RDW
7. _____ HCT
8. _____ APTT

Column B

A. An indicator of variation in red cell size

B. The average amount of hemoglobin in each RBC

C. The average amount of hemoglobin in a specific volume of blood

D. Evaluates the extrinsic and common pathways of the coagulation cascade

E. Evaluates the intrinsic and common pathways of the coagulation cascade

F. A measure of fibrinolysis

G. A measure of red blood cell mass

H. The average size of the RBCs

EXERCISE 11.3 MATCHING #2: NUCLEATED CELLS SEEN ON A BLOOD SMEAR EXAM

Instructions: Match each cell type in column A with its corresponding description in column B by writing the appropriate letter in the space provided.

Column A

1. _____ Neutrophils
2. _____ Band neutrophils
3. _____ Pelger-Huet anomaly
4. _____ Eosinophils
5. _____ Basophils
6. _____ Lymphocytes
7. _____ Reactive lymphocytes
8. _____ Neoplastic lymphocytes
9. _____ Monocytes
10. _____ Mast cells

Column B

A. Have more intensely basophilic cytoplasm and may have a perinuclear clear area

B. The predominant circulating white blood cell in dogs, cats, and horses

C. Have a twisted or irregular nucleus in dogs

D. Contain numerous purple granules and a round nucleus

E. Are also called "stabs"

F. Up to 50% may be intermediate to large size in cows

G. These cells have prominent nucleoli

H. A congenital or acquired defect most often seen in dogs

I. Have abundant gray-blue cytoplasm, possibly with clear vacuoles

J. Contain numerous, large, brightly staining granules in horses

EXERCISE 11.4 MATCHING #3: HEMOSTASIS

Instructions: Match each term related to hemostasis in column A with its corresponding description in column B by writing the appropriate letter in the space provided.

Column A

1. _____ Activated clotting time (ACT)
2. _____ Blood smear
3. _____ Coagulation cascade
4. _____ D-dimers
5. _____ Fibrin degradation products (FDP)
6. _____ Fibrinolysis
7. _____ Hemocytometer
8. _____ Plasmin
9. _____ Prothrombin time (PT)
10. _____ Refractometer

Column B

A. Activates secondary hemostasis

B. Evaluates the extrinsic and common pathways

C. Products of fibrin proteolysis that are considered to be reflective of active degradation of clots

D. A device used in the measurement of plasma protein concentration

E. This test requires use of a special tube that contains diatomaceous earth.

F. Evaluated by measuring FDPs

G. Form when fibrin undergoes proteolysis by plasmin

H. Used to evaluate platelet morphology

I. Causes proteolysis of fibrin

J. A device that can be used to manually count white blood cells

EXERCISE 11.5 MATCHING #4: ABNORMAL BODY CAVITY FLUIDS AND ASSOCIATED CAUSES

Instructions: Normal thoracic and abdominal fluid is clear and colorless in small animals but may have a yellow tint in large animals. Disease states can cause a number of color changes that give clues as to the nature of the problem. Match each description of the appearance of abnormal body fluids in column A with the common associated causes in column B by writing the appropriate letter in the space provided.

Column A

1. _____ Red or pink
2. _____ White or tan
3. _____ Brown
4. _____ Green
5. _____ Yellow

Column B

A. Hemolysis and icterus, previous hemorrhage, or ruptured bladder

B. Previous hemorrhage or leakage of bowel contents

C. Ruptured bile duct

D. Internal hemorrhage

E. Lipid or high numbers of cells

EXERCISE 11.6 PHOTO QUIZ: PHOTOGRAPHS OF RED BLOOD CELLS WITH SHAPE CHANGES

Instructions: Match each circled red blood cell in the photograph with the letter corresponding to the morphologic change.

Names

A. Acanthocyte

B. Eccentrocyte

C. Echinocyte

D. Cell with a Heinz body

E. Keratocyte

F. Apple stem cell

G. Schistocytes

H. Spherocyte

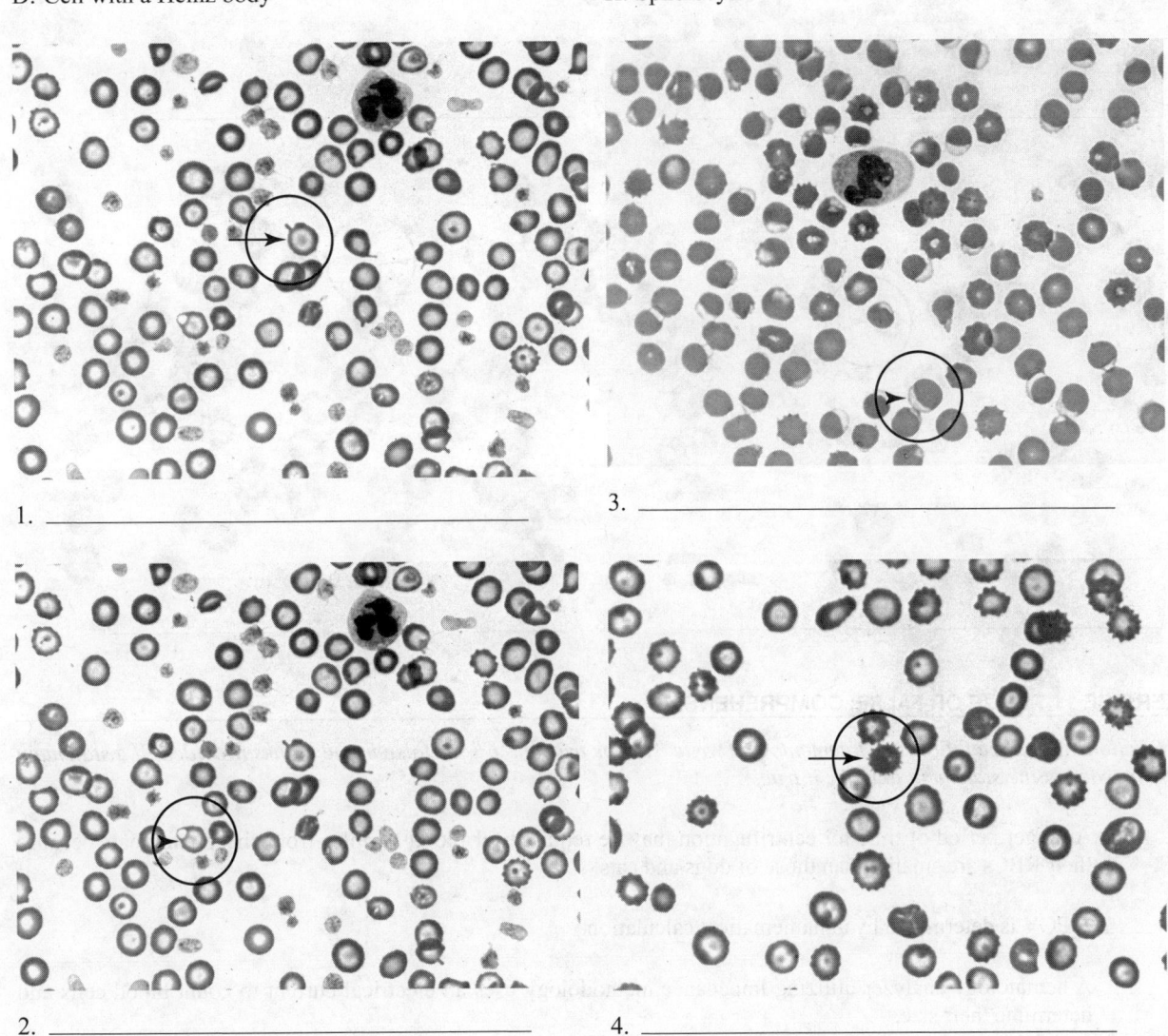

1. _____

2. _____

3. _____

4. _____

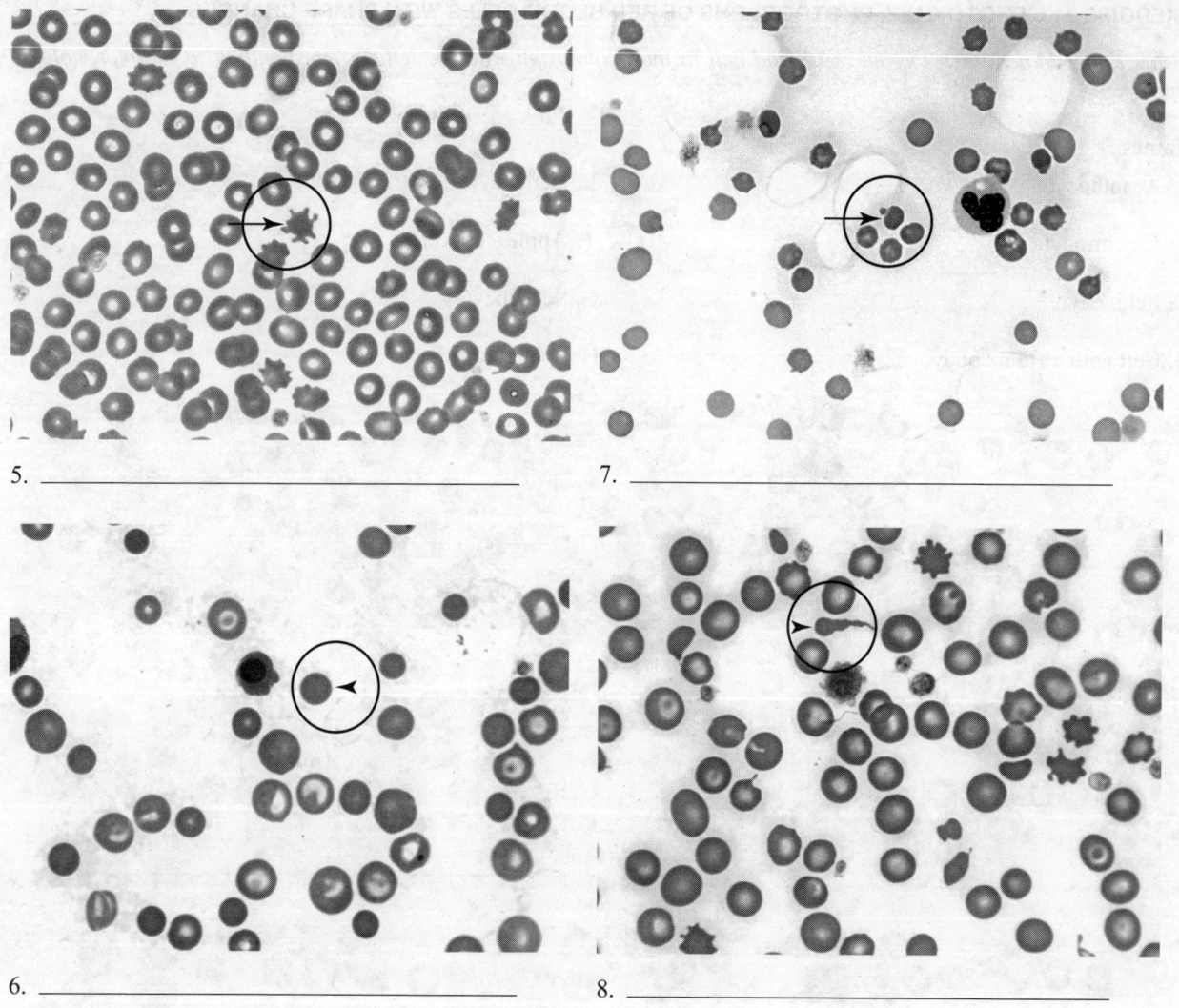

5. _____

7. _____

6. _____

8. _____

EXERCISE 11.7 TRUE OR FALSE: COMPREHENSIVE

Instructions: Read the following statements and write "T" for true or "F" for false in the blanks provided. If a statement is false, correct the statement to make it true.

1. _____ A longer period of time for centrifugation may be required for blood samples from sheep and goats because their RBCs are smaller than those of dogs and cats.

2. _____ A PCV is determined by a mathematical calculation.

3. _____ A hematology analyzer utilizing impedance methodology uses an electrical current to count blood cells and determine their size.

4. _____ WBCs are heavier than both RBCs and blood plasma and thus are found on the bottom of a microhematocrit tube following centrifugation.

5. _____ Changes in the hemoglobin concentration are generally proportional to changes in the WBC count.

6. _____ An increased red cell distribution width (RDW) indicates anisocytosis.

7. _____ Platelet clumps occur most commonly in dogs.

8. _____ Ideally, a blood smear should be stained within 24 hours.

9. _____ The substage condenser of the microscope should be in a relatively high position when evaluating a blood smear or cytology prep.

10. _____ Target cells, when noted on a blood smear, are usually seen in animals with hemangiosarcoma or heartworm disease.

11. _____ Echinocytes are most often seen in animals with lymphoma (cancer of the lymph nodes).

12. _____ Almost all RBCs look like spherocytes near the feathered edge.

13. _____ The presence of any metarubricytes on a blood smear is abnormal.

14. _____ In normal animals, up to 10% of the RBCs are polychromatophilic.

15. _____ The blood parasite *Anaplasma marginale* is easily mistaken for stain precipitate.

16. _____ If you submit a tissue sample that contains a mass, it is useful to describe the size of the mass and whether it is superficial or deep, firm or soft, and freely movable or firmly attached

17. _____ Samples collected from the horizontal portion of the ear canal should be collected using clean cotton-tipped swabs.

18. _____ When performing a differential cell count, broken cells should not be counted.

19. _____ Plasma samples for APTT and PT testing should be kept frozen until arrival at the reference lab.

20. _____ The mucin clot test is used to evaluate blood coagulation.

EXERCISE 11.8 MULTIPLE CHOICE: COMPREHENSIVE

Instructions: Circle the one correct answer to each of the following questions.

1. Citrate is the anticoagulant contained in a
   a. lavender-top tube.
   b. red-top tube.
   c. green-top tube.
   d. blue-top tube.

2. Which one of the following tests does not indicate the oxygen-carrying capacity of blood?
   a. RBC count
   b. HCT
   c. PDW
   d. PCV

3. Automated hematology analyzers determine the HCT by
   a. direct measurement.
   b. multiplying the MCV count by the RBC.
   c. dividing the PCV by the RBC count.
   d. dividing the PCV by 3.

4. MCV is often increased in patients with
   a. inflammation.
   b. chronic renal failure.
   c. primary bone marrow disease.
   d. blood loss.

5. Red blood cells in an animal with a decreased MCHC are called
   a. hypochromic.
   b. microcytic.
   c. normochromic.
   d. macrocytic.

6. Plasma is often clear and light yellow in
   a. horses and cats.
   b. dogs and cows.
   c. cats and dogs.
   d. cows and horses.

7. Rouleaux formation is most common in
   a. horses and cats.
   b. dogs and cows.
   c. cats and dogs.
   d. cows and horses.

8. Agglutination refers to irregular, variable-sized clumps of RBCs that occur most commonly in animals with
   a. liver disease.
   b. immune-mediated hemolytic anemia.
   c. lead poisoning.
   d. blood loss.

9. In which species do platelets not tend to stain as well on a blood smear as in other species?
   a. Dogs
   b. Cats
   c. Horses
   d. Cattle

10. Macroplatelets may be normal in cats and
    a. Akitas.
    b. Cavalier King Charles Spaniels.
    c. greyhounds.
    d. poodles.

11. The central pallor in RBCs is most prominent in the normal RBCs of
    a. dogs.
    b. cats.
    c. horses.
    d. cattle.

12. Anisocytosis tends to be most prevalent in _____ and least prevalent in _____.
    a. dogs; horses
    b. horses; cats
    c. cats; cows
    d. cows; dogs

13. Animals with immune-mediated hemolytic anemia often have _____ on the blood smear.
    a. spherocytes
    b. apple-stem cells
    c. eccentrocytes
    d. Heinz bodies

14. Howell-Jolly bodies are often increased in patients with
    a. liver disease.
    b. bone marrow suppression.
    c. iron-deficiency anemia.
    d. regenerative anemia.

15. A reticulocyte count is used to determine
    a. whether an anemia is regenerative or nonregenerative.
    b. whether an anemia will get better or not.
    c. the severity of an anemia.
    d. whether an anemia is longstanding.

16. Segmented neutrophils have a segmented nucleus with an average of
    a. 2 to 3 lobes.
    b. 3 to 5 lobes.
    c. 4 to 6 lobes.
    d. 5 to 7 lobes.

17. This in-house coagulation test may be used to detect abnormal platelet function.
    a. Activated clotting time
    b. Prothrombin time
    c. Bleeding time
    d. Activated partial thromboplastin time

18. This value is calculated as the TP of an unheated plasma sample minus the TP of a heated sample.
    a. Fibrinogen
    b. D-dimers
    c. PT
    d. FDPs

19. Cytologic examination of tissue masses enables evaluation of
    a. surgical margins.
    b. vascular invasion.
    c. morphology of isolated cells.
    d. association of abnormal cells with normal tissues.

20. When preparing thoracic or abdominal effusion samples for cytologic examination, direct smears are often made, but some samples require concentration of the cells. Which of the following fluids is most likely to require cell concentration?
    a. Bloody fluid
    b. Fluid with a high cell count
    c. Clear fluid
    d. Turbid fluid

EXERCISE 11.9 FILL-IN-THE-BLANK: COMPREHENSIVE

Instructions: Fill in each of the spaces provided with the missing word or words that complete the sentence.

1. EDTA prevents blood clotting by binding _____.

2. Serum protein is usually a little lower than plasma protein because there is no _____ in it.

3. The presence of increased numbers of circulating nucleated red blood cells may occur with a markedly regenerative anemia. When this occurs in the absence of anemia and is accompanied by basophilic stippling, it may indicate _____.

4. A blood smear may be too thick if, when preparing the smear, the drop of blood is too _____, the spreader slide is pushed too _____, or the angle of the spreader slide is too _____.

5. The three areas of the blood smear, in order from nearest the drop to furthest away, are the _____, the _____, and the _____.

6. Regarding the shape of nuclei of WBC, the nucleus of a neutrophil is segmented with three to five lobes, whereas the nucleus of a monocyte is round, _____, _____, or _____ in shape, and the nucleus of a lymphocyte is generally _____ in shape.

7. The RBCs of birds and reptiles differ from those of mammals in that they contain a _____ and are _____ in shape.

8. Automatic cell counters may erroneously count nRBCs as WBCs. This error will cause the WBC count to be falsely _____. A WBC count that includes nRBCs should be referred to as a total _____ cell count.

9. The differential WBC count is performed by identifying and counting a minimum of _____ cells consecutively encountered in the monolayer.

10. A state in which the number of bands exceeds the number of segmented neutrophils is referred to as a _____ left shift.

11. Primary hemostasis refers to formation of the _____.

12. Blood for a platelet count should be drawn in a tube containing _____ anticoagulant.

13. To determine viscosity of joint fluid, place a wooden applicator stick in the fluid and slowly withdraw it. If viscosity is normal, a strand _____ to _____ cm long should form.

EXERCISE 11.10 CASE STUDY: IMMUNE-MEDIATED HEMOLYTIC ANEMIA (IMHA) AND THROMBOCYTOPENIA (ITP)

Signalment: 6-year-old, spayed female Collie

History: Acute onset of severe lethargy

Physical Examination: Pale, icteric mucous membranes; tachypnea; enlarged spleen

Please examine the following CBC results *(taken from case presentation 11.1 in the text)* and answer the questions below:

CBC	Patient		Reference Interval
Plasma protein (g/dL)	7.6	H	5.7–7.2
Plasma appeared clear and moderately yellow.			
HCT (%)	17	L	36–54
Hemoglobin, g/dL	5.0	L	11.9–18.4
RBCs ($\times 10^{12}$/L)	2.2	L	4.9–8.2
MCV (fl)	80	H	64–75
MCHC (g/dL)	29.1	L	32.9–35.2
RDW	19.1	H	13.4–17.0
Reticulocytes ($\times 10^9$/L)	477.5	H	< 60

RBC Morphology: There is marked agglutination that did not disperse with saline. Moderate anisocytosis, marked polychromasia, and numerous spherocytes are observed. Numbers of Howell-Jolly bodies and nRBCs are increased.

Platelets ($\times 10^9$/L)	94	L	106–424
WBCs ($\times 10^9$/L)	34.6	H	4.1–15.2
nRBCs ($\times 10^9$/L)	10.9	H	0
Band neutrophils ($\times 10^9$/L)	8.2	H	0–0.1
Segmented neutrophils ($\times 10^9$/L)	28.2	H	3.0–10.4
Lymphocytes ($\times 10^9$/L)	1.8		1.0–4.6
Monocytes ($\times 10^9$/L)	7.3	H	0.0—1.2
Eosinophils ($\times 10^9$/L)	0		0–1.2

WBC Morphology: Moderate numbers of Döhle bodies and moderate cytoplasmic basophilia and vacuolation are interpreted as toxic change.

1. What blood collection tube would you select for this blood draw, and what anticoagulant (if any) does this tube contain?

Test	Tube top color	Anticoagulant (N/A if none)
CBC and platelet count	_____	_____

2. The hemoglobin concentration of any patient is usually proportional to the PCV or hematocrit. Using the technique for estimating hemoglobin you learned in this chapter, please estimate this patient's hemoglobin concentration in g/dL.

   Hemoglobin = _____ g/dL

3a. Are this patient's RBCs normal in size?

_____

3b. How do you know this by looking at the CBC?

_____

4. What is the term used to describe RBCs that are too large?

_____

5. Polychromasia is marked on the blood smear examination. What does this mean?

_____

6. How are polychromatophils recognized on a blood smear?

_____

7. On the blood smear, there were also about 5 platelets/100 × field. This correlates to an estimated platelet count of

_____ platelets/μL.

8. This patient had increased nRBCs. When performing a manual cell count, the presence of many nRBCs will falsely increase the total WBC count because nRBCs cannot be differentiated from other nucleated cells. However, the WBC count can be mathematically corrected.

Assume that a patient you were performing a CBC on had a total WBC count of 23,000 cells/μL, and 35 nRBCs were noted while performing the differential cell count. Using the formula you learned in this chapter, correct this patient's WBC count.

Corrected WBC count: _____ cells/μL

9. This patient also had markedly increased numbers of reticulocytes (477.5×10^9/L). What is the significance of this increase?

_____

_____

10. Calculate absolute values by considering the following scenario: You have performed a manual white blood cell count and a 100-cell differential on a patient. The results are as follows:

Total WBC count: 25,000 cell/μL
2% band neutrophils
55% segmented neutrophils
35% lymphocytes
5% monocytes
3% eosinophils

Calculate the absolute numbers of each cell.

Band neutrophils: _____ cells/μL

Segmented neutrophils: _____ cells/μL

Lymphocytes: _____ cells/μL

Monocytes: _____ cells/μL

Eosinophils: _____ cells/μL

12 Clinical Chemistry, Serology, and Urinalysis

LEARNING OBJECTIVES

When you have completed this chapter, you will be able to:
1. Pronounce, spell, and define all key terms in this chapter.
2. Do the following regarding clinical chemistry:
   - Explain the purpose of the clinical chemistry profile and list the preanalytical and analytical factors that can affect clinical chemistry testing.
   - Compare and contrast the use of chemistry analyzers in veterinary medicine and human medicine.
   - Define a calibrator and a control, and describe how they are used in quality control.
3. Describe the general principles of serologic testing and discuss the most common methods of serologic testing.
4. Do the following regarding urinalysis:
   - Describe proper collection techniques and handling of urine samples.
   - List and describe methods for the physical and biochemical evaluation of urine.
   - Describe the preparation of urine for microscopic evaluation, list the cellular elements that can be found in the urine sediment, and identify the three most common urine crystals.

EXERCISE 12.1 FILL-IN-THE-BLANK: TERMS AND DEFINITIONS

Instructions: Fill in each of the spaces provided with the missing word or words that complete the sentence.

1. To determine whether an individual control value is out of the acceptable range, it is useful to plot results on a(n) _____ chart.

2. A(n) _____ is a material that contains a known quantity of the analyte that is being measured, and is used on a regular and frequent basis to monitor performance of instruments and procedures over time.

3. _____, caused by the presence of circulating triglycerides, and _____, resulting from the rupture of RBCs, are commonly encountered preanalytical interferences.

4. Prerenal _____ is indicative of dehydration, while renal _____ indicates impaired _____ function.

5. Urine with USG in the range of 1.008 to 1.012 is _____, which means that it is not concentrated or diluted.

6. Crystals in the urine are defined as _____.

7. Urine _____ is related to the number and molecular weight of particles in urine.

8. _____ measures the bending of light as it passes through a solution and is related to fluid density.

9. Increased numbers of casts in the urine is called _____.

10. _____ can be used to detect hepatocellular injury, cholestasis, or muscle damage.

11. Enzyme-linked immunosorbent assay, more commonly known by the acronym _____, is a serologic test technique.

12. Increased numbers of leukocytes in urine indicate _____, or inflammation in the urinary tract.

13. The renal threshold for bilirubin is low in dogs, so bilirubinuria may be detected before _____ is observed.

14. This chapter provides an overview of common methods and instrumentation employed in biochemical, _____, and urinalysis testing.

15. Accurate, reliable laboratory results are much more likely when a(n) _____ system is designed and used to detect problems before test results are reported.

16. A(n) _____ contains a known, standard amount of a reference material. It is used as part of quality control to adjust an instrument so that the instrument reading matches the known amount of reference material.

17. Urine is aspirated directly from the bladder using _____ as the collection method.

18. Most analyzers found in reference laboratories use liquid reagent–based chemistry and _____ methods.

19. A(n) _____ is a detailed, step-by-step description for performing a test, performing QC, or operating an instrument.

EXERCISE 12.2 MATCHING #1: THE APPEARANCE OF NORMAL AND ABNORMAL BLOOD SERUM

Instructions: Match each description of the appearance of blood serum in column A with its associated significance in column B by writing the appropriate letter in the space provided.

Column A

1. ____ Milky
2. ____ Red
3. ____ Clear and colorless
4. ____ Light yellow
5. ____ Pink, milky
6. ____ Yellow-orange

Column B

A. Normal in large animals

B. Normal in small animals

C. Concurrent hemolysis and lipemia

D. Hemolysis

E. Bilirubin in the serum

F. Increased serum triglycerides (lipemia)

EXERCISE 12.3 MATCHING #2: ELISA SEROLOGY ASSAY

Instructions: Match each item associated with the ELISA test designed to test for patient antigens in column A with its corresponding description in column B by writing the appropriate letter in the space provided.

Column A

1. ____ Antibody
2. ____ Patient sample
3. ____ Enzyme-labeled antigen/antibody complex
4. ____ Unbound antigen and enzyme-labeled antibody
5. ____ Colorless chemical substrate
6. ____ Antigen of interest

Column B

A. Captured by the matrix-bound antibody

B. Acted on by the enzyme in the enzyme-labeled antibody

C. Bound to a solid matrix

D. In the patient sample

E. Mixed with reagent containing an enzyme-labeled antibody

F. Washed away during a washing step

EXERCISE 12.4 MATCHING #3: THE SIGNIFICANCE OF SPECIFIC GRAVITY VALUES

Instructions: Match each specific gravity in column A with its corresponding description of the significance of each value in column B by writing the appropriate letter in the space provided.

Column A

1. _____ 1.000

2. _____ 1.005

3. _____ 1.010

4. _____ 1.025

5. _____ 1.030

6. _____ 1.035

Column B

A. Indicates normal kidney function in a dehydrated cat

B. The USG should be at or above this level if a dog is dehydrated

C. Indicates kidneys are able to dilute the urine

D. The USG of distilled water

E. A minimal USG level expected in a dehydrated cow

F. Indicates the urine is neither being concentrated nor diluted by the kidneys

EXERCISE 12.5 MATCHING #4: CHEMICAL EVALUATION OF URINE

Instructions: Match each chemical constituent found on urine chemistry reagent strips in column A with the corresponding statement that applies to each in column B by writing the appropriate letter in the space provided.

Column A

1. _____ pH

2. _____ Protein

3. _____ Glucose

4. _____ Ketones

5. _____ Bilirubin

6. _____ Blood

Column B

A. Male dogs may have small amounts in concentrated urine, but not cats

B. May be false negative when the urine is exposed to formaldehyde

C. May change from positive to negative if the urine is centrifuged

D. May increase as a result of loss of carbon dioxide as urine stands

E. May appear in the urine as a consequence of glomerular disease

F. May be present in the urine in animals with starvation

EXERCISE 12.6 MATCHING #5: CONSTITUENTS OF A ROUTINE CHEMISTRY PANEL

Instructions: Match each constituent of a routine chemistry panel in column A with the corresponding statement in column B by writing the appropriate letter in the space provided.

Column A

1. _____ Glucose

2. _____ Electrolytes

3. _____ Creatinine

4. _____ Alanine aminotransferase

5. _____ Sorbitol dehydrogenase

6. _____ Creatine kinase

7. _____ Alkaline phosphatase

8. _____ Immunoglobulins

9. _____ Aspartate aminotransferase

Column B

A. May increase in patients with impaired kidney function

B. Increased levels indicate hepatocellular damage in large animals

C. Increased levels indicate either hepatocellular or muscle damage

D. Increases in the presence of inflammation

E. May decrease if the clot is left in contact with the serum for more than 1 hour

F. Increased levels indicate hepatocellular damage in small animals

G. Increased levels indicate muscle damage

H. Play(s) a role in regulating water balance and acid–base status

I. Increased from cholestasis or induced by corticosteroids

EXERCISE 12.7 PHOTO QUIZ: PHOTOGRAPHS OF URINE CRYSTALS

Instructions: Match each urine crystal (indicated by the arrow) with the name corresponding to the crystal type.

Names

A. Ammonium biurate

B. Calcium carbonate

C. Bilirubin

D. Struvite

E. Calcium oxalate dihydrate

F. Cystine

G. Calcium oxalate monohydrate

1. _____

3. _____

2. _____

4. _____

5. _____   7. _____

6. _____

EXERCISE 12.8 TRUE OR FALSE: COMPREHENSIVE

Instructions: Read the following statements and write "T" for true or "F" for false in the blanks provided. If a statement is false, correct the statement to make it true.

1. _____ The function of organs such as the liver can be measured using a routine chemistry panel.

2. _____ Increased serum bilirubin specifically indicates cholestatic disease.

3. _____ Serum calcium concentration may not accurately reflect total body content of calcium.

4. _____ Fasting is required in all domestic species prior to sample collection for a chemistry panel.

5. _____ The breed and age of a patient may affect what is considered a normal amount of each analyte in the blood.

6. _____ A disadvantage of dry reagent chemistry systems is that they are more sensitive to interference by lipemia, hemolysis, and icterus than liquid reagent systems.

7. _____ Point-of-care chemistry instruments, like the iSTAT, Alinityv, Zoetis), that use single-use, self-contained cartridges do not require in-house calibration.

8. _____ It takes approximately 1 to 3 weeks for a patient to develop an antibody response to an active infection.

9. _____ If a patient is actively infected with a pathogen, the antibody titer is expected to double over a period of 2 to 3 weeks.

10. _____ ELISA technology-based tests can be used to test for either antigens or antibodies.

11. _____ Ideally, urine should be examined within 90 minutes of collection.

12. _____ Catheterization is the preferred way of obtaining urine samples for bacterial culture.

13. _____ Specific gravity is an indicator of the concentrating ability of the kidney.

14. _____ If the kidneys are healthy, urine will be diluted in a dehydrated patient or concentrated when the patient is overhydrated.

15. _____ The presence of urease-positive bacteria in urine can cause the urine pH to decrease.

16. _____ Normal urine should not contain glucose.

17. _____ All blood collection tubes should be filled with the appropriate blood volume.

18. _____ Chemical analyzers designed for use with human samples must not be used for veterinary samples.

19. _____ Urinary casts form in the glomeruli of the kidneys.

20. _____ Urine that has been stored in the refrigerator should be brought to room temperature before undergoing chemical analysis.

EXERCISE 12.9 MULTIPLE CHOICE: COMPREHENSIVE

Instructions: Circle the one correct answer to each of the following questions.

1. Which of the following constituents of a routine chemistry panel is a calculated value?
   a. Alanine aminotransferase (ALT)
   b. Albumin
   c. Anion gap
   d. Potassium

2. Increased serum creatinine (Creat) indicates azotemia and can be caused by impaired kidney function or dehydration. To differentiate these causes, the SC must be interpreted along with
   a. albumin.
   b. urine specific gravity (USG).
   c. blood urea nitrogen (BUN).
   d. alanine aminotransferase (ALT).

3. Each of the following is a serum electrolyte except
   a. chloride.
   b. bicarbonate.
   c. creatinine.
   d. phosphorus.

4. The serum protein normally present in the highest concentrations is
   a. albumin.
   b. globulin.
   c. fibrinogen.
   d. prothrombin.

5. To avoid serum lipemia, dogs and cats should be
   a. fed.
   b. fasted for 4 hours.
   c. fasted for 8 hours.
   d. fasted for 12 hours.

6. With the exception of birds and other small pets, when sending blood to an outside lab, serum samples should be collected in a tube containing
   a. sodium citrate anticoagulant.
   b. EDTA anticoagulant.
   c. no anticoagulant.
   d. lithium heparin anticoagulant.

7. In reference to quality control, an SOP is a
   a. sample of the material used to calibrate the machine.
   b. graph used to track control results.
   c. step-by-step description for performing a test.
   d. measure of test result trends.

8. Controls must be run routinely as an integral part of good quality control. In small and large labs, they should be run at least
   a. twice a day.
   b. daily.
   c. once every other day.
   d. once a week.

9. When running controls, an acceptable variation is within ± 2 standard deviations of the mean. This means that the control may be slightly out of the acceptable range less than
   a. 2% of the time.
   b. 5% of the time.
   c. two times out of 10.
   d. every other time it is run.

10. Over time, control results may gradually progress toward the upper or lower acceptable limits. This would most likely happen if
    a. the wrong reagent is being used.
    b. the technician's technique for performing the test is incorrect.
    c. an instrument component is deteriorating.
    d. the samples are not being processed properly.

11. Serology is not commonly used to test for
    a. drugs.
    b. hormones.
    c. infectious agents.
    d. pH.

12. A single positive serologic test for antibodies to a pathogen indicates that the patient
    a. is actively infected by the pathogen.
    b. has been exposed to the pathogen either currently or in the past.
    c. has never been exposed to the pathogen.
    d. is sick from exposure to the pathogen.

13. Which of the following is *not* an example of a serologic test?
    a. IRMA
    b. GGT
    c. ELISA
    d. AGID

14. Exposure of urine to UV light may cause deterioration of
    a. ketones.
    b. protein.
    c. bilirubin.
    d. glucose.

15. Urine samples most likely to be contaminated with squamous epithelial cells are those collected by
    a. midstream void.
    b. urinary catheter.
    c. manual compression.
    d. cystocentesis.

16. The presence of RBCs, hemoglobin, or myoglobin in urine may cause it to be
    a. yellow-brown in color.
    b. amber in color.
    c. light yellow in color.
    d. reddish-brown in color.

17. Normal urine should be clear in the common domestic species of animals, except for
    a. dogs.
    b. cats.
    c. cattle.
    d. horses.

18. Reagent test pads designed strictly for human samples are
    a. ketone and leukocyte pads.
    b. leukocyte and specific gravity pads.
    c. specific gravity and bilirubin pads.
    d. bilirubin and ketone pads.

19. The protein pad on a reagent strip is most sensitive to
    a. globulins.
    b. myoglobin.
    c. albumin.
    d. mucoproteins.

20. Which ketone(s) are not detected on a reagent test strip?
    a. Beta-hydroxybutyrate
    b. Acetoacetate
    c. Acetone
    d. Acetoacetate and acetone

21. Which type of cells may appear in clusters or rafts in a urine sample?
    a. RBCs
    b. WBCs
    c. Transitional cells
    d. Squamous cells

22. Which urinary casts are normal in very low numbers (1 or fewer/LPF)?
    a. Waxy and hyaline
    b. Hyaline and granular
    c. Granular and cellular
    d. Cellular and waxy

23. Which crystal is not expected in the urine of normal dogs and cats?
    a. Hippuric acid-like calcium oxalate monohydrate
    b. Struvite
    c. Calcium phosphate
    d. Calcium oxalate dihydrate

24. Normal horses have which of the following urinary crystals in their urine?
    a. Calcium oxylate monohydrate
    b. Struvite
    c. Calcium phosphate
    d. Calcium carbonate

EXERCISE 12.10 FILL-IN-THE-BLANK: COMPREHENSIVE

Instructions: Fill in each of the spaces provided with the missing word or words that complete the sentence.

1. Corticosteroids can induce increases in the cholestatic serum enzyme _____, especially in dogs.

2. Hypoalbuminemia (decreased albumin) can cause a decrease in blood _____ because this electrolyte binds to albumin in the blood.

3. Inflammatory diseases and some lymphoid cancers may cause the blood protein _____ to increase.

4. Use of an incorrect needle size for blood collection, or excessive pressure on the syringe, can result in _____.

5. When preparing a serum sample for a chemistry profile, the blood should be allowed to clot for _____ to _____ minutes at _____ temperature, then centrifuged for _____ minutes at _____ to _____ g.

6. A SNAP test is a serologic screening test, designed to detect infectious agents, that uses _____ technology.

7. Urine should be at _____ temperature when analyzed and should be examined within _____ hour(s) of collection.

8. Collection of urine by _____ may damage or even rupture a fragile, diseased bladder.

9. A special urine collection technique for acquiring samples from bladder masses is _____.

10. Sometimes it is clinically helpful to quantify urine protein excretion by performing a urine _____ ratio.

11. When measuring USG, it is best to use a refractometer designed for veterinary patients because there is a special scale for _____.

12. Uncentrifuged urine should be used for biochemical testing unless the urine is _____.

13. The protein pad on a reagent strip may be false _____ when the urine is alkaline.

14. Glucosuria occurs when blood glucose level exceeds the _____.

15. Another name for the dipstick test for blood is _____.

16. When preparing urine samples for microscopic examination, _____ to _____ mL of urine should be centrifuged in a conical centrifuge tube at _____ to _____ rpm for _____ minutes. The supernatant should be removed by pipetting or decanting, until only _____ mL of supernatant is left with the pellet.

17. Squamous cells in urine are _____ in shape and of no clinical significance.

18. Ammonium biurate crystals may be observed in the urine of certain dogs, including the _____ breed.

EXERCISE 12.11 CASE STUDY: PRESURGICAL PANEL ON A YOUNG DOG

Signalment: 10-month-old, mixed-breed male dog

History: A presurgical chemistry panel was run prior to orthopedic surgery for hip dysplasia.

Examine the following presurgical chemistry panel *(modified from the case presentation in the text)* and answer the following questions:

	Units	Sample 2		Reference Interval
BUN	mg/dL	13		5–20
Creatinine	mg/dL	0.9		0.6–1.6
Phosphorus	mg/dL	6.4		3.2–8.1
Calcium	mg/dL	11.5		9.3–11.6
Sodium	mEq/L	152		143–153
Potassium	mEq/L	4.7		4.2–5.4
Chloride	mEq/L	111		109–120
Anion gap	mEq/L	21		15–25
Osmolality (calculated)	mOsm/kg	303		285–304
Bicarbonate	mmol/L	25		16–25
ALT	IU/L	25		10–55
AST	IU/L	28		12–40
ALP	IU/L	35		15–120
CK	IU/L	131		50–400
Cholesterol	mg/dL	166		80–315
Total bilirubin	mg/dL	0.4		0.1–0.4
Total protein	g/dL	5.4		5.1–7.1
Albumin	g/dL	3.6		2.9–4.2
Globulin	g/dL	1.8	L	2.2–2.9
A:G ratio		2.0		0.8–2.2
Glucose	mg/dL	112		77–126

A:G, albumin-to-globulin; *ALP,* alkaline phosphatase; *ALT,* alanine aminotransferase; *AST,* aspartate aminotransferase; *BUN,* blood urea nitrogen; *CK,* creatine kinase.

1a. What are the two main constituents of total serum protein?

    i. _____

    ii. _____

1b. How are albumin and globulins measured?

    _____

    _____

1c. What disease condition(s) typically cause both albumin and globulins to decrease?

    _____

1d. What disease condition(s) can cause hypoalbuminemia with normal globulins?

    _____

    _____

1e. What disease condition(s) typically cause both albumin and globulins to increase?

    _____

1f. What disease condition(s) can cause globulins to increase with no increase in albumin?

    _____

2. Which analytes indicate increased nitrogenous wastes in the blood?

    _____

    _____

3. Which analyte is generally increased in patients with diabetes mellitus and is used to diagnose this condition?

    _____

    _____

4a. Which analytes are enzymes that indicate hepatocellular damage in small animals?

    _____

    _____

4b. Why does aspartate aminotransferase (AST) have to be interpreted along with creatine kinase (CK) to accurately screen for hepatocellular damage?

_____

_____

4c. What other enzyme is measured to screen for hepatocellular damage in large animals?

_____

5. Which of the analytes are electrolytes?

_____

_____

6a. What is cholestatic disease?

_____

6b. Which analytes indicate cholestatic disease?

_____

_____

6c. Which analyte is not specific for cholestasis because it can also be increased by hemolysis?

_____

_____

13 Parasitology

LEARNING OBJECTIVES

When you have completed this chapter, you will be able to:

1. Pronounce, define, and spell all key terms in this chapter.
2. Identify the common name, affected species, key clinical signs, methods of diagnosis, life cycle, zoonotic potential, treatment, prevention, and control of ectoparasites (arthropods, flies) and endoparasites (protozoans, cestodes, nematodes, trematodes) of veterinary importance.
3. Describe the origin and clinical signs of *visceral larva migrans, ocular larva migrans, neurologic larva migrans,* and *cutaneous larva migrans,* including risk factors for and methods of preventing these zoonotic diseases.
4. Identify the common name, affected species, key clinical signs, methods of diagnosis, life cycle, zoonotic potential, treatment, prevention, and control of the pentastomes (snake parasites) of veterinary importance.
5. Do the following regarding collection and examination of fecal samples for the diagnosis of endoparasites:
   - Describe the principles of collection, storage, and examination of fecal samples and necessary safety precautions.
   - Describe indications for and procedures used to examine feces by direct fecal smear, fecal flotation, and sedimentation.
6. Do the following additional tasks regarding diagnosis of endoparasites:
   - List the special procedures used to detect the coccidian parasites *Giardia, Cryptosporidium* spp., and *Cystoisospora* spp. including safe handling.
   - Describe how necropsy findings are utilized to diagnose parasitism.
   - Explain how samples are prepared and shipped to an outside laboratory for parasite diagnosis.
   - Explain how the Baermann technique is set up and used to detect nematode larvae in feces and tissues.
   - Compare and contrast the blood examination and concentration techniques used to diagnose *Dirofilaria immitis* from other similar nematode species.

EXERCISE 13.1 FILL-IN-THE-BLANK: TERMS AND DEFINITIONS

Instructions: Fill in each of the spaces provided with the missing key term or definition that completes the sentence. Acronyms may be used when appropriate.

1. _____ is the most common intestinal parasite affecting humans.

2. *Sarcoptes scabei* belongs to a group of mites and ticks called _____.

3. The individual segments of the tapeworm are called _____.

4. Another name for a transport host is a(n) _____ host.

5. The word _____ refers to a single adult organism with the reproductive organs of both the male and the female of the species.

6. The _____ host is the host that harbors the adult, sexual, or mature stages of a parasite.

7. The term for a parasite that lives outside the body is _____.

8. _____ happens in puppies younger than three months old when roundworm larvae reach the lungs, are coughed up and swallowed, and end up maturing in the host's small intestines.

9. _____ are fast-growing organisms in developmental stages occurring as cysts in the life cycle of *Toxoplasma gondii* and other similar apicomplexan parasites.

10. In a direct blood smear, _____ of *Dirofilaria* species coil and uncoil.

11. Being in suspended animation or undergoing arrested development is the definition of _____.

12. Most of the parasitic flukes of domesticated animals are _____ flukes, meaning they have two intermediate hosts in addition to the definitive host.

13. *E. vermicularis,* the human pinworm, is really a _____ because it never infects dogs and cats.

14. _____ are parasites that live inside the host.

15. _____ eggs have a tiny door–like structure at one end that opens when the egg encounters water.

16. Within the life cycle of a parasite, the _____ host harbors the immature, asexual, or larval stage of a parasite.

17. The adult pseudo-tapeworm is sometimes referred to as the _____ tapeworm because the proglottids may divide in the middle and then reunite.

18. The type of roundworm larval migration that occurs in puppies older than 3 months where the second stage larvae encyst extraintestinally in the host's body is called _____ migration.

EXERCISE 13.2 DEFINING KEY TERMS

Instructions: Define each term in your own words.

1. Heterogonic life cycle

2. One-host tick

3. Unilocular hydatid cyst

4. Three-host tick

5. Visceral larva migrans

6. Multilocular hydatid cyst

7. Homogonic life cycle

8. Miracidium

9. Ocular larva migrans

10. Two-host tick

_____

_____

EXERCISE 13.3 MATCHING #1: TERMS AND DEFINITIONS

Instructions: Match each term in column A with its corresponding definition in column B by writing the appropriate letter in the space provided.

Column A

1. _____ Oocyst

2. _____ Merozoite

3. _____ Schistosome

4. _____ Cestode

5. _____ Acariasis

6. _____ Tachyzoite

7. _____ Parthenogenesis

8. _____ Brood capsule

9. _____ Hexacanth embryo

10. _____ Neurologic larva migrans

11. _____ Cutaneous larva migrans

Column B

A. A fast-growing organism in the developmental stage in the life cycle of _Toxoplasma gondii_

B. A blood fluke

C. A skin disease in humans caused by the larvae of hookworm parasites D. A protozoan cell that arises from parent sporozoans and may enter either the asexual or sexual phase of the life cycle

E. Six-toothed embryos

F. A disease, usually of the skin, caused by infestation with mites

G. A condition caused by the migration of the larval stage of _Baylisascaris procyonis_ through the brain and spinal cord of avian or mammalian paratenic hosts, including humans

H. The egg-like offspring produced by coccidian parasites

I. The adult stage of a tapeworm

J. A type of nonsexual reproduction in which an organism develops from an unfertilized ovum

K. A structure that is formed from the germinal membrane of a hydatid cyst

EXERCISE 13.4 MATCHING #2: TERMS AND DEFINITIONS

Instructions: Match each term in column A with its corresponding definition in column B by writing the appropriate letter in the space provided.

Column A

1. _____ Egg packet

2. _____ Aberrant parasite

3. _____ Otoacariasis

4. _____ Protozoan

5. _____ Metacercaria

6. _____ Procercoid

7. _____ Germinal membrane

8. _____ Sparganosis

9. _____ Miracidium

Column B

A. The infective stage of a digenic fluke

B. A single-cell organism

C. The thin lining of a hydatid cyst that forms brood capsules

D. A parasite found in a location in which it does not normally live

E. The ciliated, motile stage that emerges from the operculated egg of a digenetic fluke

F. The developmental stage that parasitizes the first intermediate host, usually an aquatic crustacean, in the life cycle of a pseudo-tapeworm

G. Infection of humans by the plerocercoid stage of Spirometra mansonoides, the "zipper tapeworm."

H. What is typically passed in the feces of an animal infected with Dipylidium caninum when a gravid proglottid is ruptured during defecation

I. Infestation of the external ear with mites or ticks

EXERCISE 13.5 MATCHING #3: TERMS AND DEFINITIONS

Instructions: Match each term in column A with its corresponding definition in column B by writing the appropriate letter in the space provided.

Column A

1. _____ Cercaria

2. _____ Seed ticks

3. _____ Pyrethrin

4. _____ Plerocercoid

5. _____ Metacestode

6. _____ Schistosome cercarial dermatitis

7. _____ Giardia

8. _____ Arthropoda

9. _____ Trematode

10. _____ Cysticercoid

Column B

A. The infective developmental stage that parasitizes the second intermediate host in the life cycle of a pseudo-tapeworm

B. The most common intestinal parasite intestinal parasite affecting people

C. A fluke

D. The larval stage of a tapeworm

E. The infective stage of the tapeworm

F. The six-legged larval form of the tick

G. A natural insecticide derived from plants, used to control various ectoparasites

H. This condition manifests as papular or pustular areas in the skin of humans

I. The free-swimming larva that emerges from its host snail

J. The phylum that includes all arthropods such as centipedes, millipedes, crustaceans, insects, mites, and ticks.

Instructions: Match each parasite with its corresponding name.

Names

A. *Taenia pisiformis*

B. Larval stage of *Ctenocephalides felis*

C. Adult of *Trichuris vulpis*

D. Oocysts of *Toxoplasma gondii*

E. Larval *Trombicula species*

F. Adult *Otodectes cynotis*

G. Microfilariae of *Dipylidium*

H. Adult mite, *Cheylatiella parasitivorax*

I. Infective stage of *Toxocara canis*

J. Adult *Demodex canis*

K. Anterior end of adult *Ancylostoma caninum*

L. Cyst of *Giardia species*

1. _____

2. _____

3. _____

5. _____

4. _____

6. _____

7. _____

9. _____

8. _____

10. _____

11. _____   12. _____

EXERCISE 13.7 TRUE OR FALSE: COMPREHENSIVE

Instructions: Read the following statements and write "T" for true or "F" for false in the blanks provided. If a statement is false, correct the statement to make it true.

1. _____ Parasite infections occur almost exclusively in animals younger than one year of age.

2. _____ When using a stage micrometer, 1 micron (μ) = 0.001 mm.

3. _____ Most endoparasites can be identified upon sight.

4. _____ Gross examination of a fecal sample involves noting consistency and color, and the presence of blood, mucus, or gross parasites.

5. _____ Bubonic plague is the only form of *Y. pestis* that can be spread from human to human.

6. _____ If an outbreak is suspected, *Echinococcus* species are a reportable parasite to state and federal authorities.

7. _____ The only hosts that will harbor *Toxoplasma gondii* in its sexual stages are cats and humans.

8. _____ *Cryptosporidium* species will infect all species of domestic animals, especially calves, dogs, and cats, but not rodents and humans.

9. _____ When the eggs of *Toxocara canis* are passed in the feces, they are immediately infective.

10. _____ Puppies can be infected with *Toxocara canis* while nursing.

11. _____ When a dog ingests a paratenic host infected with *Toxocara canis*, somatic migration will take place in the dog.

12. _____ *Baylisascaris procyonis* usually causes clinical disease in racoons.

13. _____ Hookworms can be a cause of anemia in young puppies.

14. _____ Humans are typically infected with hookworms via ingestion of infective larvae.

15. _____ The eggs of *Trichuris vulpis* can survive in the environment for years.

16. _____ Intestinal threadworms are best diagnosed using fecal flotation.

17. _____ Heartworm microfilariae circulating in a dog's peripheral blood will eventually mature into adult heartworms.

18. _____ Most species of mammals have their own variety of *Sarcoptes scabei*.

19. _____ Lesions associated with *Cheylatiella* are usually moist and inflamed in appearance.

20. _____ The parasite *Demodex canis* usually lives in the hair follicles of animals it infests.

21. _____ Chiggers typically burrow into the skin of infested hosts.

22. _____ *Giardia* can infect many different animal species, including humans.

23. _____ The feline is the only animal that can serve as the intermediate host for *Toxoplasma gondii*.

24. _____ *Toxoplasma gondii* infection is typically diagnosed by fecal flotation.

25. _____ A healthy host will usually be able to fight off a *Cryptosporidium* infection on its own.

26. _____ A good way for veterinary practices to save money is to reuse vials and filters used to perform fecal flotations.

27. _____ Endoparasites spend most of their life on the surface of the host body.

28. There are four developmental stages of the life cycle of the *S. scabiei*—egg, larva, nymph, and adult.

EXERCISE 13.8 MULTIPLE CHOICE: COMPREHENSIVE

Instructions: Circle the one correct answer to each of the following questions.

1. Collecting a thorough health history on all hunting hounds will help rule out or confirm
   a. *D. folliculorum.*
   b. *Otodectes cynotis.*
   c. *Giardia agilis.*
   d. *B. procyonis.*

2. During a _____, the veterinary technician uses the decanting or sieving method to recover parasites from the digestive tract.
   a. fecal sedimentation
   b. blood smear
   c. fecal flotation
   d. necropsy

3. The most important parasite of the vascular system in domestic animals in the United States is
   a. *B. procyonis.*
   b. *E. vermicularis.*
   c. *D. immitis.*
   d. *Sarcoptes scabei.*

4. Adult lice are about the size of a
   a. sesame seed.
   b. piece of rice.
   c. cucumber seed.
   d. poppy seed.

5. There are three types of proglottids:
   a. immature, intermediate, and mature.
   b. immature, mature, and gravid.
   c. gravid, parigravid, and mature.
   d. immature, aged, and postmortem.

6. Your client reports that he sees his dog frequently dragging its anus across the floor. The symptom suggests a/an _____.
   a. hookworm infection.
   b. whipworm infection.
   c. tapeworm infection.
   d. roundworm infection.

7. A client has just dropped off a fresh fecal sample on which you find several proglottids. Upon examining these proglottids under the microscope, you notice there is a pair of genital pores, which leads you to believe that these are _____ proglottids.
   a. *Multiceps*
   b. *Echinococcus*
   c. *Taenia*
   d. *Dipylidium*

8. One of the best ways to prevent *Echinococcus granulosus* infection in dogs is to
   a. prevent them from ingesting cat feces.
   b. prevent them from ingesting sheep viscera.
   c. prevent them from ingesting crayfish.
   d. use a monthly flea preventative.

9. The typical life cycle of *Spirometra mansonoides* utilizes _____ intermediate host(s).
   a. 0
   b. 1
   c. 2
   d. 3

10. Typically, if a dog younger than 3 months of age ingests a *Toxocara canis* egg containing the second-stage larva, the larva will go through
    a. tracheal migration.
    b. somatic migration.
    c. visceral migration.
    d. ocular migration.

11. The best way to diagnose ascarid infections in dogs and cats is
    a. direct smear.
    b. fecal flotation.
    c. fecal sedimentation.
    d. Baermann technique.

12. Neurologic larval migrans is a condition that can occur when a paratenic host ingests the larval stage of
    a. *Toxocara canis*.
    b. *Baylisascaris procyonis*.
    c. *Echinococcus multilocularis*.
    d. *Ancylostoma caninum*.

13. Humans can prevent cutaneous larva migrans (CLM) by
    a. avoiding skin-to-soil contact.
    b. reducing fecal-oral contact.
    c. practicing rigorous hygiene after working in kennels.
    d. abstaining from ingesting undercooked shellfish.

14. Whipworm is the common name for which one of the following parasites?
    a. *Trichuris vulpis*
    b. *Spirometra mansonoides*
    c. *Paragonimus kellicotti*
    d. *Uncinaria stenocephala*

15. From the time a dog ingests a whipworm egg containing the second-stage larva to the time that the larva is a mature, egg-producing adult is approximately
    a. 9 weeks.
    b. 10 weeks.
    c. 11 weeks.
    d. 12 weeks.

16. One of the unique aspects of intestinal threadworms is that
    a. the adult worms can live in the lungs or intestines of the host.
    b. the eggs are immediately infective when passed in feces.
    c. only the females are parasitic.
    d. only the males are parasitic.

17. In dogs and cats, adult heartworms are typically found in the
    a. pulmonary veins and left ventricle.
    b. pulmonary arteries and right ventricle.
    c. aorta and vena cava.
    d. left and right ventricles.

18. The intermediate host that is utilized during the life cycle of *Dirofilaria immitis* is the
    a. fly.
    b. tick.
    c. mosquito.
    d. flea.

19. The extreme pruritus associated with a *Sarcoptes scabei* infestation is caused by the mite
    a. chewing on the host's skin debris.
    b. piercing the host's skin with its proboscis.
    c. cementing eggs to hair shafts on the host's skin.
    d. tunneling into the host's epidermis.

20. With the *Trombicula* species, only the _____ stage of the life cycle is parasitic.
    a. pupal
    b. larval
    c. nymph
    d. adult

21. For an animal or human to become infected with *Cryptosporidium*, a(n) _____ must be ingested.
   a. oocyst
   b. merozoite
   c. sporozoite
   d. egg

22. Adult *pentastomes* are always associated with the
   a. lymph nodes.
   b. gastrointestinal tract.
   c. urogenital tract.
   d. respiratory tract.

23. When asking clients to bring in fecal samples from their dogs, you should instruct them to bring approximately _____ of feces.
   a. 1 teaspoon
   b. 2 teaspoons
   c. 1 tablespoon
   d. 2 tablespoons

24. When using a microscope to examine fecal specimens, the _____ objective is the one that is most commonly used.
   a. 4 ×
   b. 10 ×
   c. 40 ×
   d. 100 ×

25. Which one of the following flotation solutions corrodes lab equipment and can severely distort parasite eggs?
   a. Sugar solution
   b. Zinc sulfate solution
   c. Sodium nitrate solution
   d. Saturated sodium chloride solution

26. Fecal sedimentation is typically performed when _____ eggs are suspected, as they are too heavy to float in a flotation solution.
   a. hookworm
   b. roundworm
   c. fluke
   d. protozoan

27. *Enterobius vermicularis* is the most common worm infection in the United States and may be incorrectly blamed on the household pet; _____ are the primary means of transmission.
   a. fleas
   b. humans
   c. chiggers
   d. ticks

EXERCISE 13.9 CASE STUDY: PARASITE INFECTION IN A PUPPY

A client who has just obtained a new 10-week-old golden retriever puppy contacts the practice where you work as a credentialed veterinary technician. The breeder gave the puppy some dewormer when it was 6 weeks old, but the puppy has not yet been to a veterinarian to be examined. The owner indicates to you that the puppy is having some vomiting and diarrhea and also seems to have a "pot-bellied" appearance. You tell the owner that it would be a good idea to bring the puppy in to be examined by the DVM and that the owner should bring a stool sample to be examined for parasites. Please answer the following series of questions about dealing with this owner and his puppy.

1. What information should you give the owner over the phone about obtaining a fecal sample from his puppy that will result in the most accurate diagnosis?

_____

_____

_____

_____

_____

_____

2. Unfortunately, the owner arrived at the clinic and forgot to bring a stool sample. What are two possible ways that a fecal sample could be collected at the clinic?

   a. _____

   b. _____

3. Prior to performing any diagnostic tests on the stool sample, what type of examination should be completed, and what should be recorded and reported to the veterinarian?

   _____

   _____

   _____

4. You have decided to use a concentration method to examine the feces for the presence of parasite eggs. What are the two biggest advantages of using a concentration method?

   a. _____

   b. _____

5. Your clinic uses sodium nitrate as its fecal flotation solution. What is a disadvantage of using sodium nitrate?

   _____

   _____

6. When looking at the fecal sample under the microscope, you see eggs that look like the one on the right side in the picture below. Identify the genus and species of the parasite that produced this egg.

   _____

   _____

   _____

   _____

7. When you inform the owner that his golden retriever puppy has intestinal parasites, the owner is confused because the puppy was dewormed once when it was 6 weeks old. What should you tell the owner?

   _____

   _____

   _____

8. The owner then tells you there are small children in the home and asks if the children are at risk of becoming infected with *Toxocara canis*. What should you tell the owner?

_____

_____

_____

_____

_____

_____

_____

14 Clinical Microbiology

LEARNING OBJECTIVES

When you have completed this chapter, you will be able to:

1. Pronounce, define, and spell all key terms in the chapter.
2. Identify circumstances under which dangerous microorganisms (i.e., select dimorphic fungi) should not be cultured in a private practice setting.
3. Do the following regarding the collection of samples:
   - Describing methods used to collect and preserve representative samples.
   - Describe the special collection and handling procedures used to culture samples from tissues, urine, the respiratory tract, blood, joints, milk, and feces. Identify appropriate transport media and packing conditions that must be met for safe transport to an outside laboratory through shipping.
4. Do the following regarding sample processing:
   - Identify staining procedures used to for direct microscopic examination of prepared slides such as Gram stain, acid-fast stain, modified acid-fast stain, and spore staining.
5. Do the following regarding bacterial culture and identification:
   - Describe the principles of bacterial culture, including safe disposal of microbiological laboratory waste and basic equipment used for microbiological cultures.
   - Describe the differences between nutrient, enrichment, selective, and differential media, how to inoculate for biochemical testing, primary isolation of bacterial pathogens.
   - Explain how examination of growth on a culture plate is used to identify pathogens and guide clinical decisions.
   - Describe the roles that catalase, oxidase, coagulase biochemical tests and hemolysis patterns play in preliminary grouping of gram-positive and gram-negative bacteria.
   - List common bacterial flora and pathogens, identifying the classification of each and associated diseases.
6. Do the following regarding antimicrobial susceptibility testing:
   - Explain the reasons for susceptibility testing for performing and interpreting antimicrobial susceptibility tests.
   - Describe the procedures for and principles of interpretation of the broth dilution test and the disk diffusion test.
7. Do the following regarding fungal culture (mycology):
   - Describe the methods used to collect dermatophytes, inoculate dermatophyte test medium and Sabouraud dextrose agar and interpret culture results.
8. Do the following regarding the molecular detection of pathogens:
   - List the methods commonly used to detect pathogens in patient samples via enzyme-linked immunosorbent assay (ELISA), virus isolation (VI), fluorescent antibody (FA), electron microscopy (EM), immunohistochemical staining, polymerase chain reaction (PCR) and deoxyribonucleic acid (DNA) sequencing.
9. Do the following regarding nosocomial infections:
   - Demonstrate an understanding of agents and their method of causing nosocomial infections.

EXERCISE 14.1 CROSSWORD PUZZLE: TERMS AND DEFINITIONS

Across

4 Media that detects and discriminates between two organisms based on the results of a biochemical reaction.

7 The antimicrobial _____ test is used to determine whether an antimicrobial agent will kill or inhibit growth of a particular organism.

8 A stain that distinguishes bacteria that have mycolic acid incorporated in their cell walls.

9 Culture medium used to enhance the growth of specific bacteria.

11 Antibodies that recognize a single antigen.

12 Biochemical test used to differentiate *Staphyloccocus* spp. from *Streptococcus* spp.

Down

1 The lowest concentration of antimicrobial required to slow bacterial growth. (2 words)

2 Stain used to differentiate bacteria based on the composition of their cell wall.

3 Another name for the Kirby-Bauer susceptibility test. (2 words)

5 Medium that maintains bacteria in original concentrations without encouraging growth or causing death of the bacteria.

6 Biochemical test used to differentiate and identify Gram-negative bacteria.

10 Biochemical test used to differentiate pathogenic *Streptococcus* spp. and nonpathogenic *Streptococcus* spp.

EXERCISE 14.2 TERMS AND DEFINITIONS: INFECTIOUS AGENTS

Instructions: Define each term in your own words.

1. Abscess: _____

_____

2. Anaerobe: _____

_____

3. Dermatophyte: _____

_____

4. Fastidious: _____

_____

5. Hemolysis: _____

_____

6. Indigenous flora: _____

_____

7. Nosocomial infection: _____

_____

8. Opportunistic infection: _____

_____

9. Yeast: _____

_____

Instructions: Match each media in column A with its corresponding description in column B by writing the appropriate letter in the space provided.

Column A

1. _____ Blood agar plate
2. _____ Indole test media
3. _____ Hektoen enteric agar
4. _____ Selenite or tetrathionate broth
5. _____ Lysine iron agar slant
6. _____ Brucella blood agar plate
7. _____ Salt mannitol agar
8. _____ Motility media
9. _____ MacConkey's agar plate
10. _____ Christensen's urea agar slant
11. _____ Citrate test media
12. _____ Triple sugar iron agar slant

Column B

A. For direct isolation of *Salmonella* spp. from feces

B. Determining motility via flagella

C. Trypticase soy agar plate with 5% blood added

D. A selective isolation medium used to select Gram-negative organisms

E. For determining the ability of organisms to utilize glucose, sucrose, and lactose and to produce hydrogen sulfide

F. Media used to enrich samples for the detection of *Salmonella* spp.

G. Differentiates *Salmonella*

H. Determines the presence of Enterobateriaceae

I. Used to differentiate species of *Staphylococcus* based on mannitolfermentation

J. Primary isolation medium used for colony isolation

K. Determines the ability of an organism to split indole from tryptophan.

L. A medium used to determine whether an organism produces urease

EXERCISE 14.4 MATCHING #2: GRAM-POSITIVE ORGANISMS

Instructions: Match each Gram-positive organism in column A with the disease that it causes in column B by writing the appropriate letter in the space provided.

Column A

1. _____ *Erysipelothrix rhusiopathiae*

2. _____ *Corynebacterium pseudotuberculosis*

3. _____ *Trueperella*

4. _____ *Enterococcus spp.*

5. _____ *Rhodococcus equi*

6. _____ *Bacillus anthracis*

7. _____ *Streptococcus spp.*

8. _____ *Staphylococcus pseudintermedius*

9. _____ *Listeria monocytogenes*

Column B

A. Found in opportunistic infections, particularly of the urinary tract

B. A cause of septicemia in neonatal animals, abortion, and encephalitis in ruminants

C. The cause of anthraxD. In rare cases, responsible for necrotizing fasciitis

E. A cause of pneumonia in foals

F. The cause of caseous lymphadenitis in sheep and goats

G. A cause of disease in swine, turkeys, and marine mammals

H. Catalase-positive, gram-positive cocci that are normal inhabitants of the skin of dogs

I. An opportunistic pathogen common inhabitant of the skin and mucous membranes of cattle and other ruminants

EXERCISE 14.5 MATCHING #3: GRAM-NEGATIVE ORGANISMS

Instructions: Match each Gram-negative organism in column A with its corresponding description in column B by writing the appropriate letter in the space provided.

Column A

1. _____ *Escherichia coli*

2. _____ *Proteus spp.*

3. _____ *Actinobacillus spp.*

4. _____ *Bordetella bronchiseptica*

5. _____ *Pasteurella multocida*

6. _____ *Brucella spp.*

7. _____ *Aeromonas spp.*

8. _____ *Salmonella spp.*

Column B

A. A bacterial select agent that is a cause of abortion and reproductive failure

B. An important cause of diarrhea and septicemia in a variety of animal species and commonly isolated from feces of reptiles and amphibians

C. A cause of infections in aquatic animals, including fish and amphibians

D. An oxidase-positive, short, fat rod that causes rapidly progressing cellulitis in people who have been bitten by cats

E. The causative agent of canine tracheobronchitis

F. An opportunistic urinary pathogen that swarms on culture plates

G. Typically grown on MacConkey agar; often isolated from foals with septicemia or joint infections

H. An oxidase-negative member of the family Enterobacteriaceae and a cause of opportunistic infections of the urine and wounds

EXERCISE 14.6 ORDERING: ELISA TEST FOR A VIRAL PROTEIN OR ANTIGEN

Instructions: Match the steps of performing an ELISA antigen test in the proper order by placing the appropriate number (1 through 5) in the space provided.

A. _____ Add an enzyme-labeled secondary antibody to the well or membrane and incubate as directed.

B. _____ Read the color change.

C. _____ Wash the well or membrane as directed.

D. _____ Place a patient sample in the well or on the membrane and incubate for the recommended time.

E. _____ Wash the well or membrane, and add the substrate for the enzyme.

EXERCISE 14.7 TRUE OR FALSE: COMPREHENSIVE

Instructions: Read the following statements and write "T" for true or "F" for false in the blanks provided. If a statement is false, correct the statement to make it true.

1. _____ When a patient has an infection, it is best to start the patient on antibiotics right away to treat the infection and then to collect a sample for culture and sensitivity.

2. _____ When collecting microbiologic samples from an abscess, the purulent material in the abscess (pus) is the best source of material for bacterial culture.

3. _____ Urine samples collected by free-catch typically have bacteria in them from the external genitalia and skin.

4. _____ The stain used specifically to identify *Mycobacterium* spp. is the acid-fast stain.

5. _____ Acid-fast organisms stain dark blue, whereas non-acid-fast organisms and the background should stain pink.

6. _____ Broth is typically used for the initial isolation of organisms as opposed to solid agar.

7. _____ Plate media should be incubated overnight, right-side up, at 35° C to 37.5° C.

8. _____ When culturing a sample from a site like the GI tract, you should attempt to identify every organism.

9. _____ The catalase test is most commonly used to differentiate staphylococci from streptococci and enterococci.

10. _____ Gram-negative bacteria in the family *Enterobacteriaceae* are generally oxidase-positive.

11. _____ The organism *Listeria monocytogenes* is the causative agent of ulcerative lymphadenitis in horses.

12. _____ *Mycobacterium* spp. organisms are often challenging to culture because they sometimes take weeks to grow.

13. _____ The causative agent of Lyme disease is the spirochete *Borrelia burgdorferi*.

14. _____ The yeast *Cryptococcus neoformans* is often present in samples from the respiratory and gastrointestinal tract of birds.

15. _____ The pathogen in question (bacteria or virus) must be cultured and isolated before performing PCR testing.

16. _____ DNA sequencing is a way to definitively identify most organisms.

17. _____ A fomite is an animal capable of transmitting a nosocomial agent.

18. _____ A person can get a zoonotic infection from a patient, but a patient cannot get one from a person.

19. _____ Bacteria are the most common cause, and viruses are the second most common cause, of nosocomial infections.

20. _____ *Streptococcus equi* subsp. *equi (S. equi)* is frequently implicated as a nosocomial infection in veterinary patients.

EXERCISE 14.8 MULTIPLE CHOICE: COMPREHENSIVE

Instructions: Circle the one correct answer to each of the following questions.

1. Which fungal agent is designated as a "select fungal agent"?
   a. *Malassezia pachydermatis*
   b. *Blastomyces dermatitidis*
   c. *Candida albicans*
   d. *Sporothrix schenckii*

2. Most anticoagulants will interfere with bacterial culture and so cannot be used when collecting samples for culture. When collecting samples that are at risk for clotting, which of the following anticoagulants may be used because it will not interfere with bacterial culture?
   a. EDTA
   b. Sodium citrate
   c. Polyanethol sulfonate
   d. Lithium heparin

3. Which of the following organisms is a common cause of diarrhea?
   a. *Campylobacter jejuni*
   b. *Pasteurella multocida*
   c. *Bordetella bronchiseptica*
   d. *Brucella abortus*

4. Which of the following samples may be frozen prior to bacterial culture?
   a. Urine
   b. Milk
   c. Joint fluid
   d. Transtracheal wash samples

5. The stain used to identify *Nocardia* spp. is
   a. Gram stain.
   b. hematoxylin-eosin stain.
   c. Kinyoun modified Ziehl-Nielsen acid-fast stain.
   d. acid-fast stain.

6. _____ media will inhibit the growth of most organisms, while _____ media inhibits the growth of some organisms while promoting the growth of likely pathogens.
   a. Enrichment; selective
   b. Selective; differential
   c. Enrichment; differential
   d. Selective; enrichment

7. The two media most commonly used for initial inoculation and isolation of bacteria are
   a. Mueller-Hinton and TSA.
   b. TSA and MacConkey.
   c. MacConkey's and blood agar.
   d. blood agar and Mueller-Hinton.

8. Gram-negative and Gram-positive organisms are _____ in color, respectively.
   a. pink and green
   b. green and pink
   c. pink and purple
   d. purple and pink

9. Catalase-positive, gram-positive cocci include
   a. pathogenic *Streptococcus* spp.
   b. *Pasteurella* spp.
   c. *Staphylococcus* spp.
   d. *Enterococcus* spp.

10. In addition to *Salmonella, Campylobacter,* and *Clostridium*, another causative agent of diarrhea isolated from fecal culture is
    a. *Mycobacterium avium subsp. Paratuberculosis.*
    b. *Streptococcus agalactia.*
    c. *Staphylococcus aureus.*
    d. *Pseudomonas aeruginosa.*

11. When culturing urine, the colonies must be counted by performing a quantified culture. What other sample must be handled in this manner?
    a. Joint fluid
    b. Cerebral spinal fluid
    c. Blood
    d. Milk

12. Which of the following organisms is an agent of contagious mastitis in cattle?
    a. *Clostridium perfringens*
    b. *Listeria monocytogenes*
    c. *Streptococcus agalactiae*
    d. *Mycoplasma spp.*

13. Which of the following organisms are catalase-negative, Gram-positive cocci that, in rare but serious cases, cause necrotizing fasciitis?
    a. *Erysipelothrix spp.*
    b. *Streptococcus spp.*
    c. *Bordetella spp.*
    d. *Brucella spp.*

14. The Gram-positive, pleomorphic rod *Corynebacterium pseudotuberculosis* is the cause of
    _____ in sheep and goats.
    a. diamond skin disease
    b. pigeon fever
    c. contagious foot rot
    d. caseous lymphadenitis

15. Pneumonia in foals is caused by the aerobic, CAMP-positive, Gram-positive rod
    a. *Erysipelothrix rhusiopathiae.*
    b. *Rhodococcus equi.*
    c. *Actinomyces spp.*
    d. *Clostridium perfringens.*

16. The partially acid-fast organisms *Nocardia* spp. appear on microscopic examination as
    a. seagull-shaped spiral organisms.
    b. short, fat coccobacilli.
    c. rods with a "beaded" appearance.
    d. club-shaped rods.

17. An organism that is frequently isolated from fish and amphibians with infections is
    a. *Actinobacillus spp.*
    b. *Rhodococcus equi.*
    c. *Campylobacter spp.*
    d. *Aeromonas spp.*

18. The colonies of which organism are often hemolytic on blood agar, secrete a green pigment into the surrounding media, and have a metallic appearance?
    a. *Pseudomonas spp.*
    b. *Escherichia coli*
    c. *Staphylococcus spp.*
    d. *Malassezia spp.*

19. The reproductive pathogens *Brucella* spp. are a group of small, oxidase-positive
    a. Gram-positive rods.
    b. Gram-negative coccobacilli.
    c. Gram-positive cocci.
    d. Gram-positive, spore-forming rods.

20. Some important pathogens and GI-indigenous flora are Gram-negative anaerobic rods. Which of the following organisms is not a Gram-negative anaerobic rod?
    a. *Bacteroides spp.*
    b. *Fusobacterium spp.*
    c. *Prevotella spp.*
    d. *Clostridium spp.*

21. Which of the following organisms is a cause of renal disease, abortion, and infertility?
    a. *Leptospira spp.*
    b. *Borrelia burgdorferi*
    c. *Brachyspira hyodysenteriae*
    d. *Campylobacter spp.*

22. The organism *Mycoplasma* spp. is
    a. Gram-positive.
    b. Gram-negative.
    c. acid-fast-positive.
    d. not visible on Gram stain.

23. Which of the following organisms is *not* an obligate intracellular organism?
    a. *Mycoplasma*
    b. *Neorickettsia*
    c. *Chlamydia*
    d. *Ehrlichia*

24. The McFarland standard is used to
    a. set hospital policy regarding exposure to infectious agents.
    b. determine which antibiotic to use.
    c. estimate bacterial numbers.
    d. evaluate hemolytic reactions.

25. The media used to culture dermatophytes are
    a. Sabouraud dextrose agar and salt mannitol agar.
    b. salt mannitol agar and blood agar.
    c. blood agar and DTM.
    d. DTM and Sabouraud dextrose agar.

26. The pathogenic yeast that is a common cause of otitis externa is
    a. *Coccidioides immitis.*
    b. *Malassezia pachydermatis.*
    c. *Blastomyces dermatitidis.*
    d. *Cryptococcus neoformans.*

Instructions: Fill in each of the spaces provided with the missing word or words that complete the sentence.

1. Bacterial agents that are highly infectious and dangerous to the degree that they have potential use as biologic weapons are classified by the government as _____ agents and must be reported to the _____ if identified in the lab.

2. When submitting urine for bacterial culture, a minimum of _____ mL should be collected by _____ and submitted in a blood tube with a top that is _____ in color.

3. A(n) _____ infection is a local infection that spreads to multiple organs.

4. The part of the bacterium that is different in structure between Gram-negative and Gram-positive organisms, which therefore takes up stain differently, is the _____.

5. Partially acid-fast organisms stain the color _____, whereas non–acid-fast organisms and the background stain _____.

6. When attempting to identify a bacterium isolated on a culture plate, the first step is to determine its _____ and _____ as observed on a Gram stain.

7. The catalase test determines the presence or absence of this enzyme based on the ability of a bacterial organism to convert _____ to _____ and _____.

8. Hemolytic patterns are used to determine the pathogenicity of *Streptococcus* organisms. *Streptococcus* isolates are _____ flora are generally α-hemolytic, whereas _____ *Streptococcus* isolates are generally β-hemolytic.

9. Diarrhea caused by *Clostridium perfringens* and *Clostridium difficile* correlates with the presence of toxins rather than the presence of the organisms themselves. The toxins are typically detected with a(n) _____ test.

10. Each species of animal has characteristic and unique indigenous flora. Whereas the Gram-positive organism *Staphylococcus* _____ is a member of the indigenous skin flora of dogs, *Staphylococcus* _____ is a normal skin inhabitant in cats and large animals.

11. The Gram-positive, spore-forming rod *Bacillus anthracis* is the causative agent of the dangerous zoonotic disease _____ and is classified as a(n) _____ agent by the U.S. government.

12. Members of the family Enterobacteriaceae, such as *Escherichia coli, Klebsiella,* and *Salmonella,* are typically oxidase-_____.

13. An organism often associated with progressive infections in people with cat bites is _____.

14. The small, Gram-negative coccobacillus _____ is the causative agent of kennel cough, a disease also known as _____.

15. A(n) _____ agar plate is used to determine the susceptibility of an organism to an antimicrobial agent.

16. The only fungal cultures that are routinely performed in-house are _____ cultures.

17. A(n) _____ lamp is sometimes used to examine suspect dermatophyte lesions because 75% will _____ under long-wavelength ultraviolet light.

18. An infection that a hospitalized patient acquires from the hospital environment or another patient is called a(n) _____ infection. An infection that a patient is incubating at the time of admission that becomes apparent while the patient is in the hospital is called a(n) _____ infection. These infections are not to be confused with _____ infections which occur when organisms are transferred from animal patients to human persons.

EXERCISE 14.10 CASE STUDY: PERFORMING A QUANTIFIED URINE CULTURE

Tanya, a 3-year-old female Collie, was presented for urinating in the house. The owner reported that during the previous few days, Tanya urinated in the house several times, and when she was outside to "potty," she would often go four or five times in a row. Physical examination revealed no significant findings. The bladder was empty at the time of the examination. Acute cystitis with a possible bacterial infection was suspected, and urine was collected by cystocentesis for urinalysis, a quantified urine culture, and sensitivity testing. The urine was blood-tinged, and the urinalysis indicated the presence of leukocytes, red blood cells, and bacteria. Antibiotics were prescribed for 7 days while waiting for culture results.

1. Explain the procedure used to inoculate a plate for a quantified urine culture using both 1 μL and 10 μL loops.

_____

_____

_____

_____

_____

_____

_____

2. The plates were incubated at 37° C overnight, and the colonies were counted the next day. *Staphylococcus pseudointermedius* was isolated. The 1:1000 plate had approximately 90 colonies, and the 1:100 plate was covered with growth. Calculate the number of colony-forming units found on the 1:1000 plate and explain the significance of these results.

_____

_____

_____

_____

_____

15 Diagnostic Imaging

LEARNING OBJECTIVES

When you have completed this chapter, you will be able to:

1. Pronounce, define, and spell all key terms in this chapter.
2. Do the following regarding the production of X-ray:
   - Describe the properties of x-radiation.
   - Describe the parts of the X-ray tube and machine and discuss the role each part plays in generation of x-radiation.
   - Explain the production of the useful X-ray beam and scatter radiation and discuss the negative consequences of scatter radiation.
3. Do the following regarding X-ray equipment:
   - Describe the features of and uses for portable, mobile, and stationary X-ray equipment.
4. Do the following regarding image production and exposure factors:
   - Explain how *milliamperage, exposure time, kilovoltage,* and *focal–film distance* is set to produce a high-quality diagnostic radiograph.
   - Discuss the purpose of a grid, filtration, and collimation.
5. Explain the purpose for a technique chart.
6. Do the following regarding image formation with film-screen systems:
   - Explain the principles of image formation using the film screen system and the purpose of cassettes and screens.
7. Do the following regarding film processing:
   - Discuss the purpose of the darkroom in film processing and safe film handling practices.
8. Do the following regarding digital radiography:
   - Describe the features, advantages, and disadvantages of and the uses for computed radiography and digital radiography equipment.
   - Discuss the difference between computed radiography and digital radiography.
9. Describe common digital radiography artifacts, including how to identify and prevent each one.
   - Explain the roles of Digital Imaging and Communications in Medicine (DICOM), picture archiving and communication system (PACS), radiology information system (RIS), and teleradiography in the production and management of digital radiographs.
10. Do the following regarding radiographic image quality:
    - Explain how radiographic density, contrast, and detail are controlled by changing milliamperage and kilovoltage to optimize image quality.
    - Describe types of geometric distortion, such as magnification and elongation.
    - List the common technical errors and artifacts that affect image quality.
11. List and describe methods for labeling and storing radiographic images.
12. Do the following regarding radiation safety:
    - Describe the hazards of radiation and explain the role of beam filtration in minimizing its damaging effects.
    - Discuss the methods used to monitor radiation exposure and the units for measuring radiation.
    - Understand ALARA and the three main concepts of radiation safety including time, distance, and shielding.
    - Explain the principles and practices used to minimize exposure to radiation, including the use of personal protective equipment (PPE).
13. Explain the principles of patient positioning for radiographic studies, including the importance of appropriate restraint.
14. Do the following regarding radiographic contrast agents:
    - List the commonly used positive and negative radiographic contrast agents and explain how they are used in the production of a diagnostic contrast study.
    - Describe the contrast procedure used to image the upper gastrointestinal (GI) tract.
15. Do the following regarding ultrasonography:
    - Describe the indications for and characteristics of ultrasonography in diagnostic imaging.
    - Describe the basic principles of production of an ultrasound image, including the appearance of various tissues and organs on a finished image.
    - Describe how a patient is prepared for ultrasound imaging and the procedure used to conduct an ultrasound examination.
    - Discuss the equipment used to produce B-mode, M-mode, and Doppler ultrasound images.
    - Describe the appearance of an ultrasound image and the appearances and causes of common artifacts.
16. Discuss the indications and use of endoscopy along with basics of endoscope use and care.
17. Describe indications for and characteristics of, fluoroscopy, computed tomography, magnetic resonance imaging, diagnostic nuclear medicine, and positron emission tomography.

159

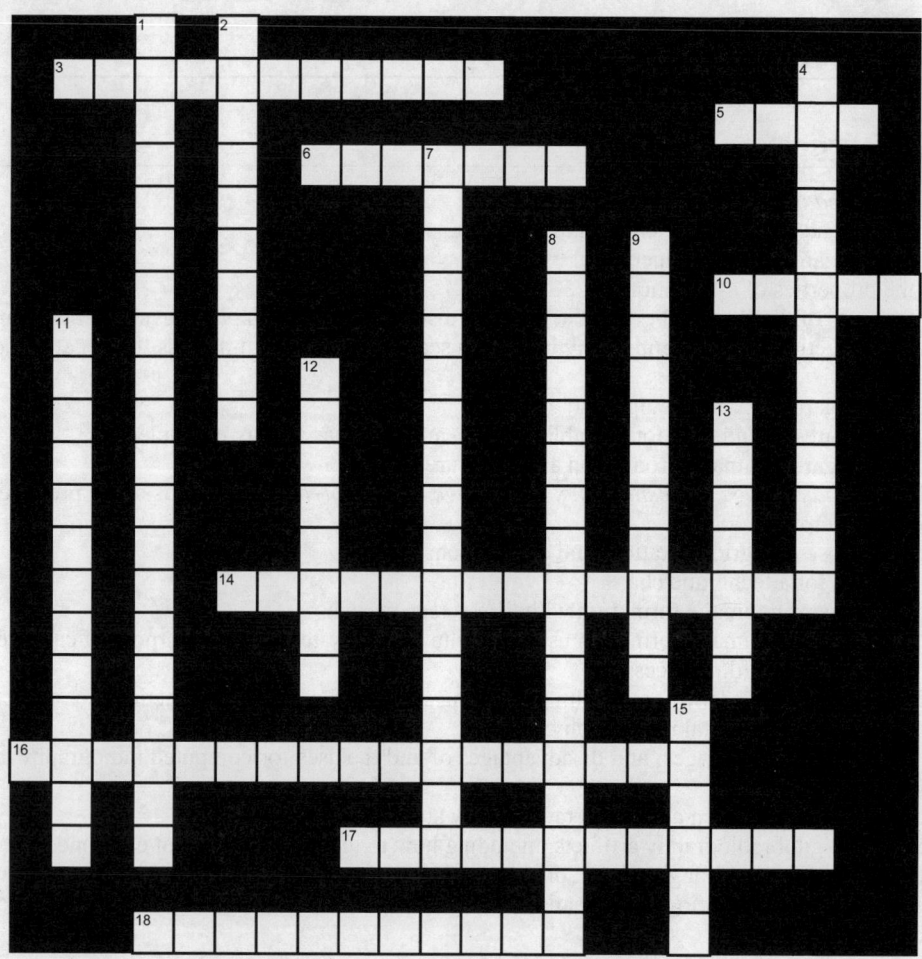

Across

3 The source of the x-ray beam in an x-ray tube. (2 words)
5 A device used to decrease scatter radiation.
6 The general amount of blackness in a radiographic image.
10 Electromagnetic radiation of shorter wavelength than light.
14 The specific type of the part that serves as the source of the x-rays in a dental or portable x-ray machine. (2 words)
16 The distance between the source of the x-rays and the image receptor. (2 words)
17 The range of gray shades, allowing both bone and soft tissues to be seen at the same exposure setting.
18 Weakening of sound waves as they travel through the body.

Down

1 A device used to make grid lines invisible. (2 words)
2 Decrease in the strength of the x-ray beam near the anode. (2 words)
4 The current applied to the cathode filament.
7 The ability to distinguish two adjacent structures on an x-ray image. (2 words)
8 Energy that breaks chemical bonds and damages DNA. (2 words)
9 Controls the speed of travel of the electrons in an x-ray tube.
11 The specific type of the part that serves as the source of the x-rays in a stationary x-ray machine. (2 words)
12 The difference between blacks and whites in a radiographic image.
13 The source of electrons in an x-ray tube.
15 The sharpness of a radiographic image.

EXERCISE 15.2 MATCHING #1: TERMS AND DEFINITIONS

Instructions: Match each term in column A with its corresponding definition in column B by writing the appropriate letter in the space provided.

Column A

1. _____ Anechoic

2. _____ Dosimetry

3. _____ B-mode

4. _____ Computed radiography

5. _____ DICOM

6. _____ Digital radiography

7. _____ Fluoroscopy

8. _____ Hyperechoic

9. _____ Hertz (Hz)

10. _____ Isoechoic

11. _____ M-mode

12. _____ PACS

13. _____ Gray

14. _____ Sievert

15. _____ Teleradiology

Column B

A. A diagnostic technique used to image moving structures

B. The computer system used to permanently store and transmit digital images to different computer workstations within a single location or between locations

C. A digital radiography method in which an X-ray detector cassette containing photostimulable phosphor is read by a processor and transferred to a computer

D. A dark structure on an ultrasound image is said to be _____.

E. A structure that has the same brightness as adjacent structures on an ultrasound image is said to be _____.

F. Measurement of a person's exposure to radiation

G. A measurement of absorbed radiation that takes into account biologic effectiveness of radiation

H. A universal digital image format that has allowed for digital images to be shared between different vendors' software

I. Allows transmission of electronic images across the Internet to referral facilities

J. Also known as "brightness mode"

K. A structure that produces more echoes than adjacent structures is said to be _____.

L. The unit of absorbed dose of ionizing radiation

M. A measurement of sound frequency

N. An imaging technique that doesn't require use of film

O. An ultrasound display used primarily for echocardiography

EXERCISE 15.3 MATCHING #2: SCREEN SPEED AND CHARACTERISTICS

Instructions: Match each characteristic in column A with its corresponding screen speed in column B by writing the appropriate letter in the space provided. Note that responses may be used more than once.

Column A

1. _____ Require less radiation

2. _____ Produce poorer detail

3. _____ Have larger crystals

4. _____ Have increased resolution

5. _____ Also called "detail screens"

6. _____ Best for imaging small exotic animals

7. _____ Regular screens

Column B

A. Fast screens

B. Slow screens

C. Intermediate screens

EXERCISE 15.4 MATCHING #3: FACTORS THAT AFFECT RADIOGRAPHIC DENSITY

Instructions: Match each action in column A (assuming no other changes are made) with the way it will affect radiographic density in column B by writing the appropriate letter in the space provided. Note that responses may be used more than once.

Column A

1. _____ Changing the kVp from 50 to 60

2. _____ Changing the object-film distance from 6 inches to 12 inches

3. _____ Changing mA from 300 to 200

4. _____ Changing the exposure time from ½ second to ¼ second

5. _____ Changing from detail screens to fast screens

6. _____ Changing the focal-film distance from 40 inches to 30 inches

7. _____ Removing the grid

Column B

A. Increases radiographic density

B. Decreases radiographic density

C. Does not change radiographic density

EXERCISE 15.5 MATCHING #4: ULTRASOUND ARTIFACTS AND INTERPRETATIONS

Instructions: Match each artifact listed in column A with its corresponding description in column B by writing the appropriate letter in the space provided.

Column A

1. _____ Reverberation artifact

2. _____ Shadowing

3. _____ Acoustic enhancement

4. _____ Edge artifact

5. _____ Mirror-image artifact

6. _____ Slice-thickness artifact

Column B

A. Refraction or redirection of the sound beam helpful in identifying smooth round structures

B. The reflection of the entire beam back to the transducer in instances when the beam encounters air or gas

C. Duplication of an image as a result of reverberation within a highly echogenic structure

D. An area or darkness resulting from inadequate sound beam penetration through a highly reflective or sound-absorptive substance

E. A layered appearance occurring when the ultrasound beam cuts through the edge of a cystic structure and solid tissue

F. Occurs when the ultrasound beam passes through a structure with low attenuation

EXERCISE 15.6 MATCHING #5: X-RAY RADIOGRAPHIC ARTIFACTS AND TECHNICAL ERRORS

Instructions: Match each of the radiographic technical errors listed in column A with its resulting artifact in column B by writing the appropriate letter in the space provided. Note that each response may be used more than once and that more than one answer may be correct.

Column A

1. _____ mAs or kV setting too high

2. _____ Dirt or debris between the film and screen

3. _____ Focal-film distance too short

4. _____ Contrast medium on tabletop, skin, or cassette

5. _____ mAs or kV setting too low

6. _____ Failure to use a grid

7. _____ Focal-film distance too long

8. _____ Defective cassette that does not close properly, exposing margins of film to light

9. _____ Anatomic part undermeasured

10. _____ Outdated film

11. _____ Crescent mark from rough handling

12. _____ Static electricity

13. _____ Anatomic part overmeasured

14. _____ Grid out of focal range or upside down

15. _____ Defect or crack in screen

16. _____ Speed of intensifying screen too slow

17. _____ Film exposed to scatter radiation

18. _____ Film stored in hot or humid environment

19. _____ Speed of intensifying screen too fast

20. _____ Gridlines

Column B

A. Increased film density

B. Decreased film density

C. Black marks

D. White marks

E. Gray film (film fog)

F. Linear artifacts

EXERCISE 15.7 PHOTO QUIZ: PARTS OF THE X-RAY TUBE

Instructions: Identify each part of an X-ray tube with the appropriate description from the list below by writing the appropriate letter in the space to the left; then name the part by writing the name in the space to the right.

Parts of the X-ray Tube

1. _____ The part through which the X-rays exit the tube

2. _____ This part produces an electron cloud when current is applied

3. _____ The high-voltage circuit controls the electrical potential between the cathode and this part

4. _____ The part that encases the other parts of the tube

5. _____ The X-rays do not emanate from this negatively charged pole

6. _____ This part directs the electrons toward the anode

7. _____ The electrons directly impact this part to produce X-rays

EXERCISE 15.8 TRUE OR FALSE: COMPREHENSIVE

Instructions: Read the following statements and write "T" for true or "F" for false in the blanks provided. If a statement is false, correct the statement to make it true.

1. _____ Radiographs are considered to be a part of a patient's legal medical record.

2. _____ X-rays are a type of electromagnetic radiation with a lower frequency than visible light, radio signals, and TV signals.

3. _____ Rotating anodes are generally used in dental machines and small portable machines.

4. _____ Scatter radiation reduces density.

5. _____ Fluoroscopy is used to study moving structures such as beating of the heart and motility of the esophagus.

6. _____ Computed radiography (CR) and digital radiography (DR) are two names for the same thing.

7. _____ One advantage of digital radiography systems is that they require less radiation to produce a diagnostic image than film/screen systems.

8. _____ CR and DR systems are not as sensitive to under- and over-exposures as conventional film/screen systems.

9. _____ A radiology information system (RIS) is a digital imaging device that is used to evaluate blood flow.

10. _____ The exposure time is related to the number of X-ray photons produced—as one goes up, the other does also.

11. _____ Endoscopy is commonly used to view internal mucosa and the intraluminal contents of hollow organs.

12. _____ The focal-film distance influences radiographic density.

13. _____ A technique chart is used to provide appropriate machine settings and must be custom-made for each machine.

14. _____ The most popular type of technique chart used by veterinarians is a variable kilovoltage chart.

15. _____ Intensifying screens should be cleaned with a 40% alcohol solution.

16. _____ X-ray film and intensifying screens must be matched for proper function.

17. _____ Barium sulfate has a low atomic number and absorbs a small amount of radiation, resulting in increased radiographic opacity.

18. _____ Automatic processors standardize, speed up, and simplify film processing and decrease the need for required maintenance.

19. _____ X-ray film is more sensitive to damage after exposure and before development than at any other time.

20. _____ Rem is an abbreviation used for the equivalent dose.

21. _____ A dosimeter should be stored outside of the X-ray room.

22. _____ Technicians should always remember that X-ray effects are cumulative.

23. _____ Nonionic organic iodides are more hypersomolar than ionic organic iodides.

24. _____ Most radiographic studies require only one view.

25. _____ When X-raying large dogs, it may be necessary to use two films per view to image the entire abdomen.

26. _____ Manual restraint of patients for radiographic studies is routine and not a safety concern as long as protective equipment is used.

27. _____ The ultrasound machine transducer both emits the sound and receives reflected waves.

28. _____ When adjacent tissues are very dissimilar in density, little of the ultrasound wave bounces off the tissue interface.

29. _____ Like radiographic artifacts, ultrasound artifacts do not contribute useful information.

30. _____ The most common use for computed tomography (CT) scans in veterinary patients is examination of the central nervous system.

31. _____ After thorough and careful cleaning, an endoscope should be stored safely in its original container.

32. _____ Pregnant woman should not participate in testing or care of patients undergoing Nuclear Scintigraphy.

33. _____ Using longer exposre times will reduce potential motion artifacts and increase the radiographic detail.

34. _____ It is not necessary to make a back up copy of digital files.

35. _____ The components for generating X-ray may vary depending on the image receptor used.

Instructions: Circle the one correct answer to each of the following questions.

1. The shorter the wavelength of X-rays,
   a. the greater the energy and the penetration.
   b. the greater the energy but the lower the penetration.
   c. the lower the energy but the greater the penetration.
   d. the lower the energy and the penetration.

2. The kilovoltage electrical circuit controls the
   a. electrical potential across the filament.
   b. number of electrons created.
   c. electrical potential between the cathode and the anode.
   d. number of the X-rays created.

3. The "target" in an X-ray tube is the area where the
   a. X-rays impact the anode.
   b. electrons impact the cathode.
   c. electrons impact the anode.
   d. X-rays impact the cathode.

4. Information regarding the maximum safe exposure time that can be used without damaging the machine may be found on the
   a. technique chart.
   b. tube rating chart.
   c. X-ray log.
   d. safe-operating procedures.

5. Which of the following factors does *not* increase scatter radiation?
   a. Thickness of the body part
   b. Size of the X-ray field
   c. Type of cassette
   d. Kilovoltage

6. The three primary machine controls that influence X-ray production are
   a. focal-film distance, kilovoltage, and milliamperage.
   b. kilovoltage, exposure time, and focal-film distance.
   c. milliamperage, exposure time, and kilovoltage.
   d. milliamperage, focal-film distance, and exposure time.

7. Which of the following X-ray machines commonly seen in small animal veterinary practices is of the 50 to 300 mA type?
   a. Dental machine-ray unit
   b. Portable machine-ray unit
   c. Mobile machine-ray unit
   d. Stationary machine-ray unit

8. Which type of unit is used to image the changing diameter of the trachea during inspiration and expiration?
   a. Mobile
   b. Portable
   c. Fluoroscope
   d. Stationary

9. Dynamic range refers to which of the following image characteristics?
   a. Range of sharpness
   b. Size
   c. General amount of blackness
   d. Number of shades of gray

10. A photostimulable phosphor plate is used to capture the image in the following type of X-ray system:
    a. computed radiography.
    b. digital radiography.
    c. film/screen.
    d. nonscreen film.

11. A digital artifact called Uberschwinger artifact appears as
    a. a grainy appearance to the image.
    b. black spots or dots on the image.
    c. loss of part of the image.
    d. a lucent halo around metal implants.

12. A universal format or standard for digital image storage, display, manipulation, and retrieval is
    a. DICOM.
    b. PACS.
    c. RIS.
    d. ALARA.

13. A computerized system used to move, transmit, and store digital images is
    a. LAN.
    b. PACS.
    c. RIS.
    d. ALARA.

14. Which is an appropriate use of radiographic contrast?
    a. Imaging the bladder of the cat
    b. Imaging the skull of the dog
    c. Imaging the thorax of the cat
    d. Imaging the leg of the dog

15. If the kilovoltage setting is increased,
    a. the radiographic density and contrast will increase.
    b. the radiographic density will increase but the contrast will decrease.
    c. the radiographic density will decrease but the contrast will increase.
    d. the radiographic density and contrast will decrease.

16. As compared with screen film, nonscreen film
    a. produces images with less detail.
    b. cannot be used for intraoral dental studies.
    c. requires a much longer exposure time to get a diagnostic image.
    d. requires the use of expensive cassettes.

17. A disadvantage of the Potter-Bucky diaphragm is that it
    a. is very loud.
    b. is very heavy.
    c. uses significantly more film per image.
    d. increases the visibility of grid lines.

18. The size of the silver halide crystals in the suspension from which X-ray film is prepared determines
    a. the expense of the film.
    b. the flexibility of the film.
    c. the speed of the film.
    d. the storage requirements of the film.

19. The primary purpose of a grid is to
    a. decrease the settings needed.
    b. minimize distortion.
    c. decrease radiation exposure.
    d. control scatter radiation.

20. Grids are placed
    a. above the patient.
    b. between the tube and the table.
    c. between the patient and the cassette.
    d. under the cassette.

21. A grid should be used when X-raying body parts that are
    a. more than 5 cm thick.
    b. less than 10 cm thick.
    c. more than 10 cm thick.
    d. more than 20 cm thick.

22. Silver can be recovered from
    a. X-ray film and fixer solution.
    b. fixer solution and developer solution.
    c. developer solution and rinse water.
    d. rinse water and X-ray film.

23. Radiographic detail is improved by
    a. using a larger focal spot.
    b. increasing the exposure time.
    c. decreasing the focal-film distance.
    d. minimizing the object-film distance.

24. Therapeutic nuclear medicine involves the administration of radioactive iodine for the treatment of
    a. sarcomas.
    b. thyroid tumors.
    c. Cushing's disease.
    d. dysplasia.

25. The machine setting that has the greatest influence on radiographic contrast is
    a. milliamperage.
    b. exposure time.
    c. focal-film distance.
    d. kilovoltage.

26. The absorbed dose of radiation is defined as the
    a. damage not seen in the lifetime of the recipient but in future generations.
    b. the energy imparted by ionizing radiation to a unit mass of irradiated material.
    c. the quantity of electrons boiled off the filament in the X-ray tube.
    d. the maximum permissible dose.

27. The benefit of Doppler ultrasound is that it can visualize and measure
    a. body cavities.
    b. bones.
    c. blood flow.
    d. heat.

28. The maximum permissible dose (MPD) is the dose of radiation a person is allowed to receive from occupational exposure over a certain time. The annual MPD for occupational personnel is
    a. 0.03 Sv/year.
    b. 0.05 Sv/year.
    c. 0.10 Sv/year.
    d. 0.15 Sv/year.

29. Protective equipment including aprons, thyroid shields, and gloves should have a(n) _____ mm lead equivalent minimum.
    a. 0.25
    b. 0.5
    c. 1
    d. 2

30. Barium sulfate is contraindicated
    a. if bowel perforation is suspected.
    b. for esophageal studies.
    c. for upper GI exams.
    d. for lower GI exams.

31. Soluble, radiopaque ionic contrast media should not be used for
    a. esophageal studies.
    b. upper GI studies.
    c. cystography.
    d. myelography.

32. Which of the following contrast studies requires that images be taken right after barium sulfate contrast is given and also 15, 30, and 60 minutes after contrast administration?
    a. Positive-contrast cystogram
    b. Upper gastrointestinal series
    c. Barium enema
    d. Myelogram

33. Which of these is not a common technical error made with automatic processors?
    a. Increased density
    b. Decreased density
    c. Gray film
    d. Scratches on film

34. An ultrasound echo is produced whenever the ultrasound beam crosses a boundary between two tissues of differing acoustic impedance (opposition to flow of the beam). The main factor that influences acoustic impedance is the
    a. speed of the sound.
    b. density of the tissue.
    c. intensity of the sound.
    d. frequency of the sound.

35. Which ultrasound display mode has little value in performing abdominal or cardiac exams and therefore is not used?
    a. A mode
    b. B mode
    c. M mode
    d. Doppler mode

36. M mode ultrasound is used primarily for
    a. abdominal ultrasonography.
    b. pregnancy exams.
    c. large animal tendon exams.
    d. echocardiography.

37. Linear array ultrasound transducers are not particularly useful for examination of the
    a. bladder from a transabdominal approach.
    b. heart from an intercostal approach.
    c. small animal uterus from a transabdominal approach.
    d. large animal reproductive tract from a transrectal approach.

38. The most appropriate transducer frequency for an ultrasound exam on a cat is
    a. 7.5 MHz.
    b. 5 MHz.
    c. 3 MHz.
    d. 1 MHz.

39. A structure on an ultrasound image that is brighter than an adjacent structure is said to be
    _____ in relation to the adjacent structure.
    a. anechoic
    b. echogenic
    c. isoechoic
    d. hyperechoic

40. Ultrasound cannot be used to image which of the following tissues?
    a. Liver
    b. Heart
    c. Brain
    d. Blood vessels

41. What alternative modality is used to treat thyroid tumors?
    a. Magnetic resonance imaging
    b. Nuclear medicine
    c. Computed tomography
    d. Ultrasonography

42. The substance technetium-99m is an agent used to perform which of the following examinations?
    a. Magnetic resonance imaging
    b. Nuclear medicine imaging
    c. Computed tomography
    d. Ultrasonography

43. Which alternative imaging technique produces an image by using a thin X-ray beam to measure X-ray attenuation?
    a. Magnetic resonance imaging
    b. Nuclear medicine imaging
    c. Computed tomography
    d. Ultrasonography

44. Some computed tomography scanners have a "helical scan mode." What is the chief advantage of this capability?
    a. It requires less radiation.
    b. It produces a better image.
    c. It does not require the patient to be still.
    d. It is faster.

45. Both magnetic resonance imaging (MRI) and computed tomography (CT) create cross-sectional views of the patient's anatomy. What is the primary difference between MRI and CT scanning in terms of the way they work?
    a. MRI does not use ionizing radiation.
    b. CT does not use X-rays.
    c. CT uses radio waves.
    d. MRI uses radionuclides.

46. Which of the following alternate imaging modalities involves use of a strong magnetic field?
    a. MRI
    b. Nuclear medicine imaging
    c. CT
    d. Ultrasonography

47. Which of the following scans is usually performed once without contrast and again with contrast?
    a. MRI
    b. Nuclear medicine
    c. Ultrasound
    d. CT

EXERCISE 15.10 FILL-IN-THE-BLANK: COMPREHENSIVE

Instructions: Fill in each of the spaces provided with the missing word or words that complete the sentence.

1. Information that must be on a diagnostic radiograph, in addition to the name of the facility where the study was taken, includes the name of the _____, the name of the _____ (or the patient ID #), _____, and the _____.

2. There are two electrical circuits in an X-ray machine. The high-voltage circuit (also known as the _____ circuit) controls the penetration of the X-ray beam. The low-voltage circuit (also known as the _____ circuit) controls the number of X-rays created.

3. Radiographic _____ refers to the degree of sharpness that defines the edge of an anatomic structure.

4. Rotating anodes have a "two-step" exposure switch. When the first step is activated, the anode starts _____, and when the second step is activated, _____ are produced.

5. Most of the energy generated by the electrons impacting the anode target is converted into heat. In fact, _____% of the energy is lost as heat, and _____% of the energy is converted to X-ray energy.

6. Scatter radiation is undesirable because it _____ film quality and _____ exposure of personnel.

7. Severe underexposure of a digital image receptor will result in a finished image with a grainy appearance, an effect known as _____ or "noise."

8. Digital radiography has a wide _____, meaning it uses many shades of gray. This allows both bone and soft tissues to be seen at the same exposure setting, which is not possible with film systems.

9. If dust, hair, or other particles are trapped in a CR cassette, _____ spots will be visible on the finished image.

10. The factors that must be set on any X-ray machine regardless of age or type are _____, _____, and _____.

11. When milliamperage (mA) is increased, radiographic density increases, or, in other words, the image gets _____. Conversely, when mA is decreased, radiographic density decreases, or the image gets _____.

12. When kilovoltage (kV) is increased, radiographic density _____. This is because the X-rays produced are more penetrating.

13. The effect of focal-film distance on the number of X-rays reaching the image receptor is governed by the "inverse square law." This law predicts that if the focal-film distance is doubled, the number of X-rays reaching the receptor will be reduced by a factor of _____.

14. Grids should be used for tissues that are greater than _____ cm in thickness.

15. The term *screen speed* refers to the ability of an intensifying screen to convert absorbed _____ energy into _____.

16. _____ does not generate visual images, but rather it detects functional or physiologic, pharmacologic, and kinetic data from the patient in the image.

17. Screen X-ray film is sensitive primarily to _____, whereas nonscreen film is more sensitive to _____.

18. Grids absorb part of the primary X-ray beam and thus require the use of _____ machine settings to produce a given film density.

19. A Potter-Bucky diaphragm moves the grid across the film during the exposure so that _____ are not visible.

20. Most ruined radiographs are owing to errors during _____.

21. The primary machine setting that affects radiographic density is _____.

22. In recent years, the old units of measurement of radiation have been replaced by international units. The "rad" has been replaced by the _____, and the "rem" has been replaced by the _____.

23. Positive-contrast agents _____ radiographic opacity, whereas negative-contrast agents _____ radiographic opacity.

24. Carbon dioxide is preferred over room air as a contrast agent because it is less likely to cause an _____, a serious, sometimes fatal, complication.

25. When a GI perforation is suspected, ionic or nonionic organic _____ should be used.

26. _____ is used almost exclusively for upper and lower GI examinations.

27. The frequency of the ultrasound waves emitted by a transducer is used to rate the output. Most transducers have an output of 2.5 to 12 megahertz (MHz). 1 Hertz (Hz) = 1 _____ per _____. Because the prefix "mega" means "million," a 5 MHz transducer emits sound at a frequency of _____ cycles/second.

28. The ultrasound transducer emits sound waves approximately _____% of the time and receives reflected waves approximately _____% of the time.

29. An ultrasound beam is weakened or _____ by absorption, reflection, scattering, refraction, and diffraction.

30. Ultrasound cannot be used to image through bone or gas because _____% of the beam is reflected off of a fat–bone interface, and 100% of the beam is reflected off of a _____ interface.

31. A patient receiving an ultrasound examination of the abdomen should be placed in lateral or _____ recumbency, and a patient receiving a cardiac examination should be placed in lateral or _____ recumbency.

32. The ultrasound transducer should be oriented in relationship to the animal's body such that when acquiring a sagittal view, the patient's head should appear on the _____ side of the screen, and when acquiring a transverse view, the patient's right side should appear on the _____ side of the screen.

33. Electromagnetic radiation that originates from radionuclides is referred to as _____ radiation.

34. The two types of diagnostic nuclear medicine used in veterinary medicine are _____ and _____.

35. The most common isotope used in PET imaging is _____.

36. The two types of personal dosimeters commonly used in veterinary medicine are _____ and _____.

EXERCISE 15.11 CASE STUDY: MINIMIZING RADIATION EXPOSURE

Your first job following graduation is as a veterinary technician in a small animal practice. This is a busy multiple-doctor practice, and you are responsible for acquiring approximately 10 to 15 sets of X-rays a day. As a good technician, you are concerned about your safety and are eager to follow protection practices to minimize your exposure to ALARA (as low as reasonably achievable). While in school, you had committed these practices to memory and now want to review them in anticipation of minimizing your risk. Review the practices as they relate to each of the following areas.

a. Collimation

_____

b. Filter

_____

c. Prevent retakes

_____

d. Exposure to the primary beam

_____

e. Use of protective equipment

_____

f. Use of accessory equipment to position the patient

_____

g. Use of chemical restraint

_____

h. Restrictions on personnel involved in the procedure

_____

i. Positioning your body while restraining the patient to limit exposure

_____

Other Important Principles:

j. Avoid dose creep

_____

k. Use fast screens

_____

l. Calibrate regularly

_____

m. Follow state radiation safety codes

_____

16 Basic Necropsy Procedures

LEARNING OBJECTIVES

When you have completed this chapter, you will be able to:

1. Pronounce, define, and spell all key terms in the chapter.
2. List and discuss the indications for a necropsy.
3. List and discuss the role of a veterinary technician in the necropsy process.
4. Explain how to write a necropsy report, including how to describe lesions.
5. Discuss sample collection for laboratory testing, including the uses for the following collections: fixed tissue, fresh tissue, swabs, and whole blood, serum, fluids, and feces, and performance of rabies procedure.
6. Discuss the public health importance of correctly shipping diagnostic specimens.
7. Describe the facilities, instruments, and supplies needed to perform a necropsy, including protective clothing and other personal protective equipment (PPE).
8. Do the following regarding the necropsy procedure for a small mammal:
   - Describe how to open the carcass.
   - Explain the principles of preliminary and external examination of the carcass.
   - Describe the initial steps of a necropsy dissection, including reflection of the skin and limbs, and examination of superficial organs and body cavities.
   - Describe the steps for dissection and examination of the skull and brain, neck and thoracic viscera, abdominal cavity, female and male urogenital tracts, abdominal aorta, rectum, and anal glands, vertebral column, and spinal cord.
   - Outline all of the steps for an entire necropsy procedure.
9. Do the following regarding necropsy variations:
   - Describe variations in necropsy procedure specific to ruminants, horses, pigs, fetuses, birds, and laboratory animals.
   - Explain the differences between a complete necropsy and a cosmetic necropsy.

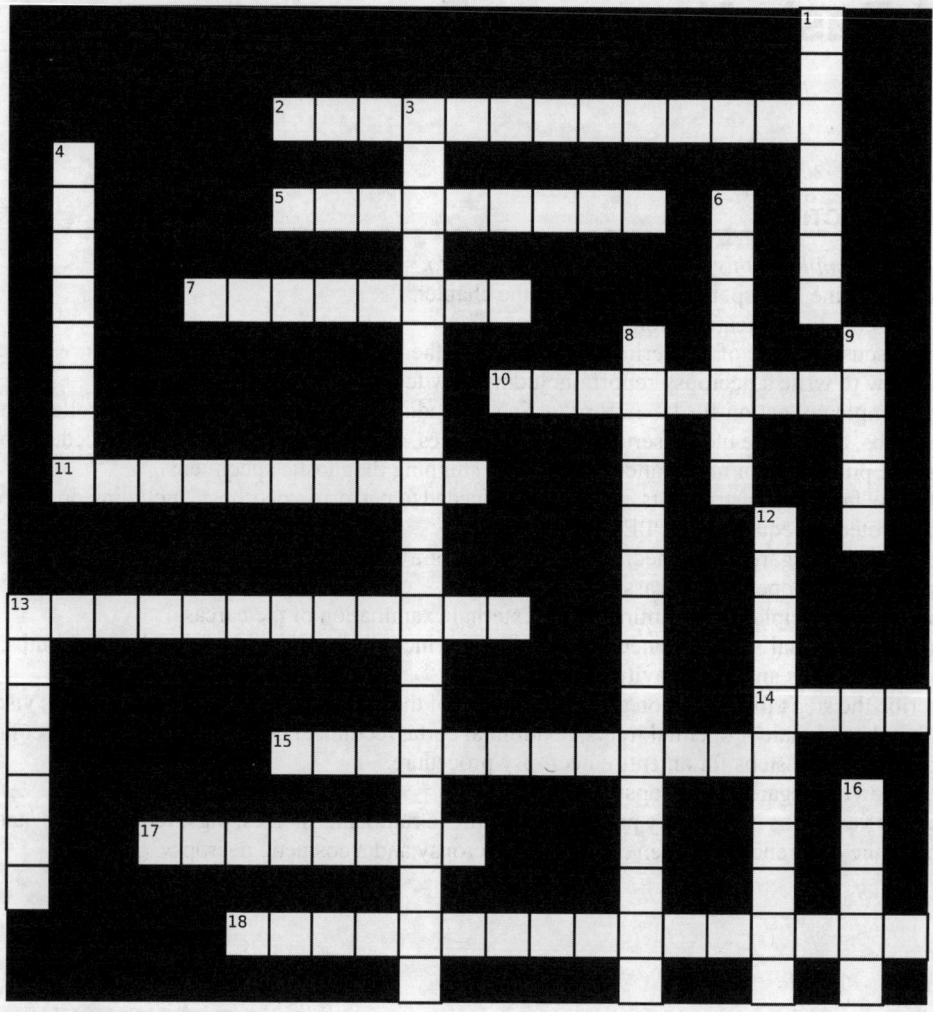

Across

2 The spinal cord exits the skull here. (2 words)
5 Contraction of the _____ causes air to be drawn into the lungs.
7 This structure is located between the stomach and the jejunum.
10 The master gland.
11 The _____ becomes diseased in cardiomyopathy.
13 You must be careful to avoid this structure when giving an IM injection in the rear limb. (2 words)
14 The second cervical vertebra.
15 All parts of the ruminant stomach except for the abomasum.
17 Membranes between the brain and calvarium.
18 The tricuspid valve is an _____ valve.

Down

1 Attachment sites within the hoof.
3 Collective term for the bones of the appendages. (2 words)
4 A cow's true stomach.
6 Part of the mesentery.
8 Takes deoxygenated blood to the lungs. (2 words)
9 The _____ bones have to be cut to remove the tongue and larynx.
12 Contains the trachea, esophagus, and heart inside the chest.
13 Attaches to the ventral aspect of the ribs.
16 A neck bone that is one half of the atlantooccipital joint.

EXERCISE 16.2 DEFINITIONS: KEY TERMS

Instructions: Define each term in your own words.

1. Necropsy: _____

_____

2. Prosector: _____

_____

3. Pathology: _____

_____

4. Gross pathology: _____

_____

5. Histopathology: _____

_____

6. Pathogenesis: _____

_____

7. Lesions: _____

_____

8. Autolysis: _____

_____

9. In situ: _____

_____

10. Hydronephrosis: _____

_____

EXERCISE 16.3 MATCHING: INSTRUMENTS AND SUPPLIES USED FOR A NECROPSY

Instructions: Match each instrument or supply in column A with its corresponding use in column B by writing the appropriate letter in the space provided.

Column A

1. _____ Stryker saw
2. _____ Pruning shears
3. _____ String
4. _____ Tissue cassettes
5. _____ Clip-on laundry tags
6. _____ Screw-top plastic containers containing formalin
7. _____ Sealable plastic bags and plastic vials
8. _____ Meat cutter's band saw

Column B

A. To hold small tissues

B. To hold refrigerated and frozen samples

C. To cut ribs

D. To hold tissues for histopathology

E. To close off bowel ends

F. To remove the brain

G. To remove the spinal cord in a horse

H. To identify tissues

EXERCISE 16.4 ORDERING: PERFORMING A NECROPSY

Instructions: To perform a complete necropsy, 36 steps must be followed that can be grouped into the following categories:

1. Examination of external and superficial structures
2. Examination of the body cavities
3. Examination of the head and CNS
4. Examination of the thoracic viscera
5. Examination of the abdominal viscera
6. Final steps

Within each category, place the steps of performing a complete necropsy in the proper order from first to last by placing the appropriate number (1, 2, 3, etc.) in the space provided.

1. **Examination of external and superficial structures** *(steps 1 through 7)*

   A. _____ Dissect and examine, section, and collect skin, lymph nodes, salivary glands, and testes or mammary glands.

   B. _____ Remove the eyes.

   C. _____ Dissect and examine, section, and collect the synovium, skeletal muscle, sciatic nerve, and bone marrow.

   D. _____ Make a midline skin incision, reflect the limbs, and extend the incision rostrally to the mandibular symphysis and caudally to the perineum.

   E. _____ Weigh the animal.

   F. _____ Open the coxofemoral, stifle, and scapulohumeral joints.

   G. _____ Perform an external examination.

2. **Examination of the body cavities** *(steps 8 through 13)*

   A. _____ Dissect and examine, section, and collect thyroid, parathyroid, and adrenal glands.

   B. _____ Examine organs and vascular structures.

   C. _____ Remove the tongue from the oral cavity and reflect the tongue, tonsils, larynx, and esophagus caudally.

   D. _____ Open the chest by cutting the ribs.

   E. _____ Open the abdomen on the midline and puncture the diaphragm.

   F. _____ Open the pericardium.

3. **Examination of the head and CNS** *(steps 14 through 19)*

   A. _____ Transect the cranial nerves and remove the brain and the pituitary gland.

   B. _____ Cut the spinal cord and vertebral column at atlantooccipital joint.

   C. _____ Section the head longitudinally and examine nasal and oral cavities.

   D. _____ Cut the calvaria and remove the caudal-dorsal portion of the calvaria and dorsal meninges.

   E. _____ Open the tympanic bullae.

   F. _____ Remove skin and muscle from calvaria.

4. **Examination of the thoracic viscera** *(steps 20 through 24)*

   A. _____ Section the lungs, saving one section from each lobe.

   B. _____ Remove the tongue, tonsils, esophagus, trachea, lungs, heart, and thoracic aorta as a unit.

   C. _____ Serially section the tongue.

   D. _____ Examine, weigh, and collect sections of the heart.

   E. _____ Open the esophagus and trachea.

5. **Examination of the abdominal viscera** *(steps 25 through 31)*

   A. _____ Serial section the spleen.

   B. _____ Weigh, section, and collect samples from the liver.

   C. _____ Remove the distal duodenum, jejunum, ileum, colon, and mesenteric lymph nodes as a unit.

   D. _____ Open the gallbladder and collect samples from the stomach, duodenum, and pancreas.

   E. _____ Open the stomach and duodenum.

   F. _____ Express the gallbladder.

   G. _____ Remove the liver, duodenum, pancreas, stomach, and spleen as a unit.

6. **Final steps** *(steps 32 through 36)*

   A. _____ Remove the spinal cord if necessary.

   B. _____ Remove the floor of the pelvis.

   C. _____ Dissect and examine, section, and collect the small intestine, colon, and mesenteric lymph nodes.

   D. _____ Dissect and examine, section, and collect tissues from all parts of the urogenital system.

   E. _____ Dissect and examine, section, and collect tissues from the rectum, anal glands, and abdominal aorta.

EXERCISE 16.5 TRUE OR FALSE: COMPREHENSIVE

Instructions: Read the following statements and write "T" for true or "F" for false in the blanks provided. If a statement is false, correct the statement to make it true.

1. _____ A body may either be frozen or refrigerated between death and the necropsy to prevent degeneration of tissues.

2. _____ Ten percent buffered formalin is a carcinogen and so should not contact skin.

3. _____ Tissues, fluids, and stomach contents that are being tested for toxins may be frozen.

4. _____ When sending in tissues for histopathologic examination, the excess formalin in the bottle should never be removed until the tissues arrive at the lab, or tissue artifacts will result.

5. ____ Formalin-fixed material should be refrigerated and then kept on ice until arrival at the lab.

6. ____ When performing a necropsy on a dog, cat, horse, or cow, the patient should be placed in right lateral recumbency.

7. ____ Unlike other soft tissues, the brain should not be sectioned until thoroughly fixed.

8. ____ The heart is removed from the thoracic cavity separately from the lungs and other viscera.

9. ____ Fluid content of the lungs can be assessed by gently squeezing them.

10. ____ After removing but before slicing each kidney, the capsule should be peeled off.

11. ____ As with other animals, a fetus should be placed in left lateral recumbency.

12. ____ Birds have only a left ovary.

13. ____ The lungs should be inflated with formalin before the lungs and heart are removed from the thorax in small rodents (mice, hamsters, and gerbils).

14. ____ Because state and federal entities regulate testing for prion disease, technicians must be certified by demonstrating that they can properly document and collect the required specimens.

15. ____ Abnormal prions cause transmissible spongiform encephalopathies (TSE).

EXERCISE 16.6 MULTIPLE CHOICE: COMPREHENSIVE

Instructions: Circle the one correct answer to each of the following questions.

1. When preserving most tissues for histopathology, which of the following fixatives should be used?
   a. 10% buffered formalin, with a fixative to tissue ratio of 10:1 by volume
   b. 50% buffered formalin with a fixative to tissue ratio of 10:1 by volume
   c. 10% buffered formalin with a fixative to tissue ratio of 1:10 by volume
   d. 50% buffered formalin with a fixative to tissue ratio of 1:10 by volume

2. Ten percent buffered formalin is made by mixing dibasic anhydrous sodium phosphate and monobasic sodium phosphate with
   a. three parts water and one part 37% to 40% formaldehyde solution.
   b. nine parts 50% formalin and one part 37% to 40% formaldehyde solution.
   c. nine parts water and one part 37% to 40% formaldehyde solution.
   d. one part 50% formalin and nine parts 37% to 40% formaldehyde solution.

3. Fifty percent formalin is made by mixing
   a. one part water and one part 37% to 40% formaldehyde solution.
   b. one part 10% formalin and one part 37% to 40% formaldehyde solution.
   c. one part water and one part 10% formalin.
   d. one part 10% formalin and five parts 37% to 40% formaldehyde solution.

4. Some tissues should be preserved in Bouin fixative because it produces less tissue shrinkage and better preservation of cellular detail. Which of the following tissues should be preserved in Bouin fixative?
   a. Brain
   b. Liver
   c. Eyes
   d. Lung

5. To avoid decomposition, a complete necropsy should begin with dissection of the
   a. lungs.
   b. liver.
   c. brain.
   d. eyes.

6. Once removed, the interior of the eye can be examined by immersion in
   a. alcohol.
   b. Bouin fixative.
   c. cool water.
   d. 10% formalin.

7. When performing a complete necropsy on a dog or cat, some joints should be routinely opened and examined. Which of the following joints should be examined in this way?
   a. Stifle joint
   b. Elbow joint
   c. Carpal joints
   d. Metacarpal–phalangeal joints

8. A "Stryker saw" is typically used to
   a. cut the ribs.
   b. open the joints.
   c. open the calvaria.
   d. cut the hyoid bones.

9. Because enteric disease is a frequent reason for necropsy of pigs, attention should be focused on collecting
   a. stomach contents.
   b. fecal matter from the colon.
   c. the gallbladder.
   d. the freshest gut tissues.

10. When performing a necropsy on very small birds such as hummingbirds and finches
    a. the same technique should be used as with other birds.
    b. the undissected body should be put in a formalin jar.
    c. the body cavities should be opened before placing the body in the formalin jar.
    d. the body should be sectioned into two halves before it is fixed.

11. In very small mammals, such as mice, hamsters, and gerbils,
    a. the entire vertebral canal with the spinal cord inside should be removed.
    b. the spinal cord should be removed as one would for a dog or cat.
    c. the spinal cord should be removed from the vertebral canal after the vertebral column is separated from the rest of the body.
    d. the spinal cord should be removed by performing a dorsal laminectomy.

12. A cosmetic necropsy is appropriate
    a. as an alternative to a complete necropsy.
    b. when the disease is limited to the abdomen and chest.
    c. when the cause of death is known before beginning.
    d. when tissues do not need to be collected.

13. Samples for prion disease may be collected with a
    a. Stryker saw.
    b. calvaria forceps.
    c. spinal tube.
    d. brain spoon.

14. Prions are classified as
    a. viruses.
    b. bacteria.
    c. proteins.
    d. parasites.

15. A transmissible spongiform encephalopathy of sheep is
    a. chronic wasting disease.
    b. scrapie.
    c. BSE.
    d. Creutzfeldt–Jakob disease.

EXERCISE 16.7 FILL-IN-THE-BLANK: COMPREHENSIVE

Instructions: Fill in each of the spaces provided with the missing word or words that complete the sentence.

1. It is important to perform a necropsy as soon as possible after death to avoid _____.

2. The fixative 50% formalin is specifically used for the following tissues: (a) _____, (b) _____, and (c) _____.

3. Tissues for virus isolation must be collected aseptically to prevent contamination and either refrigerated in a sterile container or immersed in sterile _____ buffered _____ and preserved. Fresh, refrigerated tissue immersed in _____ medium is the preferred method of tissue submission.

4. Paired organs can be cut on different planes to distinguish them. When harvesting tissue from the kidneys, to differentiate one from the other, the left kidney should be cut _____ and the right one should be cut _____.

5. Organs removed during a necropsy should be measured and/or weighed if they have an abnormal _____ or _____.

6. To free the tongue, larynx, pharynx, trachea, and esophagus, the _____ bones must be cut.

7. Patency of the bile duct can be determined by squeezing the _____.

8. The ureters should be opened and examined if they or the renal pelvis are _____.

9. Ruminoreticular contents should be examined for _____ objects and undesirable _____ material.

10. When performing a necropsy on a horse and dissecting the head and neck, special attention should be given to the _____ and _____ veins.

11. Some diseases are _____, meaning they arise suddenly, and the cause is unknown.

12. The gestational age of a large animal fetus can be estimated by _____ or _____ it.

EXERCISE 16.8 CASE STUDY: PERFORMING A NECROPSY ON A RABIES SUSPECT

Signalment: 8-year-old, castrated, male Labrador Retriever mix

History: The patient exhibits acute onset of progressive neurologic disease (seizures, ataxia, cranial nerve abnormalities, and a change in behavior) and an elevated body temperature. The patient had not seen a veterinarian in the 2 years prior to admission, and routine vaccinations, including the rabies vaccination, are 6 months overdue.

A basic diagnostic workup (blood work, parasite screen, urinalysis, and x-rays) did not reveal a cause of the neurologic illness. Over the next few days, despite supportive treatment, the neurologic signs continued to progress. Three days after presentation, in view of the severity of the condition and the significant expense that would be necessary to continue with the workup and treatment, the owners elected euthanasia and requested a necropsy. Although this patient had no known exposure to a potentially rabid animal, and a number of other differentials were being considered, infection with rabies virus could not be ruled out.

When performing a necropsy on a rabies suspect such as this patient, precautions must be taken by the prosector. Answer the following questions about the precautions you would take if involved in the necropsy of this patient.

1. Should restrictions be placed on which hospital personnel are permitted to handle this patient antemortem, handle the body postmortem, and participate in the necropsy? If so, what are they?

_____

_____

_____

_____

_____

2. It is decided that you meet the criteria to assist the doctor with the necropsy. What protective equipment should you use to minimize the risk of transmission?

_____

_____

_____

_____

_____

3. What tissue or other sample is needed to test this patient for rabies, and how is it harvested?

_____

_____

_____

_____

4. How should the tissue sample be prepared and stored between harvesting and transport to the lab?

_____

_____

_____

5. How should the carcass be handled after completion of the necropsy?

_____

_____

_____

6. How should the table, instruments, and other equipment be cleaned?

_____

_____

_____

17 Diagnostic Sampling and Therapeutic Techniques

LEARNING OBJECTIVES

When you have completed this chapter, you will be able to:
1. Pronounce, define, and spell each of the key terms in this chapter.
2. Compare and contrast patient preparation, positioning, and procedures for blood collection in small animals using venipuncture and arterial blood sampling techniques.
3. List and describe general guidelines for the collection of samples for laboratory testing and exhibit proficiency in the administration of medication to small animals:
   - Describe the indications and methods for administration of medication to cats and dogs using each of the following approaches: oral, orogastric, transdermal, ophthalmic, aural, intrarectal, intranasal, intradermal, subcutaneous, intramuscular, intravenous (IV), intratracheal, intraosseous, and intraperitoneal.
   - Compare and contrast placement of IV catheters in the peripheral and jugular veins in cats and dogs. Describe the specific steps to carry out placement of through-the-needle (TTN), over-the-needle (OTN), and multi-lumen catheters.
4. List and describe procedures for collection of urine samples in cats and dogs, including the advantages and limitations of each method.
5. Describe the indications, materials needed, and procedures for performing thoracocentesis and abdominocentesis on small animals.
6. Describe diagnostic peritoneal lavage (DPL) and list its indications and contraindications
7. Compare and contrast percutaneous and endotracheal lavage techniques.
8. Describe the indications, materials needed, and procedures for different methods of performing transtracheal wash on small animals. Explain sample handling and interpretation.
9. Define arthrocentesis and list indications for performing it in the cat or the dog, list the materials needed, and explain the procedure.
10. Explain the procedure of collecting bone marrow aspirate samples including indications, contraindications, and potential complications; compare and contrast the procedure if the sample is obtained from the ilium, humerus, or femur; and explain how the procedure of fine-needle aspiration differs from other procedures.
11. Describe the methods of orally administering medication to large animal species.
12. Compare and contrast the procedures for administering large volumes of medication via nasogastric tubes in horses and orogastric tubes in ruminants and swine.
13. Do the following regarding IV administration of medication in the large animal:
    - Describe the procedures in the horse for IV administration of medications using the jugular vein and IV catheterization utilizing the cephalic vein and the lateral thoracic vein.
    - List the indications for the use of specific veins for IV administration of medication in ruminants and swine.
    - Compare and contrast the materials needed and procedures for placing IV catheters in camelids and food animal species.
14. List the possible sites of intramuscular administration for each large animal species and describe limitations and contraindications.
15. Compare and contrast the methods used for administration of medication to horses and food animal species using each of the following approaches: subcutaneous, intradermal, intraperitoneal, intranasal, intramammary (cows only), ophthalmic, epidural, transdermal, intrasynovial, rectal and intramuscular, including limitations and contraindications in food animals.
16. Compare and contrast venous and arterial blood collection techniques in equine, camelid, and food animal species.
17. List and describe procedures for collecting urine and fecal samples in equine, camelid, and food animal species and list the advantages and limitations of each method.
18. Describe procedures for collection and evaluation of milk samples from dairy animals.
19. Describe procedures for collection of rumen fluid in large animals.
20. Describe the indications, materials needed, and procedures for performing a thoracocentesis, transtracheal wash, bronchoalveolar lavage (BAL), abdominocentesis, and cerebrospinal fluid collection in equine, camelids, and food animal species.

183

Instructions: Fill in each of the spaces provided with the missing word or words that complete the sentence.

1. In order to properly collect blood from the marginal ear vein, the patient's ear is warmed to promote
   _____.

2. Leakage of something out of its container or normal location, such as a drug out of a vein, is called
   _____.

3. Fecal samples are collected for gross visual inspection, for microscopic examination, and for microbiological culture
   or _____ assay.

4. Pressure is often applied to a venipuncture site after removal of the needle. This helps prevent a(n)
   _____ from forming.

5. When IV catheterization is not possible or cannot be performed rapidly, needles can be placed directly into
   the bone marrow cavity to deliver fluids, drugs, and blood products. This route of administration is called
   _____.

6. _____ is the term for a condition characterized by an abnormally high total number of
   circulating white blood cells.

7. Two methods for performing equine transtracheal aspiration are endoscopic, which is noninvasive, and
   _____, which is invasive.

8. Severe _____ is a relative contraindication for bone marrow aspiration and may require
   the administration of plasma or platelet-rich plasma before the procedure is begun.

9. _____ is the aspiration of fluid from a joint.

10. The clinical term for loss of appetite or absence of food, especially when prolonged, is _____.

11. Vigorous mixing of a collected blood sample and the tube's contents, as well as forcefully ejecting the collected
    blood though the needle of the collection device, may cause _____, yielding inaccurate
    results.

12. _____ fluid is collected and analyzed for diagnosis of diseases of the forestomachs.

13. The condition characterized by an abnormal decrease in the number of the most common type of white blood cells
    in the blood is called _____.

14. The act of striking the chest wall rhythmically with cupped hands is _____.

15. When performing a retention enema, a well-lubricated _____ catheter with balloon is
    inserted into the rectum.

16. Fluids or drugs that have a(n) _____ greater than 600 mOsm/L should be administered
    through the jugular vein.

17. Catheter-induced pathology includes phlebitis, infection, and _____, the latter of which is indicated by a cord-like feeling in the vein, or the vein standing on its own.

18. _____ is the percutaneous aspiration of urine from the bladder.

19. _____ consists of infusion of fluid into the abdomen followed by retrieval of the fluid for laboratory analysis.

20. _____ is a procedure that involves aspiration of 5–7 mL/kg of fluid from the abdominal cavity for diagnostic and therapeutic purposes.

21. Mastitis, or _____, of the mammary gland, may be present without a bacterial component if the teat or udder has received a traumatic injury.

22. A decrease to below normal in the concentration of the three major blood cell types is termed

_____.

EXERCISE 17.2 MATCHING #1: INDICATIONS FOR CLINICAL PROCEDURES

Instructions: Match each clinical procedure in column A with its corresponding indication in column B by writing the appropriate letter in the space provided.

Column A

1. _____ Cystocentesis
2. _____ Thoracentesis
3. _____ Milk sample collection
4. _____ Abdominocentesis
5. _____ Epidural
6. _____ Bone marrow aspirate
7. _____ Arthrocentesis
8. _____ Fine-needle aspiration
9. _____ Bronchoalveolar lavage
10. _____ Cerebrospinal fluid tap

Column B

A. Analgesia

B. Chronic productive cough

C. Skin mass

D. Seizure

E. Mastitis

F. Lameness

G. Pleural effusion

H. Hematuria

I. Ascites

J. Pancytopenia

EXERCISE 17.3 MATCHING #2: SUPPLIES FOR CLINICAL PROCEDURES

Instructions: Match each clinical procedure in column A with the corresponding list of supplies in column B by writing the appropriate letter in the space provided.

Column A

1. _____ Fine-needle aspiration
2. _____ Transtracheal wash
3. _____ Abdominocentesis
4. _____ Sterile milk collection

Column B

A. 16-gauge catheter, 3.5-French polypropylene urinary catheter, 20-mL syringe filled with sterile saline

B. Teat cannula, scalpel blade

C. Clean hands, culture collection tubes

D. 3-mL syringe with a 22-gauge needle, microscope slides

EXERCISE 17.4 MATCHING #3: URINE COLLECTION IN LARGE ANIMALS

Instructions: Match each large animal species in column A with the corresponding technique used to collect urine by free-catch in column B by writing the appropriate letter in the space provided.

Column A

1. _____ Horse

2. _____ Male pig

3. _____ Cow

4. _____ Alpaca

5. _____ Female goat

Column B

A. Wait for the animal to rise after a period of recumbency

B. Take the animal to the dung pile

C. Stroke prepuce with soft brush

D. Stroke the skin beneath the vulva

E. Place fresh bedding in the stall

EXERCISE 17.5 MATCHING #4: SITES FOR SUBCUTANEOUS INJECTION

Instructions: Match each species in column A with its corresponding site for subcutaneous injection of medication in column B by writing the appropriate letter in the space provided.

Column A

1. _____ Dog

2. _____ Pig

3. _____ Goat

4. _____ Horse

5. _____ Cow

Column B

A. Base of ear

B. Behind the elbow

C. Base of neck

D. Axillary region

E. Lateral hip

EXERCISE 17.6 TABLE #1: ROUTES OF MEDICATION ADMINISTRATION IN SMALL ANIMALS

Instructions: For each route of medication administration in the left column, indicate an associated important potential complication and the action you should take to prevent it.

Route of Medication Administration in the Small Animal Patient	Important Potential Complication	Actions Taken to *Prevent* the Complication
Oral administration of liquid suspension		
Oral administration of a capsule		
Intramuscular injection		
Administration of topical ophthalmic ointment		
Intravenous administration of a chemotherapeutic agent		

Instructions: Indicate the rationale for each statement. The first statement and rationale are completed as an example.

Statement	Rationale
Venipuncture should only be attempted if the vessel is clearly delineated	Blind venipuncture often fails and leads to unnecessary patient discomfort.
Cephalic venipuncture should be the last site of choice for collection of diagnostic samples.	
Even though they are smaller than other arteries, the dorsal pedal and dorsal metatarsal arteries are the most common sites for arterial blood gas sample acquisition.	
The needle used to collect blood for coagulation profiles should penetrate the vessel on the first attempt, with minimal tissue trauma.	
If an animal coughs during orogastric intubation, the tube should be removed.	
A fentanyl patch should not be applied to skin that will be in contact with a heating pad, a heat lamp, or another external heat source.	
The ear must be cleared of debris before medication is applied.	
The dorsal region of the neck and back should be avoided when performing subcutaneous injections in small animals.	
If a "clean stick" is not achieved on the first placement attempt of an IV chemotherapy catheter, a different vein should be used.	
When cystocentesis is performed, most, but not all, of the urine should be removed from the bladder.	
Caution should be exercised when performing diagnostic peritoneal lavage in patients with respiratory distress.	

Instructions: Read the following instructions for peripheral vein catheterization in the small animal patient. In the first table, circle the incorrect steps in the left column, and write the corrected procedural step in the right column. In the second table, enter the number of each incorrect step you circled, and describe the complications that could arise if the procedural step was performed as written.

1. Generously clip the fur from the area.	
2. Spray alcohol once over the area.	
3. Occlude the vein upstream of the insertion site with a tourniquet or the help of an assistant.	
4. Extend the leg to visualize the vein.	
5. Use your thumb to stabilize the vein.	
6. With the bevel up, insert the catheter through the skin at a 45-degree angle.	
7. Advance the catheter into the vessel.	
8. When blood appears in the flash chamber (hub), the needle and the catheter are advanced together as a unit for an additional 4 to 6 mm.	
9. Advance the catheter off the needle and into the vessel lumen.	
10. Cap the catheter with a T-connector or injection cap, and flush with heparinized saline.	
11. Secure the catheter to the leg with adhesive tape.	
12. Place a 2 × 2-inch gauze pad over the insertion site.	
13. A 1-inch (2.54-cm) second piece of tape is placed sticky side down underneath the catheter before wrapping around the leg.	
14. Roll gauze is wrapped around the catheter and leg proximal and distal to the insertion site.	

Step #	Complication

EXERCISE 17.9 TABLE #4: ARTERIAL BLOOD SAMPLE COLLECTION

Instructions: Read the following protocol for arterial blood sample collection in the small or large animal patient using a regular needle and syringe. In the first table, circle the incorrect steps in the left column, and write the corrected procedural steps in the right column. In the second table, enter the number of each incorrect step you circled, and describe the patient complication or erroneous blood gas analysis result(s) that could arise if the procedural step was performed as written.

1. Choose a site and locate the artery by palpating the pulse.	
2. Clean the site using the appropriate aseptic technique.	
3. Attach an appropriate-sized needle to a syringe and draw a small amount of heparin into the syringe. Expel this small amount of heparin from the syringe into the needle, which is then ready for use.	
4. Occlude the artery.	
5. Insert the needle into the artery, and firmly pull back on the syringe plunger multiple times to aspirate blood into the syringe.	
6. Withdraw the needle, and have the assistant hold off on the puncture site for 20 to 30 seconds.	
7. Expel any air bubbles from the syringe and replace the needle cap onto the needle.	
8. Roll the syringe between your hands to distribute the anticoagulant throughout the sample.	
9. Immediately perform blood gas analysis.	

Step #	Complication

Instructions: Name the procedure being performed in each photo.

1. _____

2. _____

3. _____

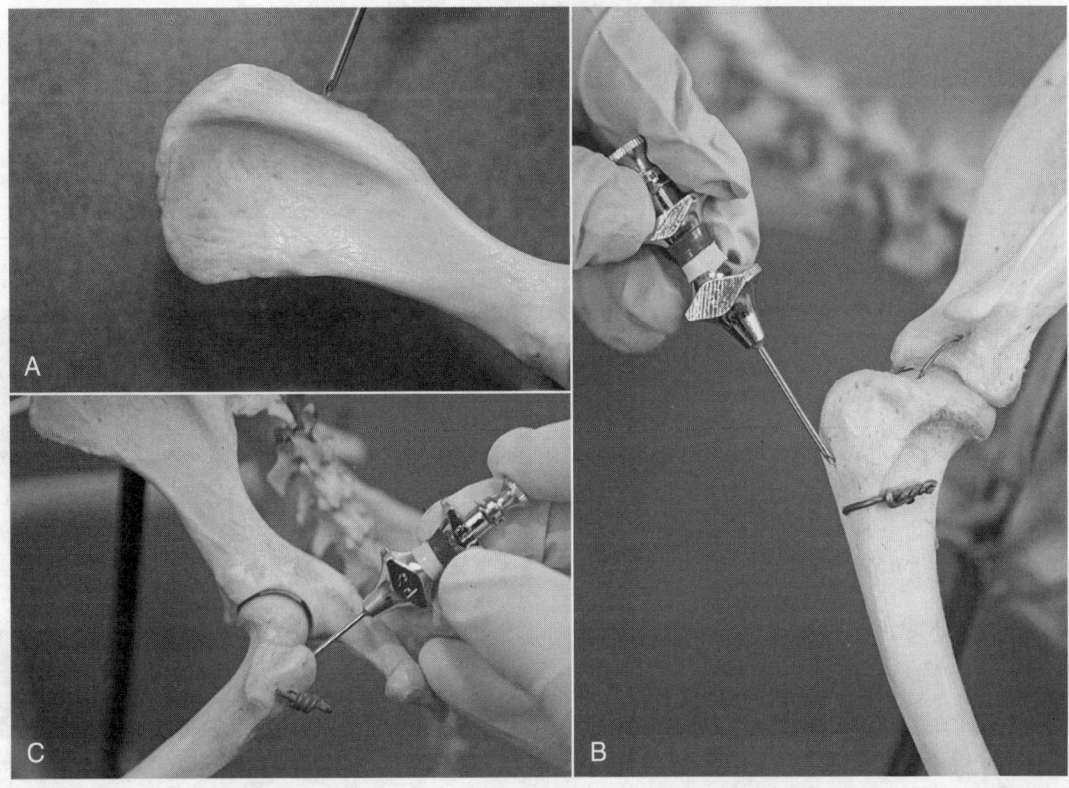

4. _____

Chapter **17** **Diagnostic Sampling and Therapeutic Techniques**

5. _____

6. _____ 7. _____

8.

10. _____

9. _____

EXERCISE 17.11 PHOTO QUIZ #2: INTRAVENOUS CATHETERS

Instructions: Answer the following questions by writing the appropriate letter in the space provided. (Note that each letter will be used only once.)

1. _____ Which IV catheter can be used to administer multiple yet separate infusions?

2. _____ Which IV catheter is commonly used for a quick, one-time administration of medication?

3. _____ Which IV catheter is commonly placed as an indwelling catheter in the cephalic vein?

4. _____ Which IV catheter is commonly placed as an indwelling catheter in the jugular vein?

EXERCISE 17.12 TRUE OR FALSE: COMPREHENSIVE

Instructions: Read the following statements and write "T" for true or "F" for false in the blanks provided. If a statement is false, correct the statement to make it true.

1. _____ If antiseizure medication cannot be administered to a convulsing dog by the intravenous route, it may be given intranasally or intrarectally.

2. _____ To prevent the needle from penetrating both sides of the skin while giving a subcutaneous injection, it is important to insert the needle perpendicular to the long axis of the skin fold.

3. _____ In a severely dehydrated patient, intravenous administration of medications or isotonic fluids is preferred over subcutaneous administration.

4. _____ When placing a jugular catheter in a dog, the catheter is always placed with the tip of the catheter directed toward the heart.

5. _____ Marginal ear venipuncture is used exclusively for assessing blood glucose levels.

6. _____ Male dogs may not require sedation for the placement of a urinary catheter, whereas male cats are usually sedated for this procedure.

7. _____ The seal of the syringe's plunger should never be broken prior to performing venipuncture.

8. _____ When performing a cranial vena cava venipuncture on a pig, it is preferred to use the left side because it reduces the risk of damaging the phrenic nerve.

9. _____ When instilling both an ophthalmic ointment and solution into a patient's eye, the correct order of administration is to apply the ointment first, wait 3–5 minutes, and then apply the solution.

10. _____ When performing an equine abdominocentesis, at least 0.5 mL of fluid must be collected to ensure an accurate analysis of the abdominal fluid.

EXERCISE 17.13 MULTIPLE CHOICE: COMPREHENSIVE

Instructions: Circle the one correct answer to each of the following questions.

1. An indication for placing an orogastric tube in a small animal patient is to
   a. obtain a sample of stomach contents for analysis.
   b. administer activated charcoal to absorb an ingested toxin.
   c. administer water to correct severe dehydration.
   d. obtain a sample of tracheal secretions for analysis.

2. Trauma to the sciatic nerve is a potential complication when administering an intramuscular injection into which of the following muscles?
   a. Triceps muscle
   b. Lumbosacral muscle
   c. Cranial thigh muscle
   d. Semimembranosus muscle

3. Jugular vein catheterization is preferred over peripheral vein catheterization in the small animal patient for which of the following treatment scenarios?
   a. Single administration of an IV medication
   b. Administration of fluids that have an osmolality of greater than 600 mosm/L
   c. Administration of total parenteral nutrition
   d. Administration of blood products for a transfusion

4. The Seldinger guide wire technique refers to the placement of
   a. a spinal needle during a cerebrospinal tap.
   b. a foley catheter during a urinary catheter placement.
   c. a multilumen catheter during a jugular catheter placement.
   d. an over-the-needle catheter during a transtracheal wash.

5. Which of the following small animal procedures requires strict adherence to aseptic technique, including the placement of a surgical drape over the exposed area of the patient?
   a. Cystocentesis
   b. Bone marrow aspiration
   c. Nasoesophageal feeding tube placement
   d. Dorsal metatarsal artery puncture

6. Your patient is a 2-week-old female DSH brown tabby who is severely dehydrated as the result of an *Isospora* (coccidia) infection that has caused profuse diarrhea. Administration of fluids is ordered. You are unable to place an intravenous catheter. Which of the following routes of administration would be the next best choice?
   a. Oral
   b. Intrarectal
   c. Intraosseous
   d. Subcutaneous

7. The doctor has ordered a urine culture and sensitivity to be collected and submitted on your next patient, a neutered male Boston Terrier named Kyle. Which of the following collection methods is preferred for this test?
   a. Free catch
   b. Bladder expression
   c. Cystocentesis
   d. Urinary catheterization

8. Fecal examination in veterinary practices is commonly used to detect
   a. mucus, blood, intestinal parasites, and pus.
   b. viruses, blood, bacteria, and pus.
   c. mucus, blood, intestinal parasites, and ova.
   d. bacteria, blood, intestinal parasites, and ova.

9. It is often necessary to monitor urine production in a small animal patient with an indwelling urinary catheter. For a normovolemic dog weighing 27 pounds, 8 ounces, how much urine should be produced in 24 hours?
   a. 25 mL
   b. 55 mL
   c. 600 mL
   d. 1300 mL

10. Bone marrow aspirates are very painful. Which part of the procedure is responsible for causing the most amount of pain to the patient?
    a. Infiltrating the skin with 2% lidocaine
    b. Making the stab incision into the skin with a scalpel blade
    c. Inserting the stylet into the bone
    d. Aspirating the bone marrow fluid

11. Which of the following needles is most appropriate for performing a jugular venipuncture in a cow?
    a. 18-gauge
    b. 20-gauge
    c. 22-gauge
    d. 25-gauge

12. Jugular venipuncture is contradicted in patients that
    a. have a cough.
    b. weigh less than 25 pounds.
    c. are suspected of having Cushing's disease.
    d. have possible head trauma.

13. In the llama, which cervical vertebra is used as the landmark for low neck jugular venipuncture?
    a. Fourth
    b. Fifth
    c. Sixth
    d. Seventh

14. Placement of an intravenous catheter in the auricular vein is appropriate for repeat sampling in which species?
    a. Cat
    b. Horse
    c. Cow
    d. Pig

15. Which of the following muscles is appropriate to use for medication administration in the cow and pig?
    a. Gluteal muscle
    b. Cervical (neck) muscle
    c. Semimembranosus muscle
    d. Shoulder muscle

16. The most common reason for catheterizing a male cat is
    a. to obtain a urine specimen for bacterial culture.
    b. to relieve a urethral obstruction.
    c. to avoid cystocentesis.
    d. to administer medication for a bladder infection.

17. Meningitis is a potential complication associated with
    a. cerebrospinal fluid tap.
    b. pleural tap.
    c. diagnostic peritoneal lavage.
    d. arthrocentesis.

18. In which of the following patients is it correct to use a balling gun to administer oral tablets?
    a. A foal
    b. A pig
    c. A horse
    d. A steer

19. The most appropriate method for administering mineral oil to a horse is
    a. through a nasogastric tube.
    b. through an orogastric tube.
    c. via drenching.
    d. mixing it in with feed.

20. What is the purpose of a subpalpebral lavage system?
    a. To facilitate gastric lavage
    b. To administer ophthalmic medications
    c. To facilitate joint lavage
    d. To administer rectal medications

EXERCISE 17.14 CASE STUDY:RESPIRATORY DISTRESS IN A CAT

Patient name: Louie Hansen
Signalment: 2-year-old, neutered male DSH brown tabby; indoor-outdoor cat
Presenting complaint: Trouble breathing; seems to be in pain
Relevant triage physical examination findings: Patient is in respiratory distress as evidenced by tachypnea and open-mouthed breathing with abdominal effort. Patient is cyanotic.

1. After completing the triage examination, what should you do next? *(Choose the correct response.)*
    a. Complete a full examination to discover what is causing the respiratory distress.
    b. Bring the patient to the radiology suite for radiographs.
    c. Place an IV catheter and administer shock doses of an isotonic fluid.
    d. Bring the patient into the treatment area and administer oxygen.

As you are completing this, the doctor comes in to listen to Louie's chest. As she is putting her stethoscope into her ears, she discusses with you her concern that Louie may have pleural effusion or a pneumothorax.

2. Define pleural effusion.

_____

_____

3. Define pneumothorax.

_____

Based on the chest auscultation, the doctor believes that Louie has pleural effusion and wants to proceed with a thoracocentesis.

4. Define thoracocentesis.

_____

_____

5. Describe the purpose of each of the following supplies needed for this procedure.

    a. Butterfly catheter: _____

_____

    b. Three-way stopcock: _____

_____

    c. 20-mL syringe: _____

_____

The thoracocentesis site has been aseptically prepared.

6. Based on the doctor's assessment, describe where you insert the needle to perform the thoracocentesis.

_____

_____

The thoracocentesis was successful, with 70 mL of fluid drained from the left side and 130 mL drained from the right side. The fluid sample is packaged and awaiting courier pickup from the lab.

_____

Louie's breathing has returned to normal, and his mucous membranes are returning to a healthy pink color. He appears to be comfortable in his oxygen cage. However, even though he appears stable at the moment, you know his status can change quickly if he develops any complications following the procedure or if the fluid builds back up in the pleural space.

7. What should you monitor in your patient to assess his respiratory function?

_____

_____

_____

Now that Louie is stable, the doctor orders a complete blood count, chemistry panel, serum thyroid level, and urinalysis. You know that minimizing stress during restraint is important for Louie since he has respiratory compromise.

8. With this in mind, describe which venipuncture approach you will choose and why.

_____

_____

_____

The pleural fluid analysis reveals that Louie's pleural effusion is pus. He has pyothorax (pus in the thoracic cavity). Louie is being admitted to the hospital to have bilateral chest tubes placed to drain the pus from his chest. He will be given intravenous analgesics, antibiotics, and fluids.

_____

It is the next morning, and you are giving Louie his morning treatments. You notice the bandage around his IV catheter is soaking wet.

9. What problems may have occurred with his IV catheter to cause his bandage to become wet?

_____

_____

_____

As you are changing Louie's bandage to inspect the catheter and catheter site, you also assess the area for phlebitis.

10. Define phlebitis.

_____

11. What are the signs of phlebitis?

_____

_____

_____

You discover and fix the cause of Louie's catheter malfunction, confirm he does not have phlebitis, and rebandage his catheter.

_____

After 7 days of intensive nursing care, Louie is finally ready to go home! Louie has been prescribed two oral antibiotic pills he will need to take for the next 2 weeks.

12. Explain to Mrs. Hansen how to administer an oral tablet to Louie using common language.

_____

_____

_____

_____

_____

Mrs. Hansen looks horrified as she listens to you and watches you demonstrate administering a tablet to Louie. When you finish, she asks, "Wouldn't it be easier to just put the pill in some food and feed it to him? That is the way we gave antibiotic pills to our dog, Chester, last year when he had that skin infection, remember? That was so easy!"

13. What is your reply to Mrs. Hansen's question?

_____

_____

_____

_____

18 Small Animal Medical Nursing

LEARNING OBJECTIVES

When you have completed this chapter, you will be able to:
1. Pronounce, define, and spell all key terms in this chapter.
2. Explain the relationship between the "Five Freedoms of Animal Welfare" and the veterinary technician's responsibilities.
3. List in order the four steps that constitute the veterinary technician practice model and describe what is involved in carrying out each step of the nursing process.
   - List the four steps of SBAR and explain the importance of a clear and concise communication method and how it supports patient care.
4. Explain the relationship between etiology, pathogenesis, and clinical signs; list and describe the most common forms seen in cats and dogs regarding:
   - Respiratory diseases. Explain the clinical relevance of upper versus lower disease and the role of inflammation in clinical signs.
   - Cardiovascular diseases. Explain the significance of determining if a patient has situational, idiopathic, or secondary hypertension.
   - Gastrointestinal and hepatobiliary diseases. Define vomiting versus regurgitation and list the clinical signs associated with small versus large bowel diarrhea.
   - Urinary diseases. Explain the differences between acute kidney injury (AKI) and chronic kidney disease (CKD); and the importance of IRIS staging/grading in patient care.
   - Endocrine disease. Explain the importance of client education and support for successful long-term disease management.
   - Immune-mediated disease. Explain the importance of client education and support for successful long-term disease management.
5. Do the following regarding infectious diseases in dogs and cats:
   - Discuss the etiology and pathogenesis of infectious diseases.
   - List and describe special protocols needed to provide nursing care for dogs and cats with infectious diseases.
   - Explain how to educate clients about stopping the spread of infectious diseases.

EXERCISE 18.1 FILL-IN-THE-BLANK #1: TERMS AND DEFINITIONS

Instructions: Fill in each of the spaces provided with the missing word or words that complete the sentence.

1. The term for a large, dilated esophagus is _____.

2. _____ is inflammation of the stomach mucosa often caused by ingestion of spoiled food, toxic plants, or foreign objects.

3. Corneal _____ are a clinical sign of feline herpes virus.

4. Medical management of _____ symptoms includes limited fasting, fluid therapy, dietary therapy, probiotic therapy, antiemetics, and antacids, among other measures.

5. The weight loss, loss of muscle mass, and general debilitation that may accompany chronic disease is called _____.

6. _____ is the study of the causation or origination of disease.

7. Inflammation of the intestinal mucosa often caused by infectious agents (viral, bacterial, parasitic), dietary changes, or indiscretions, is known as _____.

8. A cough may be _____, meaning that mucus, fluid, or blood is brought up from the airway (and usually swallowed).

9. _____ is characterized by increased thickness of the left ventricle wall and a small ventricular lumen, and is the most common form of feline cardiomyopathy.

10. _____ is defined as deficient oxygenation of tissues.

11. _____ is excessive production of urine.

12. _____ is inflammation of the esophagus.

13. _____ is the passive expulsion of material from the mouth, pharynx, or esophagus. Nausea and abdominal contractions are not typically seen.

14. The first step in the Veterinary Technician Practice Model is _____.

15. _____ is the term for inflammation of the tissue under the lid margins and surrounding the visible globe.

16. Diagnostic imaging for respiratory diseases includes _____, _____, computed tomography (CT), and magnetic resonance imaging (MRI).

17. Clinical signs of diabetes in dogs include excessive thirst or _____, along with polyuria, weight loss, increased appetite, and cataracts.

18. Rabies is an example of a(n) _____, an infectious disease that is transmitted directly from animals to humans.

EXERCISE 18.2 DEFINITIONS: KEY TERMS

Instructions: Define each term in your own words.

1. Pathogenesis: _____

_____

2. Nasal and sinus congestion: _____

_____

3. Stertor: _____

_____

4. Stridor: _____

_____

5. Cough: _____

_____

6. Hemoptysis: _____

_____

7. Pleural effusion: _____

_____

8. Dyspnea: _____

_____

9. Orthopnea: _____

_____

10. Hypoxemia: _____

_____

11. Cardiomyopathy: _____

_____

12. Systemic hypertension: _____

_____

13. Azotemia: _____

_____

14. Vomiting: _____

_____

15. Hematemesis: _____

_____

16. Hematochezia: _____

_____

17. Melena: _____

_____

18. Tenesmus: _____

_____

19. Hyperthermia: _____

_____

20. Barrier nursing: _____

_____

21. Hepatic encephalopathy: _____

_____

22. Diarrhea: _____

_____

23. Constipation: _____

_____

24. Colitis: _____

_____

EXERCISE 18.3 MATCHING #1: TERMS AND DEFINITIONS

Instructions: Match each term in column A with the corresponding definition in column B by writing the appropriate letter in the space provided.

Column A

1. _____ Diarrhea
2. _____ Hepatitis
3. _____ Nausea
4. _____ Secondary immune-mediated hemolytic anemia (IMHA)
5. _____ Serous
6. _____ *Escherichia coli*
7. _____ Hypoxia
8. _____ Constipation
9. _____ Mucopurulent
10. _____ Mucoid
11. _____ Hemorrhagic
12. _____ Portosystemic shunts
13. _____ Feline lower urinary tract disease
14. _____ Primary immune-mediated hemolytic anemia

Column B

A. Clear liquid discharge

B. Opaque and sticky nasal discharge

C. Green-yellow and mucoid nasal discharge

D. Bloody discharge

E. A sign that often precedes vomiting; characterized by anxiety, hypersalivation, vocalization, and lip smacking

F. A symptom characterized by frequent passage of loose, unformed, and often watery stool

G. A condition characterized by infrequent and often difficult passage of hard stool

H. Inadequate oxygenation

I. Inflammation of the liver parenchyma

J. Extrahepatic or intrahepatic vascular abnormalities that connect the systemic and portal circulations

K. The most common cause of bacterial cystitis in small animals

L. The term used to describe the constellation of signs indicating bladder and urethra irritation in the cat

M. A type of IMHA in which the immune system develops autoantibodies against components of the red blood cell membrane

N. A type of IMHA in which an underlying cause for the massive immune response is identified and can be often treated

EXERCISE 18.4 MATCHING #2: DISEASES AND CONDITIONS

Instructions: Match each disease or condition in column A with its corresponding description in column B by writing the appropriate letter in the space provided.

Column A

1. _____ Heartworm disease

2. _____ Hypoadrenocorticism

3. _____ Hyperthyroidism

4. _____ Hepatic lipidosis

5. _____ Myasthenia gravis

6. _____ Hemolytic anemia

7. _____ Hepatic encephalopathy

8. _____ Hyperadrenocorticism

9. _____ Kidney disease

10. _____ Diabetes mellitus

11. _____ Immune-mediated disease

12. _____ Acute cholangitis

Column B

A. Mosquito-borne infectious disease affecting dogs and cats

B. The disease of cats caused by a derangement of lipid metabolism associated with prolonged anorexia

C. The acute disease of the bile ducts caused by an ascending bacterial infection from the small intestines and characterized by neutrophilic inflammation

D. A disease characterized by irreversible, progressive loss of renal function

E. A disease that affects cats in which the thyroid gland is overactive, producing abnormally large amounts of thyroid hormones

F. A disease caused by either insufficient production of insulin by the pancreatic beta cells or by insulin resistance characterized by the body's inability to respond properly to endogenous insulin

G. A disease that primarily affects dogs and is characterized by elevated circulating levels of cortisol produced by the adrenal cortex

H. A disease caused by adrenal gland atrophy or destruction resulting in inadequate secretion of glucocorticoids and mineralocorticoids

I. A disease in which the immune system has lost tolerance of self and damages organs

J. A disease characterized by RBC destruction

K. A disorder of neuromuscular transmission that causes muscle weakness

L. A condition resulting from exposure of the brain to GI toxins

EXERCISE 18.5 TRUE OR FALSE: COMPREHENSIVE

Instructions: Read the following statements and write "T" for true or "F" for false in the blanks provided. If a statement is false, correct the statement to make it true.

1. _____ Etiology is defined as the cause of a disease.

2. _____ Anorexia is loss of appetite or absence of food, especially when prolonged.

3. _____ Hypovolemia is an increase of intravascular fluid.

4. _____ Regurgitation is the forceful expulsion of contents from the stomach and/or intestines.

5. _____ The use of anti-inflammatory drugs in the treatment of lower respiratory disease specifically targets the airways.

6. _____ In dogs, sneezing is most commonly associated with upper respiratory viral infections, whereas sneezing in cats is usually the result of inhalation of foreign material.

7. _____ Cats do not normally pant, so the presence of open-mouth breathing with noticeable chest movements indicates dyspnea.

8. _____ Coughing is a common sign of CHF in cats.

9. _____ Treatment of feline heartworm disease is unrewarding because a safe and effective adulticide protocol has yet to be found.

10. _____ In dogs, exocrine pancreatic insufficiency is commonly caused by chronic pancreatitis.

11. _____ A urolith is a pathologic stone formed from mineral salts in the urinary tract.

12. _____ In resistant or recurrent UTI cases, a 2-week course of antibiotics is needed.

13. _____ Hypothyroidism primarily affects dogs, although a rare congenital form can be seen in kittens.

14. _____ Dogs tend to develop type-2 diabetes mellitus, whereas cats are more prone to type-1 diabetes mellitus.

15. _____ Diabetes mellitus will often progress to a condition called diabetic ketoacidosis despite diagnosis and treatment.

16. _____ Immune-mediated diseases are those in which the immune system has failed to protect the patient from invasion by microorganisms.

17. _____ Acquired myasthenia gravis is more common in cats than it is in dogs.

18. _____ Vaccination, maintenance of proper health, and proper nutrition strengthen host defense systems.

19. _____ Unduly stressing a patient with dyspnea can cause respiratory arrest.

20. _____ One of the first signs that heart disease has progressed to heart failure is tachycardia.

21. _____ Systemic hypertension is often secondary to another disease, such as chronic kidney disease.

EXERCISE 18.6 MULTIPLE CHOICE: COMPREHENSIVE

Instructions: Circle the one correct answer to each of the following questions.

1. The Five Freedoms of Animal Welfare include all of the following except
   a. Freedom from Captivity
   b. Freedom from Fear and Distress.
   c. Freedom from Discomfort.
   d. Freedom to Express Normal Behavior.

2. A disease of the heart muscle seen in cats that is characterized by an increase in the thickness of the left ventricle wall and a small ventricular lumen is classified as
   a. dilated.
   b. hypertrophic.
   c. arrhythmogenic.
   d. restrictive.

3. Diagnosing heart disease relies partly on diagnostic procedures, including all of the following except
   a. diagnostic ultrasonography.
   b. radiographs.
   c. endoscopy.
   d. electrocardiography.

4. Dilated cardiomyopathy is the most common canine cardiomyopathy. It is characterized primarily by
   a. extreme atrial and ventricular dilatation with decreased contractility.
   b. thromboembolism with increased contractility.
   c. increased contractility and ventricular arrhythmias.
   d. atrial enlargement with normal ventricular function.

5. Treatment of canine heartworm disease may include any of the following except
   a. adulticide therapy.
   b. microfilaracide therapy 3 to 4 weeks later.
   c. surgical removal of worms.
   d. a gradual increase in activity over 3 to 4 weeks.

6. Which is not an intervention for patients suffering from regurgitation?
   a. Elevating food and water bowls
   b. Keeping the patient's head and forelimbs elevated for 10 minutes postmeal
   c. Changing the form of food and monitoring for signs of aspiration
   d. The use of antiemetics

7. The premature activation of trypsin in the pancreas is associated with what condition?
   a. Tenesmus
   b. Exocrine pancreatic insufficiency
   c. Pancreatitis
   d. Hepatic lipidosis

8. Clinical signs associated with feline pancreatitis typically include
   a. vomiting, weight gain, hyperthermia, lethargy, and hypotension.
   b. hypothermia, diarrhea, anorexia, vomiting, and hypotension.
   c. vomiting, diarrhea, regurgitation, and hypothermia.
   d. vomiting, lethargy, weight loss, anorexia, and hypothermia.

9. Management of acute hepatic encephalopathy includes all of the following except
   a. fluid therapy.
   b. correcting electrolyte imbalances.
   c. analgesia.
   d. treatment of seizures.

10. Chronic hepatitis indicates a history of liver disease for a prolonged period of time, usually greater than
    a. 2 to 3 weeks.
    b. 6 to 8 weeks.
    c. 2 to 3 months.
    d. 4 to 6 months.

11. Cholangitis refers to
    a. inflammation of the bile ducts.
    b. inflammation of the liver.
    c. inflammation of the pancreas.
    d. inflammation of the gallbladder.

12. Medical management of chronic kidney disease focuses on all of the following except
    a. slowing the progression.
    b. treating concurrent diseases.
    c. partial removal of kidneys.
    d. correcting electrolyte imbalances.

13. UTI is a common secondary complication in all of the following except
    a. diabetes mellitus.
    b. chronic kidney disease.
    c. hyperadrenocorticism.
    d. hypothyroidism.

14. Feline lower urinary tract disease is typically classified as
    a. nonhemorrhagic or hemorrhagic.
    b. nonobstructive or obstructive.
    c. noninvasive or invasive.
    d. nonpainful or painful.

15. Clinical signs of hyperthyroidism include
    a. increased activity.
    b. weight gain.
    c. decreased appetite.
    d. decreased urine output.

16. Treatment of feline hyperthyroidism falls into two categories:
    a. curative and palliative.
    b. symptomatic and supportive.
    c. acute and chronic.
    d. primary and secondary.

17. The treatment of diabetes mellitus is different for dogs and cats. Dogs require lifelong treatment that includes the administration of insulin, glucose-monitoring, and a high-fiber diet. In contrast, a high-protein/lower-fat diet is recommended for cats. In addition, which of the following is true of cats?
    a. Aggressive treatment with insulin is often associated with spontaneous remission within 3 to 4 months.
    b. Cats require lifelong treatment with insulin and lifelong daily glucose monitoring.
    c. Blood glucose is monitored and insulin therapy is incorporated as needed.
    d. Most cats respond well long term to the administration of oral hypoglycemics.

18. Hyperadrenocorticism or Cushing syndrome can be caused by
    a. a functional adrenal gland tumor.
    b. a functional anterior pituitary tumor.
    c. immune damage of the adrenal gland.
    d. Either A or B
    e. Either B or C

19. Feline Cushing syndrome is rare and, when diagnosed, is often seen concurrently with
    a. mastitis.
    b. osteosarcoma.
    c. pancreatitis.
    d. diabetes mellitus.

20. Which of the following is not typically a sign of hypoadrenocorticism (Addison disease)?
    a. Diarrhea
    b. Vomiting
    c. Polydipsia
    d. Hyperactivity

21. Secondary immune-mediated disease can result from
    a. infection.
    b. interaction with other immune-altered animals.
    c. interaction with immune-altered humans.
    d. stress.

22. If a patient with myasthenia gravis has megaesophagus, common presenting signs are
    a. dry mouth and vomiting.
    b. vomiting and diarrhea.
    c. diarrhea and hypersalivation.
    d. hypersalivation and regurgitation.

23. Which of the following is contagious directly between animals or indirectly through fomites?
    a. Canine heartworm disease
    b. Borrelia burgdorferi
    c. Feline calicivirus
    d. Rocky Mountain spotted fever

24. The correct order for the tasks involved in the Veterinary Technician Practice Model is
    a. Evaluation, Planning, Assessment, Implementation.
    b. Assessment, Planning, Implementation, Evaluation.
    c. Evaluation, Planning, Implementation, Assessment.
    d. Planning, Evaluation, Assessment, Implementation.

25. The obstructive form of feline lower urinary tract disease is a(n)
    a. endocrine disorder.
    b. common, easily diagnosed condition.
    c. medical emergency.
    d. disorder found primarily in female cats.

26. In lung auscultation, "crackles" are associated with
    a. bronchial and pleural disease.
    b. pleural and pulmonary disease.
    c. pulmonary disease and effusion.
    d. effusion and bronchial disease.

27. An increased PCV and TP indicates
    a. dehydration.
    b. hypovolemia caused by blood loss.
    c. hypothermia.
    d. cardiac insufficiency.

28. Which of the following is *not* associated with restoration of normovolemia?
    a. Pink/dry mucous membranes
    b. Normal CRT
    c. Normal cardiac function
    d. Normal blood pressure

29. A temperature less than 99° F, shivering, prolonged CRT, bradycardia, cyanosis, and decreased respirations are symptoms of
    a. pain.
    b. hypothermia.
    c. electrolyte imbalance.
    d. cardiac insufficiency.

30. Symptoms of cardiac insufficiency include all of the following except
    a. hyperactivity.
    b. tachycardia.
    c. prolonged CRT.
    d. tachypnea.

31. A body condition score of 4 or higher out of 5 indicates
    a. overweight.
    b. overhydration.
    c. neurologic depression.
    d. decreased muscle mass.

32. Malnutrition leads to all of the following except
    a. multisystemic organ dysfunction.
    b. electrolyte imbalance.
    c. dehydration.
    d. pancreatitis.

33. Loss of gag and swallow reflexes commonly occur in all of the following except
    a. sedation or anesthesia.
    b. megaesophagus.
    c. damage to cranial nerves.
    d. hyperadrenocorticism.

34. Clinical signs of feline bronchitis include all of the following except
    a. cough.
    b. stridor.
    c. wheezing.
    d. dyspnea.

EXERCISE 18.7 FILL-IN-THE-BLANK #2: COMPREHENSIVE

Instructions: Fill in each of the spaces provided with the missing word or words that complete the sentence.

1. Nasal discharge results from irritation or inflammation of the nasal mucosa and can be described as _____ (green-yellow and mucoid), _____ (bloody), _____ (clear liquid), or _____ (opaque and sticky).

2. A patient with nasal discharge, sneezing, and/or congestion should be closely examined for facial _____ that can accompany some causative diseases such as fungal infections, tooth root abscess, and neoplasms.

3. A cough may be _____, meaning fluid, mucus, or blood is brought up from the airway.

4. A _____ cough is sometimes referred to as a "dry cough."

5. The presence of pleural effusion can be confirmed via _____, ultrasonography, or radiography.

6. In an extreme situation, stressing a dyspneic patient can result in _____.

7. Heart disease can be caused by a pathologic abnormality affecting the _____, _____, rhythm conduction, or the overall structure of the heart.

8. The first respiratory sign that heart disease has progressed to heart failure is often _____.

9. Degenerative atrioventricular valve disease affects the cardiac valve _____ or _____ and is characterized by thickening of the tissue.

10. Patients with high heartworm burdens and severe cardiopulmonary disease are at high risk for pulmonary _____ and must be stabilized prior to the administration of adulticide for heartworm treatment.

11. For both dogs and cats, the key to avoiding heartworm disease is to _____ infection. This is achieved through the use of approved _____ class preventatives.

12. Once high blood pressure is diagnosed, treatment with _____ medication is begun immediately.

13. Systemic hypertension is often secondary to another disease such as chronic _____ disease, _____, _____, or diabetes mellitus.

14. Difficulty eating is also referred to as _____.

15. _____ material typically consists of undigested or partially digested food.

16. Vomiting patients are prone to _____ and _____ imbalances, so monitoring for and treating these secondary problems is of importance when providing complete patient care.

17. Hematochezia usually indicates a problem with the _____ or _____.

18. Tenesmus of GI origin is usually the result of _____ disease and often accompanies diarrhea or constipation.

19. Pancreatitis occurs when the digestive enzyme _____ is prematurely activated within the _____ tissue instead of within the duodenum.

20. Pancreatitis may be chronic or acute in nature. The frequency of each type varies among species. Chronic cases are seen more commonly in _____, whereas acute cases are seen more commonly in _____.

21. Chronic pancreatitis can lead to _____ or _____.

22. _____ is caused by insufficient production and secretion of digestive enzymes by the pancreas.

23. In dogs, EPI is most commonly the result of pancreatic acinar _____.

24. The loss of digestive enzymes leads to maldigestion and malabsorption of ingested nutrients causing clinical signs of polyphagia, _____, and chronic pale, fatty, and voluminous diarrhea.

25. Patients with severe hepatobiliary disease may develop _____ as a result of exposure of the brain to GI toxins.

26. Symptomatic treatment of HE focuses on decreasing the amount of _____ in the systemic circulation, which can be achieved by decreasing production within the _____.

27. Feline hepatic lipidosis is caused by a derangement of lipid _____ associated with _____.

28. _____ portosystemic shunts are congenital and typically involve one or two vessels that connect the portal vein to the vena cava.

29. _____ portosystemic shunts can be congenital or acquired secondary to portal hypertension and are multiple shunts within the hepatic parenchyma.

30. Chronic feline cholangitis is characterized by _____ inflammation. The cause of this condition is _____.

EXERCISE 18.8 CASE STUDY #1: DISEASES AFFECTING THE THYROID GLAND

Signalment: Petunia, a 10-year-old, spayed female domestic long hair cat
Chief complaint: The owner reports that Petunia has been losing weight gradually over the past several months.
Minimum database: Petunia's appetite is good, but she is acting more lethargic lately. The physical examination confirms weight loss (body weight of 5.7 pounds and a body condition score of 2/5), an elevated heart rate, an unkempt hair coat, and a palpable thyroid nodule. Blood testing revealed an elevated serum T_4 level, along with a number of other changes in chemistry values. The attending veterinarian diagnosed hyperthyroidism.

1. Briefly describe hyperthyroidism. Specifically explain the causes of this condition, how it is diagnosed, common clinical signs, and treatment options.

   a. Brief description of hyperthyroidism: _____

   _____

   _____

   b. Causes: _____

   _____

   c. Diagnosis: _____

   _____

   _____

   d. Clinical signs: _____

   _____

   e. Treatment options: _____

   _____

   _____

   _____

2. Unlike cats, which much more frequently develop hyperthyroidism, dogs much more frequently develop hypothyroidism.

These diseases differ greatly and are in many ways opposites. Explain the causes of hypothyroidism, how it is diagnosed, common clinical signs, and treatment options.

a. Brief description of hypothyroidism:_____

_____

_____

b. Causes: _____

c. Diagnosis: _____

_____

_____

d. Clinical signs: _____

_____

e. Treatment options: _____

_____

_____

_____

3. Finally, explain the key differences between these diseases of the thyroid gland.

_____

_____

_____

_____

_____

_____

_____

_____

Signalment: Molly, a 10-year-old, spayed female terrier mix-breed dog

Chief complaint: The owner reports that Molly has been coughing lately, doesn't have much energy, and tires quickly after going on walks.

Database: After gathering a complete history and performing a physical examination, the doctor orders a complete workup to evaluate Molly's heart, including blood work and thoracic radiographs. He is concerned about valvular heart disease but wants more data before a treatment plan is developed. Consider the following facts gleaned from Molly's patient database.

Physical findings:

- Tachycardia and tachypnea
- Open-mouth breathing, increased respiratory effort, and slight cyanosis
- Grade V/VI systolic heart murmur
- Increased lung sounds (crackles)

Diagnostic workup:

- Radiographs reveal left-sided heart enlargement and evidence of fluid in the lungs (pulmonary edema).
- Blood work results are unremarkable.

The doctor believes Molly may have degenerative A-V valve disease and secondary congestive heart failure. In animals with this condition, the heart valves degenerate and thicken, allowing blood to flow backwards from the ventricles into the atria. This causes a backup of blood in the heart and subsequent development of fluid in the lungs, as well as a decrease in forward flow. The cause of this disease is unknown, although there may be a genetic predisposition, as dogs of certain breeds are especially prone to this condition.

1. Any disease, including this one, can be defined by its etiology, pathogenesis, associated lesions, and clinical signs.

   a. Define each of these terms.

      i. Etiology:_____

      _____

      ii Pathogenesis:_____

      _____

      iii. Lesion:_____

      _____

      iv. Clinical signs:_____

      _____

   b. What is the relationship between each of these elements? _____

   _____

   _____

   _____

   c. What are Molly's main clinical signs? _____

   _____

   _____

   _____

2. Use of the veterinary technician practice model in this case will ensure that Molly is provided with consistently excellent care. The first step is to help gather patient data, which you have already done.

   a. What would be the next steps? _____

_____

_____

   b. List two technician evaluations shown in Table 18.4 that would apply to Molly. What evidence do you have that each of these evaluations applies?

      i. _____

_____

      ii. _____

_____

_____

_____

   c. What technician interventions would be indicated to help Molly? _____

_____

_____

_____

_____

_____

   d. How will you know that Molly is responding to your interventions? _____

_____

_____

_____

_____

_____

19 Large Animal Medical Nursing

LEARNING OBJECTIVES

When you have completed this chapter, you will be able to:

1. Pronounce, define, and spell all key terms in the chapter.
2. Explain the importance of a thorough physical examination and medical record for large animal patients.
3. List and describe the most common diseases and conditions of the horse for the gastrointestinal, musculoskeletal, respiratory, hemolymphatic, cardiovascular, neurologic, ophthalmologic, dermatologic, endocrine, and urinary systems, including the causes and pathogenesis of each.
4. Discuss the care of the hospitalized equine patient, including biosecurity, patient monitoring, supportive care, and laboratory diagnostics.
5. List and describe the most common diseases and conditions of ruminants for the digestive, respiratory, reproductive/ mammary gland, metabolic, hemolymphatic, cardiovascular, nervous, ophthalmologic, musculoskeletal, dermatologic, and urinary systems, including special care and conditions of the neonate.
6. List and describe the most common diseases and conditions of swine for the gastrointestinal, respiratory, reproductive, nervous, and musculoskeletal systems, including abnormal behaviors.
7. List and describe the common diseases and conditions of camelids, including special care and conditions of the neonate.

Across

2 Adjective describing a pathologic condition in which the body forms few or no antibodies
7 A bacterial toxin that has been weakened by heat or chemical treatment
8 Lower-than-normal levels of blood glucose
9 Condition characterized by altered function of the central nervous system in which brain swelling and inflammation lead to necrosis of brain tissue
10 A common reproductive condition in goats that may develop in does with or without exposure to a buck
11 An antibody that neutralizes a specific biologic toxin. The antibody is produced in response to a particular toxin such as tetanus
12 First milk containing antibodies
14 Slow or difficult labor or delivery of a newborn
15 Necrosis of a large area of a mammary gland or glands secondary to infection (2 words)
16 Invasion of the bloodstream by microorganism (usually bacteria) from a focus of infection
17 Inflammation of muscle
18 A condition that is characterized by the formation or presence of calculi in the urinary tract

Down

1 Deficient levels of antibodies absorbed by the gut in animals dependent upon colostrum for immunologic protection (4 words)
3 A neurologic deficit in which the animal loses awareness of body position and movement in space (2 words)
4 A cancer of lymphocytes and lymphoid tissues that is the third most common cancer diagnosed in dogs
5 Condition that occurs in ewes during the last few weeks of pregnancy when there is a sudden demand for energy by fast-growing fetuses (2 words)
6 Abnormal position of the eyes
13 Inflammation of the mammary gland

EXERCISE 19.2 MATCHING #1: TERMS AND DEFINITIONS

Instructions: Match each term in column A with its corresponding definition in column B by writing the appropriate letter in the space provided.

Column A

1. _____ Endotoxemia
2. _____ Epistaxis
3. _____ Keratoconjunctivitis
4. _____ Ketosis
5. _____ Pericarditis
6. _____ Persistent infection
7. _____ Hepatic lipidosis
8. _____ Serous
9. _____ Stranguria

Column B

A. Inflammation of the pericardial membrane surrounding the heart

B. Bleeding from the nose

C. Straining to urinate

D. Condition in high-producing dairy cows caused by the buildup in the blood of products of fat breakdown

E. Chronic infection that does not resolve despite the use of antimicrobials

F. Of, relating to, producing, or resembling serum

G. A group of clinical signs caused by bacteria-associated toxins circulating through the bloodstream

H. Fatty liver disease

I. Combined inflammation of the cornea and conjunctiva

EXERCISE 19.3 MATCHING #2: DISEASES OF RUMINANTS

Instructions: Match each disease or causative organism of disease in column A with the primary body system that it affects in column B by writing the appropriate letter in the space provided. (Note that responses may be used more than once.)

Column A

1. _____ Grain overload
2. _____ Nervous ketosis
3. _____ BVD
4. _____ Listeriosis
5. _____ Infectious bovine rhinotracheitis
6. _____ Traumatic reticuloperitonitis
7. _____ *Pasteurella multocida*
8. _____ Caprine arthritis encephalitis
9. _____ *Mycoplasma bovis*
10. _____ Salmonellosis
11. _____ Rabies
12. _____ Coronavirus

Column B

A. Central nervous system

B. Respiratory system

C. Gastrointestinal system

EXERCISE 19.4 MATCHING #3: DISEASES OF PIGS

Instructions: Match each description in column A with its corresponding disease of pigs in column B by writing the appropriate letter in the space provided. (Note that responses may be used more than once, and some responses may not be used.)

Column A

1. _____ Infection causes a high fever and may produce characteristic diamond skin lesions

2. _____ Infection in baby pigs results in the development of neurologic signs and, in some cases, vomiting and diarrhea

3. _____ Infection results in pneumonia

4. _____ Weaning and growing pigs exhibit fever; pneumonia; a dry, nonproductive cough; and flu-like signs

5. _____ Respiratory signs include labored breathing, increased secondary respiratory infections, increased postweaning mortality, and decreased rate of gain and feed efficiency

6. _____ Infection in adults may cause reproductive problems, including early embryonic death, abortion, or stillbirths, in pregnant sows or gilts

7. _____ Reproductive signs include abortion, stillbirths, fetal mummies, and the birth of weak piglets

Column B

A. Rhinotracheitis

B. Pseudorabies

C. Erysipelas

D. Rabies

E. Porcine reproductive and respiratory syndrome

EXERCISE 19.5 MATCHING #4: BODY CONDITION SCORE (BCS) FOR SHEEP

Instructions: Match each description in column A with its corresponding body condition score for sheep in column B by writing the appropriate number in the space provided.

Column A

A. _____ Slight bulging (convexity) between the dorsal and transverse spinous processes

B. _____ Mild concavity between the dorsal and transverse spinous processes

C. _____ Absence of lumbar musculature and subcutaneous fat, leaving a profound depression between the tips of the dorsal and transverse spinous processes

D. _____ No depression (straight line) between the dorsal and transverse spinous processes

E. _____ Moderate concavity between the dorsal and transverse spinous processes

F. _____ Profound convexity between the dorsal and transverse spinous processes (cannot palpate spinous processes)

Column B

0

1

2

3

4

5

Instructions: Read the following statements and write "T" for true or "F" for false in the blanks provided. If a statement is false, correct the statement to make it true.

1. _____ Llamas and alpacas are herd animals and, therefore, need to live with at least one other llama or alpaca.

2. _____ Strangles is characterized by the development of one or more abscess.

3. _____ A life-threatening side effect of guttural pouch infections can be the growth of plaque over the internal carotid artery.

4. _____ Heaves is one of the more commonly encountered GI diseases in horses.

5. _____ Second-degree atrioventricular (AV) block is an arrhythmia in horses that is a medical emergency.

6. _____ Horses are predisposed to atrial fibrillation because of the small atria and high vagal tone.

7. _____ Equine contagious arteritis is a bacterial disease that produces limb swelling, conjunctivitis, abortion, and respiratory disease in horses.

8. _____ Choke is an indication of a tracheal obstruction.

9. _____ Eastern, Western, and West Nile equine encephalitis vaccines are highly effective, and vaccinated horses rarely get sick.

10. _____ Equine patients with Wobbler syndrome are more likely to be female than male.

11. _____ Horses with equine herpes virus must be isolated to stop the spread of the disease.

12. _____ Addison disease in the horse is a common cause of polyuria and polydipsia.

13. _____ IV catheters in hospitalized horses should be flushed with heparinized saline flush every 12 hours and monitored for heat, swelling, and pain.

14. _____ Bovine respiratory disease syndrome (BRDS) is caused by a single organism, *Pasteurella multocida*.

15. _____ BRDS in feedlot cattle is often referred to as shipping fever.

16. _____ Milk fever predominantly occurs in first-calf heifers.

17. _____ Pregnancy toxemia in ewes occurs in late gestation.

18. _____ Goats are more prone to copper toxicity than sheep.

19. _____ Small ruminants are susceptible to tetanus and should receive toxoid/antitoxin prior to surgery.

20. _____ Most cases of lameness in ruminants occur in the foot as opposed to the upper limb.

21. _____ Orf is treated with antibiotics, as it is caused by a bacterium.

22. _____ Neonatal pigs easily become hyperthermic, and care must be taken to keep them cool and comfortable.

Instructions: Circle the one correct answer to each of the following questions.

1. Normal temperature for the adult horse is
   a. 89° F to 91.5° F.
   b. 96° F to 101.5° F.
   c. 99° F to 101.5° F.
   d. 100° F to 103.5° F.

2. A normal pulse in the adult horse is
   a. 18 to 34 bpm.
   b. 28 to 44 bpm.
   c. 38 to 54 bpm.
   d. 48 to 64 bpm.

3. Normal respiration for the adult horse is
   a. 4 to 8 breaths/min.
   b. 8 to 20 breaths/min.
   c. 16 to 26 breaths/min.
   d. 34 to 48 breaths/min.

4. Strangles is caused by the bacterial pathogen
   a. *Neorickettsia risticii*.
   b. *Clostridium perfringens*.
   c. *Salmonellosis equi*.
   d. *Streptococcus equi*.

5. The most common cause of a fungal infection of the guttural pouches is
   a. *Aspergillus* spp.
   b. *Salmonellosis* spp.
   c. *Streptococcus* spp.
   d. *Neorickettsia* spp.

6. Which is not a condition associated with camelids?
   a. Heat stress
   b. Hepatic lipidosis
   c. Meningeal worm infestation
   d. Strangles

7. PPID is the most common disease condition in horses that are
   a. older than 2 years of age.
   b. older than 5 years of age.
   c. older than 10 years of age.
   d. older than 15 years of age.

8. Potomac horse fever is caused by
   a. *Salmonella* spp.
   b. *Neorickettsia risticii*.
   c. *Clostridium perfringens*.
   d. larval cyathostomiasis.

9. The secondary hosts of the causative agent of equine protozoal myelitis (EPM) are
   a. raccoons.
   b. opossums.
   c. birds.
   d. mice.

10. Which ophthalmic disease is the most common cause of blindness in horses?
    a. Corneal ulceration
    b. Recurrent uveitis
    c. Entropion
    d. Glaucoma

11. Monitoring of the equine patient with an infectious disease should occur
    a. every 1 to 2 hours.
    b. every 3 to 4 hours.
    c. every 4 to 6 hours.
    d. every 8 to 12 hours.

12. Equine patients unable to defecate because of recumbency should have the feces manually removed
    a. once per day.
    b. twice per day.
    c. three times per day.
    d. only when the patient is uncomfortable.

13. The recumbent equine patient should be repositioned every
    a. 2 hours.
    b. 4 hours.
    c. 6 hours.
    d. 8 hours.

14. What is not a typical cause of reproductive failure or abortion in swine?
    a. PRV infection
    b. Fibroblastic sarcoids
    c. Brucellosis
    d. Leptospirosis

15. The normal range for the PCV in the equine patient is
    a. 12% to 17%.
    b. 19% to 32%.
    c. 32% to 45%.
    d. 45% to 57%.

16. Endotoxins can cause margination and sequestration of the
    a. white blood cells.
    b. red blood cells.
    c. platelets.
    d. plasma.

17. The equine patient has a yellow tint to the blood serum because
    a. it doesn't have a gallbladder.
    b. of the large cecum.
    c. of the large muscle mass.
    d. the liver is small in comparison to the patient's size.

18. What chemistry test is an indicator of muscle damage?
    a. Phosphate
    b. Blood urea nitrogen
    c. Albumin
    d. Creatine phosphokinase

19. Normal equine urine pH is
    a. 2 to 4.
    b. 5 to 7.
    c. 7 to 9.
    d. 9 to 10.

20. Small ruminants should be vaccinated for enterotoxemia
    a. every 2 months.
    b. every 4 months.
    c. every 6 months.
    d. once a year.

21. The normal pH of the rumen is
    a. 6.0 to 6.4.
    b. 6.5 to 6.8.
    c. 7.2 to 7.8.
    d. 7.5 to 8.8.

22. Which disease affects both cattle and small ruminants?
    a. Johne's
    b. BVD
    c. Nervous ketosis
    d. BRDS

23. In the ruminant foot, which claws bear the most weight?
    a. Front lateral and hind lateral claws
    b. Front medial and hind lateral claws
    c. Front medial and hind medial claws
    d. Front lateral and hind medial claws

24. PPV causes death and mummification of the fetus
    a. at less than 30 days of gestation.
    b. between 30 and 70 days of gestation.
    c. after 70 days of gestation.
    d. at any stage of gestation.

25. PPV causes death and resorption of the fetus
    a. at less than 30 days of gestation.
    b. between 30 and 70 days of gestation.
    c. after 70 days of gestation.
    d. at any stage of gestation.

26. Which animals listed below are classified as Old World camelids? (*Choose all that apply.*)
    a. Guanaco
    b. Bactrian camels
    c. Vicuña
    d. Dromedary camels
    e. Llama
    f. Alpaca

27. Which animals listed below are classified as New World camelids? (*Choose all that apply.*)
    a. Guanaco
    b. Bactrian camels
    c. Vicuña
    d. Dromedary camels
    e. Llama
    f. Alpaca

28. Which animal is the normal host of *Parelaphostrongylus tenuis*?
    a. Llama
    b. White-tailed deer
    c. Mule deer
    d. Alpaca

EXERCISE 19.8 CASE STUDY #1: EQUINE INFECTIOUS ANEMIA

Your client, Mrs. Ratcliff, has called the clinic and asked why it is important to test her horses for equine infectious anemia (EIA) and why everyone thinks it is such a serious issue.

1. What do you tell her?

_____

_____

_____

_____

_____

_____

_____

EXERCISE 19.9 CASE STUDY #2: EQUINE GASTRIC ULCERS

Mr. Fredrickson received a call from his farm manager. Many of the young horses on his farm are developing gastric problems, and they think it is ulcers. Mr. Fredrickson calls you to discuss the predisposing factors in horses that may contribute to the formation of gastric ulcers and what signs to be aware of so that he can address this issue with the farm manager. He would also like to know about treatment and prevention.

1. What do you tell him?

_____

_____

_____

_____

_____

_____

EXERCISE 19.10 CASE STUDY #3: DERMATOPHILOSIS AND CULICOIDES HYPERSENSITIVITY

Dr. Rainy has been to see the horses at Ms. Lawler's barn. Several of them have dermatophilosis, and a couple of her older mares have *Culicoides* hypersensitivity.

Dr. Rainy prescribed medication for the affected horses and directed Ms. Lawler to call you so you could talk to her about what she could do with regard to the environment to help these horses recover and not become affected each year.

1. What do you tell Ms. Lawler when she calls?

_____

_____

_____

_____

_____

_____

_____

_____

_____

_____

_____

_____

EXERCISE 19.11 CASE STUDY #4: REARING LAMBS

Mrs. Rogers has just started a small sheep operation, and she is interested in raising lambs. She has contacted your clinic to ask questions about how best to make sure her lambs are born healthy, how to prevent lamb rejection, and how to prevent lamb stealing by ewes. Your DVM has indicated that you can share the standard protocol the clinic recommends with Mrs. Rogers and that she should also schedule a herd wellness check prior to breeding season.

1. What do you tell her?

_____

_____

_____

_____

_____

_____

_____

_____

_____

_____

_____

_____

_____

_____

_____

_____

_____

_____

_____

EXERCISE 19.12 CASE STUDY #5: CARE OF NEONATAL CRIAS

Mrs. Jones has just purchased a pair of llamas, and the female is pregnant. Mrs. Jones is concerned about the birth of the cria and what she needs to do to make sure that everything goes well after the birth. She also asks what to look for, which would warn her that the cria is in trouble.

1. What information will you share with Mrs. Jones?

_____

_____

_____

_____

_____

_____

_____

_____

_____

_____

_____

20 Veterinary Oncology

LEARNING OBJECTIVES

When you have completed this chapter, you will be able to:
1. Pronounce, define, and spell all key terms in this chapter.
2. Discuss the pathogenesis of cancer, including the following:
3. Define oncology and explain mechanisms by which tumors cause clinical signs.
4. Differentiate between malignant and benign tumors.
5. List the classifications of tumors by tissue origin and provide examples of each.
6. Describe the difference between staging and grading and explain how each can be used to make treatment decisions.
7. Discuss the epidemiology of cancer, including the following:
8. List and describe common tumor types.
9. List clinical warning signs that can be associated with cancer.
10. Describe general staging diagnostics for patients with cancer, including the following:
11. Describe what is involved in an initial database for a patient.
12. Discuss how imaging can be used to evaluate a patient.
13. Describe the difference between cytology and histology and list the advantages and limitations of each.
14. Discuss the process of staging cancer.
15. Describe therapeutic options in veterinary oncology, including surgery, radiation, chemotherapy, and palliative and comfort care and discuss safety concerns and side effects related to administration and use of both oral and IV chemotherapy, along with ways to address such concerns and ways to reduce risks of side effects.
16. Discuss complementary, alternative, and integrative therapy and explain why oncologists usually reject alternative medicine but embrace complementary and integrative therapies.
17. List and discuss the common tumors of horses and cattle.

EXERCISE 20.1 MATCHING #1: IDENTIFYING TYPES OF TUMORS

Instructions: Match each term in column A with its corresponding definition in column B by writing the appropriate letter in the space provided.

Column A

1. _____ Neoplasm

2. _____ Lymphoma

3. _____ Mast cell tumor

4. _____ Osteosarcoma

5. _____ Carcinomas

6. _____ Oral tumors

7. _____ Hemangiosarcoma

Column B

A. Primarily affects bones of the appendicular skeleton

B. Characterized by unrestrained proliferation of abnormal cells

C. Common in larger, middle-aged to older dogs; commonly found on the skin, heart, liver, and spleen

D. The most common malignant skin tumors in dogs

E. Affects primarily older animals

F. Cancer of immune system cells

G. Tumors of epithelial tissues

EXERCISE 20.2 MATCHING #2: TYPES OF MEDICINE

Instructions: Match each description in column A with its corresponding type of medicine practice in column B by writing the appropriate letter in the space provided. (Note that responses may be used more than once.)

Column A

1. _____ Approach that makes use of complementary, holistic, and conventional treatments

2. _____ Used synonymously with "comfort care"

3. _____ Use of nonstandard treatments in place of standard therapy

4. _____ The goal of treatment is to improve the patient's quality of life with less regard for longevity

5. _____ Examples include I'm-Yunity, Yunnan Baiyao, and nutritional management

6. _____ Uses nonstandard treatments in combination with standard therapy

Column B

A. Complementary medicine

B. Integrative medicine

C. Alternative medicine

D. Palliative care

EXERCISE 20.3 FUNDAMENTAL CHARACTERISTICS OF CANCER CELLS

Instructions: Identify 5 of the 8 characteristics of cancer cells.

1. _____

2. _____

3. _____

4. _____

5. _____

EXERCISE 20.4 MATCHING #3: TUMOR CLASSIFICATION

Instructions: Match each item in column A with the appropriate tissue of origin in column B.

Column A

1. _____ Osteosarcoma

2. _____ Lymphosarcoma

3. _____ Adenoma

4. _____ Leiomyosarcoma

5. _____ Sarcoma

6. _____ Liposarcoma

Column B

A. Glandular tissue

B. Mesenchymal tissue

C. Lymph cells

D. Smooth muscle tissue

E. Bone

F. Fat cells

EXERCISE 20.5 FILL-IN-THE-BLANK: CHARACTERISTICS OF COMMON TUMORS

Instructions: Fill in each of the spaces provided with the missing word or words listed below and complete the sentence. Terms may be used more than once.

Lymphoma
Mast cell tumor
Osteosarcoma
Melanoma
Hemangiosarcoma
Carcinomas
Squamous cell carcinoma

1. _____ is a tumors of epithelial tissue that arise from many sites.

2. A patient with _____ often presents an emergency with pale gums, poor or snappy pulses, distended abdomens, and extreme lethargy.

3. _____ is the most common oral tumor in dogs.

4. When lameness is presented, radiographs are recommended to rule out the presence of_____.

5. _____ is typically found under the tongue in cats.

6. Cells of a _____ tumor are filled with vesicles containing histamine.

7. A dog with a _____ most commonly presents with an acute history of collapse and abdominal swelling.

8. The most common presentation of _____ in dogs is multiple, nonpainful, enlarged lymph nodes.

9. The most common presentation of _____ in cats is a subacute to chronic history of weight loss, possible vomiting, decreased appetite, and diarrhea.

EXERCISE 20.6 TRUE OR FALSE: COMPREHENSIVE

Instructions: Read the following statements and write "T" for true or "F" for false in the blanks provided. If a statement is false, correct the statement to make it true.

1. _____ Neoplasm is another term for new blood.

2. _____ Patients undergoing a CT must be either anesthetized or sedated.

3. _____ The term neoplasia describes only malignant tissue.

4. _____ Cytology slides should be fixed with formalin.

5. _____ The absence of cancer cells in a cytology sample does not always rule out cancer.

6. _____ A tumor that grows large and causes discomfort is likely malignant.

7. _____ The grade of a tumor can only be determined by a pathologist.

8. _____ Tumor size and how far it has spread are part of the grade of the tumor.

9. _____ One of the leading causes of disease-related deaths in the small animal species is coronary artery disease.

10. _____ Radiography is the best choice to guide the percutaneous collection of biopsy samples and body cavity effusions.

11. _____ Morphine should be used in patients with confirmed or suspected mast cell tumors because these tumors can be quite painful.

12. _____ The most common feline presentation of lymphoma is in the kitten.

13. _____ The most common malignant skin tumor in dogs is melanoma.

14. _____ Sarcomas most commonly spread through the bloodstream alone.

15. _____ Tissue biopsy is the only definitive proof of hemangiosarcoma.

16. _____ Pain medication is of little use in the dog.

17. _____ "Watch and wait" is the best approach during early diagnosis procedures.

18. _____ Tumor grade is determined by diagnostic tests, such as caliper measurements, abdominal ultrasonography, thoracic radiography, computed tomography (CT), blood work, urinalysis, magnetic resonance imaging (MRI), and lymph node cytology or biopsy.

19. _____ Canine and human cancers often exhibit remarkably different clinical presentations, pathology, treatment responses, and molecular underpinnings.

20. _____ Elspar is used to treat thyroid adenocarcinoma and melanoma.

21. _____ Staging a tumor is essential for planning appropriate and effective treatment.

22. _____ The primary goal of treatment in veterinary oncology is to prolong the life of the animal.

23. _____ Rarely is surgery recommended for a patient with metastasis.

24. _____ A form of radiation therapy frequently used in veterinary medicine is the placement of radioactive "seeds" in the body.

25. _____ Radiation does not specifically target cancer cells.

26. _____ Severe reactions to radiation are common.

27. _____ Leukotrachia is common following radiation therapy.

28. _____ Chemotherapeutic drugs all work to target cell replication.

29. _____ Chemotherapy is not useful in treating every type of cancer, and not all chemotherapy has negative side effects.

30. _____ Chronic exposure to chemotherapeutic agents is of particular concern for pregnant veterinary staff.

31. _____ ATLS is usually fatal unless treatment is immediate.

32. _____ The nadir of neutrophil count is approximately 5 to 7 days following the administration of chemotherapy.

33. _____ Home-cooked meals provide the best balance to meet the long-term feeding needs of pets.

228

34. ＿＿ Canned pumpkin is a good addition to the diet to help with loose stools.

35. ＿＿ Cat owners should be aware that anorexia for short periods is common and poses no significant threat to a cat's wellbeing.

EXERCISE 20.7 FILL-IN-THE-BLANK: COMPREHENSIVE

Fill in each blank with the missing information to form a correct statement.

1. ＿＿＿＿＿＿＿＿＿＿＿＿ is the most common type of skin tumor in horses; it is locally invasive but rarely metastatic.

2. ＿＿＿＿＿＿＿＿＿＿＿＿ tumors are associated with prolonged exposure to the sun and are therefore more commonly seen in open-ranged cattle.

3. ＿＿＿＿＿＿＿＿＿＿＿＿ tumors are cutaneous tumors derived from melanocytes.

4. ＿＿＿＿＿＿＿＿＿＿＿＿ is one of the most common tumors in the frog of a horse's foot.

5. Cutaneous tumors are common in horses and are often found on ＿＿＿＿＿＿＿＿＿＿＿＿, ＿＿＿＿＿＿＿＿＿＿＿＿, ＿＿＿＿＿＿＿＿＿＿＿＿, ＿＿＿＿＿＿＿＿＿＿＿＿, ＿＿＿＿＿＿＿＿＿＿＿＿-＿＿＿＿＿＿＿＿＿＿＿＿, and ＿＿＿＿＿＿＿＿＿＿＿＿ ＿＿＿＿＿＿＿＿＿＿＿＿.

6. The diet recommended over the use of generic brands is a(n) ＿＿＿＿＿＿＿＿＿＿＿＿ -approved diet.

7. An all-natural herbal supplement known to stop bleeding, used by herbalists and acupuncturists, is ＿＿＿＿＿＿＿＿＿＿＿＿.

8. Non-mainstream therapies used instead of standard medical treatments are known as ＿＿＿＿＿＿＿＿＿＿＿＿ treatments.

9. ＿＿＿＿＿＿＿＿＿＿＿＿ therapy is treatment given in addition to primary treatment.

10. Most common side effects of ＿＿＿＿＿＿＿＿＿＿＿＿ include skin reactions, such as hair loss or moist dermatitis, which occur toward the middle-to-end of the treatment period.

11. ＿＿＿＿＿＿＿＿＿＿＿＿ is an antibiotic antineoplastic used to treat lymphoma, carcinoma, leukemia, and sarcoma.

12. The components of the Quality of Life (HHHHHMM) include these criteria: ＿＿＿＿＿＿＿＿＿＿＿＿, ＿＿＿＿＿＿＿＿＿＿＿＿, ＿＿＿＿＿＿＿＿＿＿＿＿, ＿＿＿＿＿＿＿＿＿＿＿＿, ＿＿＿＿＿＿＿＿＿＿＿＿, and ＿＿＿＿＿＿＿＿＿＿＿＿.

13. The most abundant type of WBC with a short half-life and rapid turnover is the ＿＿＿＿＿＿＿＿＿＿＿＿.

14. A serious and potentially life-threatening allergic reaction is known as ＿＿＿＿＿＿＿＿＿＿＿＿.

15. Dogs with four white feet may carry the ＿＿＿＿＿＿＿＿＿＿＿＿ mutation, making them more likely to have a toxicity reaction to chemotherapeutic agents.

16. In the scale produced by the VCOG that standardizes the reporting of adverse drug events, a grade 1 and 2 toxicity is considered to be ＿＿＿＿＿＿＿＿＿＿＿＿.

17. The most common side effects of chemotherapy are _____

_____, _____, _____, _____, and

_____.

18. PPEs that should be worn when working with chemotherapeutic drugs include _____,

_____, _____, _____,

_____, and _____.

19. Traditionally, chemotherapy is given at the _____ possible dose for relatively

_____ periods, with intervals of recovery when no chemotherapy is given.

20. Some chemotherapy agents, called _____, cause severe tissue irritation, blistering, and

sloughing of skin and tissue if they are _____.

21. Doses of chemotherapeutic drugs should be checked _____ times to avoid overdose.

22. The Patient Management Check List for Veterinary Technicians in Oncology includes six main areas:

_____, _____, _____,

_____, _____, and _____.

23. Radiation causes damage to DNA _____ and _____

through the formation of highly charged particles (called free radicals) that damage DNA.

24. Practically, chemotherapy involves a diverse array of therapies that include _____,

nonsteroidal anti-inflammatory drugs, _____, traditional chemotherapy,

_____, and targeted therapies.

25. Histologic examination requires a sample of tissue obtained through either _____ or

_____ of the mass.

26. Cancer should be considered in patients with one or more of the following signs: _____

that persist or grow; _____ wounds; weight _____; loss of

_____; bleeding or discharge from _____; reluctance to

exercise or _____; persistent _____ or stiffness; difficulty

breathing; _____; or _____.

27. To assess cell morphology and to confirm that proper technique was used during blood collection and handling, a

_____ should be performed.

28. The standard of care for cancer patients that may undergo treatment includes _____,

_____, and _____.

29. Two of the most important factors for long-term treatment success are _____ and

_____.

30. It is estimated that _____ million dogs and cats are annually diagnosed with cancer.

230

EXERCISE 20.8 CASE STUDY: BLADDER CANCER IN BUFFY, A MIXED-BREED DOG

Buffy, a cocker spaniel mix, age 14, has been brought to the clinic. The owner reports that Buffy has been urinating frequently, and he has seen blood in Buffy's urine on and off for about 2 weeks. Buffy appears to strain a bit upon urination and has been urinating more frequently than in the past, but otherwise seems "normal, but maybe not quite himself, you know, a little tired," according to the owner. The HHHHHMM score is 40. The initial examination involved palpation and a rectal examination, and an initial suspicion of bladder cancer was suggested.

1. The veterinarian asks you to prepare the tests for an initial cancer evaluation. What tests need to be provided for Buffy?

   _____

   _____

   _____

   _____

2. As you prepare to take a blood draw from the jugular vein, an assistant in the practice pulls you aside and asks, "Why are we taking a blood draw from the jugular vein?" You respond:

   _____

   _____

   _____

   _____

3. The vet asks that you not use cystocentesis when collecting urine from Buffy. Why would such a request be made?

   _____

   _____

   _____

   _____

4. The vet also orders a thoracic radiograph. You know that the thoracic CT scan is more sensitive than radiographs and more likely to detect smaller and more subtle lesions. Why do you think radiographs are always recommended prior to taking a CT scan?

   _____

   _____

   _____

   _____

5. A fine-needle biopsy is completed on Buffy, during which no cancer cells are noted. The cells have been sent to a pathologist for verification. Is it appropriate to tell the owner, "Good news! The tumor is benign."?

_____

_____

_____

_____

6. What four aspects should be considered during the process of staging a cancer?

_____

_____

_____

_____

7. The pathology report confirms transitional cell carcinoma (TCC). Due to the grade of the tumor, the course of chemotherapy that has been elected by the veterinarian and agreed to by Buffy's owner will include several weeks of therapy during which a drug of low-vesicant potential and effective in the treatment of TCC will be used. If mitoxantrone is the drug selected, what side effects can be expected, and what is the nadir?

_____

_____

_____

_____

8. The vet has asked you to assist in post-administration care for Buffy. You review the Post-Administration portion of the Patient Management Checklist for Veterinary Technicians in Oncology. What are the ten questions to ask yourself from this portion of the checklist?

_____

_____

_____

_____

_____

_____

_____

_____

9. Buffy's owner asks about nutrition and wants to begin an organic, all-natural diet for him. The owner says, "He is such a member of our family; he deserves home-cooked meals, like the rest of us." How would you respond?

_____

_____

_____

_____

_____

_____

_____

_____

10. The veterinary assistant wonders if the drugs are safe for staff to handle. What do you tell her about safe handling?

_____

_____

_____

_____

_____

_____

_____

_____

_____

_____

_____

_____

_____

_____

_____

_____

11. The veterinarian is considering a metronomic approach to dosing and asks if you know what this means. You respond:

_____

_____

_____

_____

21 Neonatal Care of Puppies, Kittens, and Foals

LEARNING OBJECTIVES

When you have completed this chapter, you will be able to:

1. Pronounce, define, and spell all key terms in this chapter.
2. Define the neonatal period for puppies and kittens, obtain an accurate and thorough clinical history for all littermates and parents, and describe the procedure for physical examination of a neonate, including equipment needed and potential abnormalities.
3. Explain the timeline of normal development in neonatal puppies and kittens.
4. Do the following regarding performance of diagnostic procedures and routine maintenance in neonatal puppies and kittens:
   - Discuss how to perform diagnostic procedures on a neonatal puppy or a kitten.
   - Discuss appropriate times to administer medical treatments to neonatal puppies and kittens and explain proper nutrition, preventive medicine, and behavior to the owner.
5. Do the following regarding common concerns and disorders in puppies and kittens:
   - Explain common concerns of neonatal puppies and kittens, such as hypothermia, dehydration, hypoglycemia, malnutrition, fading puppy or kitten syndrome, and neonatal isoerythrolysis in kittens.
   - Discuss proper care of an orphaned neonatal puppy or kitten and common complications involved with orphaned neonates.
6. Do the following regarding the perinatal period and the high-risk mare:
   - Differentiate between normal and abnormal perinatal periods in the mare and explain how to care for a high-risk mare.
   - Identify the stages of labor in a mare and describe how to treat any complications that may arise at each stage.
7. Describe the normal development of a neonatal foal that occurs during the first 24 hours after birth and identify normal vital signs and behavior.
8. Do the following regarding care of the sick foal:
   - List the signs of a critically ill foal, including symptoms of prematurity and dysmaturity and classic early clinical signs of disease.
   - Identify common sites and procedures for venous and arterial blood collection and the appropriate needles, syringes, and restraint techniques to be used in the neonatal foal.
   - Identify parameters that should be monitored in the hospitalized foal and describe complications that may arise during hospitalization.
   - Describe proper nursing care for the foal to prevent contamination, including washing of hands and injection sites, changing of intravenous (IV) fluid lines, and maintenance of IV and jugular catheters.
   - Explain appropriate physical therapy for the recumbent foal, the necessity for keeping it in sternal position and frequent changes in recumbency, and the proper restraint techniques that can be used for the ambulatory foal.
9. Explain alternative methods that can be used to ensure that nutritional needs are met if a foal is unable to nurse from the mare.

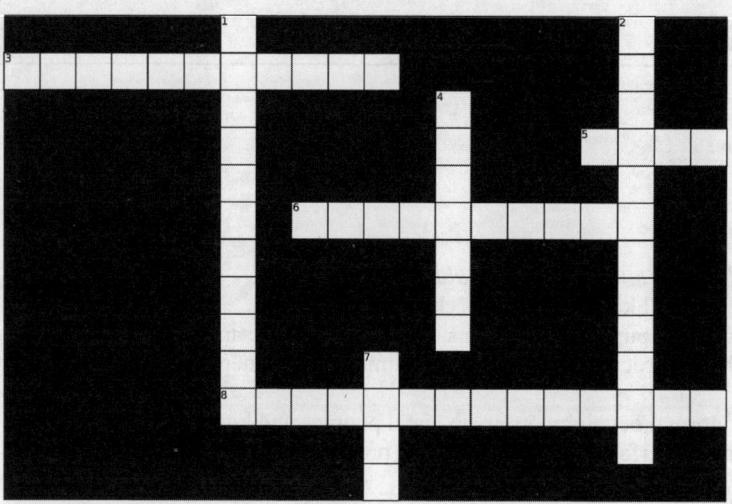

Across

3 Abnormally low body temperature. The measured body temperature must be compared with what is normal for the age group because neonates have lower body temperatures than adults.

5 A juvenile horse nursing from its mother

6 Born with a specific condition. Can be genetic or environmentally induced

8 In puppies and kittens, the first 2 to 4 weeks of life are characterized by complete dependence on the mother because of incomplete neurologic functions, such as audio and visual abilities and proper spinal reflexes.

Down

1 Abnormal depletion of body fluids

2 Lower than normal levels of blood glucose resulting in lack of fuel to the brain and other organ systems

4 When one parent or both parents transmit disease-causing genes to the offspring, that disease is described as_____.

7 Adult female horse

EXERCISE 21.2 DEFINITIONS: COMMON DISEASES AND CONDITIONS OF NEONATAL FOALS

Instructions: Define each disease or condition of neonatal foals in your own words.

1. Sepsis or septic shock: _____

   _____

2. Neonatal encephalopathy: _____

   _____

3. Failure of passive transfer (FPT): _____

   _____

4. Neonatal nephropathy: _____

   _____

5. Neonatal isoerythrolysis: _____

   _____

6. Dysmaturity: _____

   _____

7. Neonatal gastroenteropathy: _____

   _____

8. Colitis: _____

   _____

9. Musculoskeletal abnormalities: _____

   _____

10. Patent urachus: _____

    _____

11. Ruptured bladder: _____

    _____

12. Entropion: _____

    _____

13. Septic arthritis or septic physitis: _____

_____

14. Meconium retention: _____

_____

15. Prematurity: _____

_____

EXERCISE 21.3 MATCHING: THE NEONATAL FOAL

Instructions: Match each word in column A with its corresponding definition in column B by writing the appropriate letter in the space provided.

Column A

1. _____ Patent urachus
2. _____ Neonatal encephalopathy
3. _____ Neonatal ophthalmia
4. _____ Bacteremia
5. _____ Petechiae
6. _____ Omphalitis
7. _____ Placentitis
8. _____ Colostrum
9. _____ Hypovolemia
10. _____ Foaling
11. _____ Icterus
12. _____ Chorioallantoic membrane rupture
13. _____ "Bagging up"
14. _____ Holosystolic flow murmur
15. _____ Hypoxemia
16. _____ Wax-up
17. _____ Telemetry
18. _____ Glycosuria
19. _____ Bucket baby
20. _____ Primiparous
21. _____ Injected
22. _____ Miotic

Column B

A. Parturition in a mare

B. The accumulation of pre-foaling secretions on the teats

C. Another name for a maiden mare

D. First milk, which contains antibodies

E. Results in the releasing allantoic fluid, signaling the end of Stage 1 labor

F. Low blood oxygen levels

G. A foal raised as an orphan

H. The term for the pre-parturition change in the mare of udder enlargement

I. Infection in the bloodstream

J. A normal finding during neonate heart auscultation in an otherwise healthy foal

K. The word used to describe mucous membranes with prominent vessels is often dark purple.

L. Yellow discoloration of tissues, serum, or plasma caused by the presence of bilirubin

M. Small areas of hemorrhaging

N. A common infection of the umbilicus

O. A method of monitoring heart rates in high-risk mares

P. Decreased circulating blood volume

Q. A term used to describe constricted pupils

R. A leading high-risk complication in the mare that can present with vaginal discharge, premature udder development, and lactation

S. Sugar present in the urine

T. Condition that can cause urine to leak from the navel

U. Bulging eyes behind closed eyelids

V. Also called "dummy foal" or neonatal maladjustment syndrome

EXERCISE 21.4 TRUE OR FALSE: COMPREHENSIVE

Instructions: Read the following statements and write "T" for true or "F" for false in the blanks provided. If a statement is false, correct the statement to make it true.

1. _____ The history taken for neonatal puppies and kittens should include the number of ill animals in the litter, the method by which they were raised, and the queen or bitch's vaccination history.

2. _____ Because the neonate can have a body temperature lower than 94° F (34.4° C), a digital thermometer that measures as low as 85° F (29.4° C) is necessary.

3. _____ To evaluate a neonate's hydration status, its skin turgor is evaluated by gently pinching the skin on its neck.

4. _____ By 3 days of age, kittens and puppies should be able to crawl in a coordinated manner.

5. _____ Normal neonatal puppies and kittens often have sparse hair coats.

6. _____ Bluish or dark red skin may be normal in a neonatal puppy or kitten.

7. _____ A bloated abdomen in a neonatal puppy is a typical finding.

8. _____ Gloves should be worn at all times when directly handling the neonate foal, administering medications, changing fluids or IV lines, etc.

9. _____ Normal neonates may have irregular heart and respiratory rates.

10. _____ When neonates are born, they are capable of maintaining their body temperature.

11. _____ The abdominal component of breathing is absent in neonatal puppies and kittens.

12. _____ Dog testicles do not descend until 6 to 8 weeks of age.

13. _____ When a neonate is brought in as an emergency, priority should be placed on obtaining all samples necessary for accurate diagnosis.

14. _____ Orphan neonates must be weighed four times a day or more.

15. _____ A vast array of antibodies are transferred in utero to canine and feline fetuses, and they are born immunologically mature.

16. _____ Fluid requirements are high in neonates, but the total volumes that can be given are low.

17. _____ There is less risk of aspiration associated with tube feeding than with syringe and bottle feeding in neonates.

18. _____ The most common causes of diarrhea in the orphaned neonate are overfeeding and inappropriate dilutions of milk replacer.

19. _____ Foals are born without a menace response.

20. _____ The packed cell volume (PCV) of the normal foal during the first 24 hours of life is less than half that of an adult horse.

EXERCISE 21.5 MULTIPLE CHOICE: COMPREHENSIVE

Instructions: Circle the one correct answer to each of the following questions.

1. The time period of a puppy or kitten's life that is considered to be the neonatal period is
   a. 1 to 2 weeks.
   b. 2 to 4 weeks.
   c. 4 to 6 weeks.
   d. 6 to 8 weeks.

2. Neonatal puppies and kittens are unable to regulate their own body temperature during the first _____ weeks of life.
   a. 2
   b. 3
   c. 4
   d. 6

3. Normal developing puppies and kittens will nurse as frequently as every _____ during their first week of life.
   a. 1 to 2 hours
   b. 2 to 4 hours
   c. 3 to 6 hours
   d. 3 to 5 hours

4. The age at which puppies and kittens should be able to lift their head is
   a. 1 day.
   b. 2 days.
   c. 3 days.
   d. 4 days.

5. The age at which puppies and kittens begin to crawl in a coordinated manner is
   a. 1 week.
   b. 2 weeks.
   c. 3 weeks.
   d. 4 weeks.

6. The term neonate encompasses foals
   a. from birth to one month of age.
   b. from one month to three months of age.
   c. from birth to six months of age.
   d. from one month to six months of age.

7. Kittens and puppies begin to open their eyes at the age of
   a. 3 to 7 days.
   b. 5 to 10 days.
   c. 7 to 12 days.
   d. 10 to 14 days.

8. The external ear canals of puppies and kittens will open at the age of
   a. 10 to 12 days.
   b. 12 to 14 days.
   c. 14 to 16 days.
   d. 16 to 18 days.

9. When obtaining blood from a neonate, the percentage of the circulating blood volume obtained over the course of 1 week should not exceed
   a. 5%.
   b. 10%.
   c. 15%.
   d. 20%.

10. If possible a hospitalized foal should be weighed
    a. biweekly.
    b. hourly.
    c. daily.
    d. twice daily.

11. Blood can easily be obtained from neonates by using the
    a. cephalic vein.
    b. jugular vein.
    c. saphenous vein.
    d. femoral artery.

12. Puppies and kittens are able to stand with good postural reflexes at the end of the week
    a. 2.
    b. 3.
    c. 4.
    d. 5.

13. If a neonatal puppy or kitten weighs 300 g, the maximum volume of blood that can be drawn in the course of 1 week would be
    a. 1.5 cc.
    b. 2.0 cc.
    c. 3.0 cc.
    d. 3.5 cc.

14. To obtain urine samples in the neonate,
    a. use an ultrasound.
    b. perform cystocentesis.
    c. stimulate the bladder by gently rubbing the genital area with a moistened cotton ball.
    d. forcefully express the bladder.

15. Because neonatal animals have immature kidneys, it is considered normal to find urine with a specific gravity between
    a. 1.010 and 1.015.
    b. 1.012 and 1.020.
    c. 1.015 and 1.025.
    d. 1.020 and 1.030.

16. Healthy neonatal puppies and kittens born to healthy mothers with good maternal instincts require
    a. routine check-ins every 2–4 hours.
    b. almost no care during the first weeks of life.
    c. frequent handling to ensure proper socialization.
    d. frequent monitoring of interaction between mother and offspring at all times.

17. A neonate is considered hypothermic if, at birth, the body temperature drops below
    a. 90° F.
    b. 92° F.
    c. 94° F.
    d. 97° F.

18. When treating hypothermic neonatal puppies, it is important to withhold the administration of oral food until the animal has
    a. audible gut sounds and is appropriately rewarmed.
    b. audible gut sounds and a bowel movement.
    c. no gut sounds but is moderately rewarmed.
    d. no gut sounds but is fully rewarmed.

19. Any disease process or fluid or electrolyte imbalance in neonatal animals will quickly lead to
    a. hypothermia.
    b. colic.
    c. lethargy.
    d. dehydration.

20. The acceptable route(s) of fluid administration in the neonate is/are
    a. IV only.
    b. IV or IO only.
    c. IV, IO, and PO.
    d. IV or PO only.

21. When administering fluids intraosseously to a neonate, a 20- or 22-gauge needle can be placed in the
    a. proximal tibia or proximal femur.
    b. proximal tibia or distal femur.
    c. distal tibia or distal femur.
    d. distal tibia or proximal femur.

22. _____ in neonatal puppies and kittens can be the cause of seizures.
    a. Dehydration
    b. Neonatal isoerythrolysis
    c. Malnutrition
    d. Hypoglycemia

23. Dextrose solutions should never be administered _____, as they may cause tissue damage.
    a. intravenously
    b. subcutaneously
    c. intraosseously
    d. intraperitoneally

24. Occasionally, a mare will develop a problem during late-term pregnancy. These mares are referred to as
    a. primiparous mares.
    b. high-risk mares.
    c. late-term mares.
    d. problem mares.

25. The average gestational length for the mare is
    a. 200 days.
    b. 240 days.
    c. 300 days.
    d. 340 days.

26. The veterinarian will perform a rectal examination and transrectal ultrasound on a pregnant mare at approximately
    a. 15 days and 30 days.
    b. 15 days, 30 days, and 90 days.
    c. 30 days and 90 days.
    d. 30 days, 90 days, and 120 days.

27. During the first week of life, healthy foals
    a. socialize with other foals intermittently.
    b. keep a distance of approximately 3–15 feet from the mare unless nursing.
    c. nurse often and stay within close proximity of the mare.
    d. be quiet, sleepy, and uninterested in anything but the mare.

28. Mares often foal
    a. mid-morning.
    b. in the afternoon.
    c. in the early evening.
    d. at night.

29. Agitation, pacing, turning and biting at sides, and posturing to urinate or defecate are signs of which stage of labor in the mare?
   a. Stage 1
   b. Stage 2
   c. Stage 3
   d. Stage 4

30. Sweating around the shoulders of a mare in labor is indicative of
   a. dystocia.
   b. foaling within 30 minutes.
   c. colic.
   d. overheating.

31. The mare will pass her placenta during _____ of labor.
   a. Stage 1
   b. Stage 2
   c. Stage 3
   d. Stage 4

EXERCISE 21.6 FILL-IN-THE-BLANK: NEONATOLOGY OF PUPPIES AND KITTENS

Instructions: Fill in each of the spaces provided with the missing word or words that complete the sentence.

1. When performing a physical examination on a neonate, the use of a(n) _____ with a 2-cm bell is helpful.

2. When a neonate is born, hair will be present on most of the body, excluding the _____.

3. The only motor skills present in a neonatal puppy or kitten are _____, _____, _____, and distress _____.

4. Urination and defecation of neonates is initiated by the bitch or queen licking the _____ area.

5. The body temperature of puppies and kittens at birth will be lower than in adult animals and will rise to 94.7° F to 100.1° F during their first _____ of life.

6. A neonate's umbilical cord will dry out during its first day of life and is expected to fall off by day _____ to _____.

7. The flexor tone present at birth in puppies will switch over to the _____ after the _____ day of life.

8. Neonates generally tolerate a(n) _____ examination better than a radiography examination when imaging techniques are used.

9. At the beginning of week _____ of life, puppies and kittens should receive their first deworming treatment of pyrantel pamoate.

10. Deworming treatment in puppies and kittens is aimed mainly toward eliminating a common intestinal parasite called _____.

11. Healthy kittens and puppies will have doubled their birth weight by _____ and _____ days, respectively.

12. A neonate is considered hypothermic if its body temperature drops below _____.

13. Feeding a hypothermic neonate can cause milk replacer to be regurgitated and aspirated, resulting in _____, or stomach contents may ferment, leading to _____.

14. Clinical signs in a chilled neonate with a body temperature above 88° F include restlessness, continuous crying, _____ mucous membranes, and skin that feels _____ to the touch.

15. When the body temperature of a small animal neonate falls into the range of _____ ° F to _____ ° F, the neonate appears lethargic and uncoordinated but responsive.

16. When the body temperature of a small animal neonate is below _____ ° F, the animal will appear to be dead.

17. _____ also contributes significantly to hypothermia in the neonate, thus proper ventilation or oxygen should be administered when possible.

18. Warm air and _____ in a human neonatal incubator is optimal for rewarming hypothermic animal neonates.

19. _____ rewarming of a neonate will result in heat prostration with increased respiratory rate and effort.

20. Raising the body temperature of a neonate more than _____ ° F is usually fatal because of delayed organ failure.

21. The hydration status of a neonate is best checked by looking at the oral _____.

22. All fluids should be warmed to _____ before administration to the neonate unless the neonate is substantially colder.

23. Tacky or dry mucous membranes in a neonate indicate _____% dehydration.

24. When a neonate has reached _____% dehydration, the oral mucous membranes will be dry, with a noticeable decrease in skin elasticity.

25. To rehydrate a neonate, boluses can be given at _____ per 100 g of the neonate's weight over _____ minutes.

26. When administering intravenous fluids to a neonate, it is often easiest to place a short 23- or 25-gauge catheter in the _____ vein.

27. If a nasogastric tube with pre-marked measurements is not available for a neonate requiring tube feeding, a _____ may be used.

28. _____ and _____ are the first indications that a neonate is not doing well.

29. Hypoglycemic neonates will have serum glucose less than _____ mg/dL.

30. A _____ solution is used to treat a neonate with hypoglycemia.

31. One of the most common causes of seizures in neonatal puppies and kittens is _____.

EXERCISE 21.7 CASE STUDY: POSTPARTUM EXAMINATION OF A LITTER OF PUPPIES

Signalment: Roxanne, a 3-year-old female Rottweiler with her litter of six 4-day-old puppies

Chief Complaint: Roxanne and her puppies are presented for a routine postpartum examination, including puppy tail docking and dewclaw removal. The owner reports that Roxanne delivered the six puppies uneventfully 4 days prior to presentation. This is Roxanne's second pregnancy, and she is accepting and caring for the puppies. All of the puppies seem to be nursing vigorously and gaining weight. Answer the following questions regarding this case.

a. What are the ways in which the examination of neonates differs from the examination of adult animals?

_____

_____

_____

_____

b. What special equipment is needed when examining neonates?

_____

_____

_____

_____

c. What are the components of a complete neonatal examination, including specific abnormalities you would look for?

_____

_____

_____

_____

_____

_____

_____

_____

22 Care of Birds, Reptiles, and Small Mammals

LEARNING OBJECTIVES

When you have completed this chapter, you will be able to:
1. Define and spell all key terms in this chapter.
2. Do the following regarding the intake process and examination of birds:
   - Collect an accurate and thorough clinical history for an avian patient and explain proper capture and restraint techniques for an effective and timely examination with minimal stress to the patient.
   - Discuss proper nutrition and husbandry of pet birds.
   - Discuss the physical examination process.
3. Explain sample collections and diagnostic procedures commonly used in birds and describe proper anesthetic techniques.
4. Describe the common routes for administering medication to birds, gavage, hand-feeding, and grooming.
5. Discuss avian nutrition.
6. Manage the hospitalized avian patient.
7. List the materials needed to properly treat and handle reptiles in the veterinary hospital in regards to zoonotic diseases, transmission and precention of Salmonella and understanding of the information needed for an accurate and thorough clinical history of a reptile patient.
8. Describe sample collections, and diagnostic procedures commonly used in reptiles.
9. Understand anesthesia and intubation recommendations for the chelonian, snake, and lizard.
10. Describe husbandry requirements for the reptilian patient, including nutrition, temperature, humidity, lighting, and substrate requirements.
11. Explain the proper care of ferrets including: handling, grooming, phlebotomy, anesthesia, nursing management, and nutritional requirements.
12. Discuss the common presenting complaints of ferrets.
13. Explain the proper care of rabbits including: housing, nutritional requirements, anesthetic techniques, and intravenous access.
14. Describe some common presenting complaints in pet rabbits.
15. Explain the proper care of rodents, including antibiotic therapy, anesthetic techniques, antiparasitic agents, and nutritional requirements, specifically for guinea pigs, hamsters, gerbils, rats, and chinchillas.
16. Describe the proper care of hedgehogs and sugar gliders, including husbandry requirements, dietary requirements, and common disease conditions.

EXERCISE 22.1 DEFINITIONS: KEY TERMS

Instructions: Define each term in your own words, including the species or general type of animal to which it applies.

1. Cloaca:_____

_____

2. Ecdysis:_____

_____

3. Conjunctivitis: _____

_____

4. Colonic wash: _____

_____

5. Medial metatarsal vein: _____

_____

EXERCISE 22.2 FILL-IN-THE-BLANK: TERMS AND DEFINITIONS

Instructions: Fill in each of the spaces provided with the missing term that completes the sentence.

1. The use of penicillin antibiotics in guinea pigs often causes _____ to occur.

2. The _____ is an outpouching of the esophagus located above a bird's sternum, where food is stored prior to digestion.

3. _____ is a general term used to refer to diarrhea in the hamster.

4. A turtle is an example of a(n) _____.

EXERCISE 22.3 MATCHING: TERMS AND DEFINITIONS

Instructions: Match each term in column A with its corresponding definition in column B by writing the appropriate letter in the space provided.

Column A

1. _____ *Giardia*

2. _____ glottis

3. _____ palpebral edema

4. _____ *Mycoplasma spp.*

5. _____ gram-positive organisms

6. _____ basilic vein

Column B

A. Located on the wing of birds

B. Inflammation of the eyelid

C. Organisms inhabiting the digestive system in most pet bird species

D. The opening into the trachea

E. A pathogen that causes respiratory infections in rats

F. A protozoan GI parasite that affects birds

Instructions: Read the following statements and write "T" for true or "F" for false in the blanks provided. If a statement is false, correct the statement to make it true.

1. ____ Most medical problems in exotic pets are caused by the owner's lack of knowledge about basic nutrition and proper husbandry.

2. ____ Psittacosis, caused by *C. psittaci*, is a disease transmissible to humans.

3. ____ The left jugular vein is recommended for venipuncture in most, if not all, companion avian species.

4. ____ Injectable anesthetics are most commonly used to restrain birds for radiography.

5. ____ Clipping flight feathers to prevent birds from flying should only involve the feathers of the right wing.

6. ____ The best method to medicate birds is by putting their drugs in their water.

7. ____ Most pet birds should be weighed on a gram scale.

8. ____ Vitamin A deficiency is common in turtles.

9. ____ Seed diets are acceptable for smaller psittacine birds.

10. ____ Birds do not have sweat glands.

11. ____ Rabbits should have cool stone or tiles, ample fresh water, and cool hiding areas when the temperature exceeds 90° F.

12. ____ The African hedgehog is a crepuscular, social animal that requires social interaction to maintain physical and emotional health.

13. ____ NSHP is the most common of the metabolic bone diseases that are prevalent in captive reptiles.

14. ____ It is vital that clients use full spectrum lights for reptiles.

15. ____ Guinea pigs are primarily herbivores.

16. ____ Hypovitaminosis in chelonians can be prevented by providing a diet that supplies earthworms, small fish, and orange or yellow vegetables.

17. ____ Lizards are strict carnivores.

18. ____ Ferrets are induced ovulators.

19. ____ Rabbits are nocturnal (most active at night).

20. ____ Ferrets are very susceptible to vaccine reactions.

21. ____ Routine bathing will help alleviate the musky odor that ferrets possess.

22. ____ Guinea pigs should be fed a diet high in calcium.

23. ____ Wire cage bottoms may cause footpad ulcers in guinea pigs.

24. ____ Guinea pigs lack the enzyme L-gulonolactone oxidase.

247

25. _____ Hamsters should be housed separately.

26. _____ Gerbils can be safely picked up by grasping the tail firmly.

27. _____ Nasal discharges in rats may turn red, but this is not usually caused by blood.

28. _____ Hedgehogs in captivity are prone to obesity.

29. _____ Sugar gliders need to consume large quantities of fruit.

EXERCISE 22.5 MULTIPLE CHOICE: COMPREHENSIVE

Instructions: Circle the one correct answer to each of the following questions.

1. Which is a protozoan parasite that might be found in a crop sample taken from a crop wash?
   a. *Candida*
   b. *Capillaria*
   c. *Giardia*
   d. *Trichomonas*

2. What should bird owners bring to the veterinary office when arriving for an examination?
   a. Sample of droppings
   b. The toys the bird plays with
   c. The label from the bird's primary food/diet
   d. The health records of other pets in the house

3. Which muscles are most commonly used for injections in birds?
   a. Pectoral
   b. Epaxial
   c. Gluteal
   d. Biceps

4. Which is the recommended site for placing an intraosseous catheter in a bird?
   a. Distal humerus
   b. Distal tibia
   c. Distal femur
   d. Distal ulna

5. Which pet population is growing steadily, requiring high-quality veterinary care?
   a. Cat
   b. Rat
   c. Reptile
   d. Rabbit

6. What is the proper size of rodent to feed a snake?
   a. Twice the diameter of the snake's body
   b. About the same diameter as the snake's body
   c. No more than 4 inches long
   d. Length and size are not important

7. Which radiographic view is used routinely in turtles but not in snakes, lizards, or birds?
   a. Lateral
   b. Hanging VD
   c. AP (or frontal)
   d. Lateral oblique

8. How often does a snake feed?
   a. Once every 1 to 2 weeks
   b. Every 3 to 6 days
   c. Once a month
   d. Every 48 to 56 hours

9. Safe blood collection volumes from birds should never be greater than what percentage of the bird's body weight?
   a. 5%
   b. 3%
   c. 1%
   d. 0.5%

10. It is very important that owners know that _____ is toxic to birds and, therefore, should never be offered to them.
    a. kale
    b. papaya
    c. avocado
    d. crickets

11. Which is the best place for IV access in the rabbit?
    a. Ear
    b. Foot
    c. Jugular vein
    d. Saphenous vein

12. Human influenza is seen in which of the following animals?
    a. Hedgehog
    b. Prairie dog
    c. Ferret
    d. Guinea pig

13. Which mite most commonly affects the fur of rabbits?
    a. *Sarcoptes*
    b. *Microsporum*
    c. *Demodex*
    d. *Cheyletiella*

14. Which animal produces precocious young?
    a. Ferret
    b. Rabbit
    c. Guinea pig
    d. Sugar glider

15. Which antibiotic is least likely to cause dysbiosis in rabbits and rodents?
    a. Amoxicillin
    b. Streptomycin
    c. Oxytetracycline
    d. Ciprofloxacin

16. An adult female ferret with a swollen vulva and hair loss is most likely to have which disorder?
    a. Hyperadrenocorticism
    b. Hypothyroidism
    c. Ovarian neoplasia
    d. Hyperthyroidism

17. Which animal requires vitamin C in its diet?
    a. Rabbit
    b. Sugar glider
    c. Hedgehog
    d. Guinea pig

18. Which of the following is a social animal and needs special attention if housed singly?
    a. Guinea pig
    b. Sugar glider
    c. Hamster
    d. Rabbit

19. The cranial vena cava is often the preferred site for blood collection in which animal?
    a. Rabbit
    b. Ferret
    c. Parrot
    d. Snake

20. Clinical dermatologic diseases are common in reptilian species and often result from
    a. contact with other reptiles.
    b. contact with humans.
    c. UVB exposure.
    d. inappropriate humidity.

21. Ferrets should be vaccinated against which disease?
    a. Feline panleukopenia
    b. Canine distemper
    c. Measles
    d. Leptospirosis

22. Which of the following animals has cheek pouches that it can stuff with food?
    a. Sugar glider
    b. Guinea pig
    c. Ferret
    d. Hamster

23. Seizures are an inherited disorder seen in which of the following?
    a. Gerbils
    b. Hamsters
    c. Rabbits
    d. Ferrets

24. Which animal originally comes from Australia?
    a. Gerbil
    b. Sugar glider
    c. Hedgehog
    d. Hamster

25. The enclosure of all poikilotherms should be kept at their POTZ or
    a. pressure-optimized temperature zone.
    b. poikilotherm optimal temperature zone.
    c. preferred optimum temperature zone.
    d. probable optimal temperature zone.

26. Which of the following should be fed an insectivore diet?
    a. Hedgehog
    b. Prairie dog
    c. Sugar glider
    d. Iguana

27. Which of the following rodents has hypsodontic teeth?
    a. Hamster
    b. Rabbit
    c. Guinea pig
    d. Gerbil

28. Which of the following animals should be examined for dental malocclusion, trichobezoars, and dehydration?
    a. Anorexic rabbit
    b. Obese guinea pig
    c. Bulimic turtle
    d. Stressed bird

29. Which of the following animals should be on heartworm preventive medication if kept outdoors in an area with a high prevalence of heartworm?
    a. Rabbit
    b. Prairie dog
    c. Sugar glider
    d. Ferret

30. Which animal should be housed in a tall wire enclosure with branches and places to hide?
    a. Hedgehog
    b. Sugar glider
    c. Guinea pig
    d. Prairie dog

EXERCISE 22.6 CASE STUDY: GUINEA PIG NUTRITION, HUSBANDRY, AND PREVENTIVE CARE

1. A client calls and states that her daughter received an adult guinea pig for Christmas but does not have any knowledge of what or how to feed it. On further questioning, she mentions that she is feeding it the same diet she feeds her rabbit. What advice should you give her?

_____

_____

_____

_____

_____

_____

_____

_____

_____

_____

_____

23 Rehabilitation and Integrative Medical Nursing

LEARNING OBJECTIVES

When you have completed this chapter, you will be able to:

1. Pronounce, define, and spell all key terms in this chapter.
2. List the common indications for veterinary rehabilitation.
3. Understand the principals and implementation of therapeutic exercise and manual therapies
4. Compare and contrast the therapeutic modalities used in veterinary rehabilitation, including, electrical- and magnet-based therapies, light and sound–based therapies, and superficial thermal therapies.
5. List supportive and assistive devices commonly used for animal patients.
6. List commonly used nutraceuticals and chondro-protectants and describe their therapeutic uses.
7. Explain the principles and techniques of acupuncture and describe the role of the veterinary technician in acupuncture therapy.
8. Describe how veterinary spinal manipulative therapy can benefit animal patients and explain the role of the veterinary technician.
9. Describe the role of veterinary herbal medicine:

Instructions: Define each term in your own words.

1. Glucosamine: _____

   _____

2. Chondroprotectants: _____

   _____

3. Ayurvedic medicine: _____

   _____

4. Goniometer: _____

   _____

5. Chondroitin: _____

   _____

6. Nutraceuticals: _____

   _____

7. Rehabilitation: _____

   _____

8. Hyaluronic acid: _____

   _____

9. Modality: _____

   _____

10. Polysulfated glycosaminoglycans: _____

   _____

EXERCISE 23.2 MATCHING #1: KEY TERMS AND DEFINITIONS

Instructions: Match each term in column A with its corresponding description in column B by writing the appropriate letter in the space provided.

Column A

1. _____ Thermotherapy

2. _____ Acupressure

3. _____ Passive range of motion (PROM)

4. _____ Hydrotherapy

5. _____ Massage

6. _____ Cryotherapy

7. _____ Low-level laser therapy (LLLT)

8. _____ Myotherapy

9. _____ Neuromuscular electrical stimulation (NMES)

10. _____ Ultrasound (therapeutic)

11. _____ TENS

12. _____ Acupuncture

13. _____ Orthotic

Column B

A. Relief of soft-tissue pain resulting from muscle tension or "knots"

B. Applying firm digital pressure to an acupuncture point for a specific length of time

C. A device used when a patient requires rigid support or needs support in a joint that is not commonly braced

D. The stimulation of tissue with light to achieve a therapeutic effect

E. Stimulation of a specific point on the body to produce a physiologic effect

F. The application of cold to the body to decrease pain and inflammation

G. The use of stretching

H. A systematic and scientific manipulation of the soft tissues of the body for the purpose of obtaining or maintaining health

I. The application of electrical current to elicit a muscle contraction

J. The use of electric current to stimulate the nerves to release endogenous opioids

K. Application of heat to the body to reduce pain

L. The use of sound waves to treat tissue

M. The use of water to promote physical activity

EXERCISE 23.3 MATCHING #2: ALTERNATIVE THERAPIES

Instructions: For the following alternative therapies, identify whether each condition is an indication or contraindication for that therapy by writing an "I" for indication or "C" for contraindication in the space provided.

1. Alternative therapy: Neuromuscular electrical stimulation
   a. _____ Infection
   b. _____ Thrombophlebitis
   c. _____ Mast cell tumor
   d. _____ Muscle atrophy following surgery

2. Alternative therapy: Low-level laser therapy
   a. _____ Degenerative joint disease
   b. _____ Intervertebral disc disease
   c. _____ Soft tissue injury
   d. _____ Treatment of trigger points

3. Alternative therapy: Massage therapy
   a. _____ Bite wound abscess
   b. _____ Toning atrophied muscle
   c. _____ Tendonitis
   d. _____ Surgical site

EXERCISE 23.4 MATCHING #3: REHABILITATION—PHYSICAL DYSFUNCTIONS

Instructions: Match each physical dysfunction in column A with its corresponding description in column B by writing the appropriate letter in the space provided.

Column A

1. _____ Osteoarthritis
2. _____ Inflammation
3. _____ Reduced range of motion
4. _____ Arthrodesis
5. _____ Intervertebral disk disease
6. _____ Muscle tightness or spasm
7. _____ Trigger points
8. _____ Scar tissue
9. _____ Hip dysplasia
10. _____ Ataxia
11. _____ Balance and proprioception
12. _____ Wound healing

Column B

A. A response to tissue injury characterized by pain, swelling, redness, and heat

B. Treated with a balance board exercise

C. Treated with ischemic compression

D. A condition in which discs between the vertebrae of the spine herniate into the space occupied by the spinal cord

E. A decrease in the parameter measured by goniometry

F. Often treated with myotherapy

G. A condition marked by the wearing away of cartilage in a joint

H. Developmental orthopedic disease treated with acupuncture and land treadmill

I. Friction is a massage technique that is used to break up this type of tissue

J. Treated with a clinical application of ultrasound

K. Uncoordinated gait

L. Surgical fusing of a joint together such that all motion at the joint is lost

EXERCISE 23.5 MATCHING #4: REHABILITATION—THERAPEUTIC EXERCISES

Instructions: Match each of the therapeutic exercises in column A with its corresponding benefit in column B by writing the appropriate letter in the space provided.

Column A

1. Proprioceptive exercises

2. Endurance exercises

3. Neuromuscular re-education exercises

4. Balance exercises

5. Strengthening exercises

Column B

A. To decrease muscle atrophy

B. For the cardiovascular system

C. To improve stability

D. To correct posture and gait

E. To improve body awareness

EXERCISE 23.6 TRUE OR FALSE: COMPREHENSIVE

Instructions: Read the following statements and write "T" for true or "F" for false in the blanks provided. If a statement is false, correct the statement to make it true.

1. _____ Complementary and alternative medicine is now mainstream and conventional.

2. _____ Ayurvedic herbal medicines are typically formulated with a single herb.

3. _____ The main advantage of using herbal supplements is that, unlike drugs, they are safe and do not cause side effects.

4. _____ Bulk herbs are most commonly used for herbivores.

5. _____ It is important that herbs are purchased from a reputable source that emphasizes quality control.

6. _____ Capsules and tables are more often used for carnivores.

7. _____ A standardized extract is unlike a drug in that a specific amount of active ingredient is measured instead of measuring the herb itself.

8. _____ Similar to drugs, some herbs have a low margin of safety.

9. _____ At this time, there is no official specialty in veterinary rehabilitation.

10. _____ The least invasive form of acupuncture is dry-needle insertion.

11. _____ A chiropractic vertebral subluxation is most often detected on X-rays.

12. _____ Swimming is the best treatment for strengthening both forelimbs and hindlimbs.

13. _____ When using the underwater treadmill, maximum strengthening is achieved when the water is at the level of the shoulder.

14. _____ Benefits of a land treadmill are greatest when going up- or downhill.

15. _____ Extracorporeal shockwave is high energy focused on an entire muscle group or zone.

16. _____ One of the most common uses for LLLT is to enhance wound healing.

17. _____ Cryotherapy and thermotherapy can be used over areas without sensation as long as the application time is limited to 5 minutes or less.

18. _____ Bruising is reduced by cryotherapy.

19. _____ Complications resulting from the use of assistive devices include skin irritation and ulceration, chewing, breakdown and wear, and lack of patient acceptance.

20. _____ Wheelchairs, while helpful, are not typically well accepted by the patient or client.

EXERCISE 23.7 MULTIPLE CHOICE: COMPREHENSIVE

Instructions: Circle the one correct answer to each of the following questions.

1. Alternative medicine is used
   a. in conjunction with conventional medicine.
   b. in place of conventional medicine.
   c. in place of complementary medicine.
   d. in conjunction with complementary medicine.

2. Chondroitin sulfate has a synergistic effect with
   a. ginger.
   b. aloe.
   c. glucosamine.
   d. echinacea.

3. Herbs are more likely to be toxic to
   a. humans.
   b. dogs.
   c. pigs.
   d. cats.

4. In many veterinary rehabilitation practices, the technician is
   a. relegated to the role of assistant.
   b. required to have completed certification.
   c. limited to restraining animals while manipulations are performed.
   d. the primary caregiver.

5. The most commonly practiced form of herbal medicine in veterinary medicine is
   a. Ayurvedic.
   b. Chinese.
   c. Western.
   d. Native American.

6. Western herbal medicine can be traced back to
   a. China.
   b. Turkey.
   c. Greece.
   d. France.

7. Which Ayurvedic herb is used to treat digestive disorders?
   a. Boswellia
   b. Cinnamon
   c. Licorice
   d. Neem

8. Which of the following is a clinical indication for the use of *Taraxacum officinale*?
   a. To increase mental alertness
   b. To support heart function
   c. As a diuretic
   d. To prevent anxiety

9. Which Chinese herb is used to treat nausea?
   a. Red peony
   b. Ginger
   c. Maitake
   d. Coptis

10. The commonly used Western herb to treat skin irritation is
    a. aloe.
    b. echinacea.
    c. hawthorne.
    d. milk thistle.

11. Research shows that most acupuncture points are located in
    a. peripheral nerves.
    b. joints.
    c. areas of decreased electrical resistance or increased electrical conductivity.
    d. highly vascular tissue.

12. Rehabilitation is primarily used to
   a. treat the physical aspects of a disability.
   b. encompass lifestyle management and physical intervention.
   c. address the physical aspects of a disorder.
   d. cure pulmonary and cardiac disorders.

13. Which of the following modalities would typically not be part of a comprehensive rehabilitation plan?
   a. Hydrotherapy
   b. Laser and ultrasound therapy
   c. Chiropractic
   d. Aromatherapy

14. The massage stroke most commonly used to loosen phlegm congestion in the lungs is
   a. Petrissage
   b. Effleurage
   c. Tapotement
   d. Coupage

15. The massage stroke most commonly used to stimulate nerve endings is
   a. petrissage.
   b. effleurage.
   c. tapotement.
   d. coupage.

16. Pneumo-acupuncture is used solely used to treat
   a. muscle spasms.
   b. inflammation.
   c. atrophy.
   d. pain.

17. It is felt that therapeutic ultrasound works by producing
   a. sound waves.
   b. a magnetic field.
   c. electrical impulses.
   d. vibration.

18. A contraindication for electro-acupuncture is
   a. a history of seizures.
   b. spondylomyelopathy.
   c. renal disease.
   d. electrolyte imbalance.

EXERCISE 23.8 FILL-IN-THE-BLANK: COMPREHENSIVE

Instructions: Fill in each of the spaces provided with the missing word or words that complete the sentence.

1. Information about herbs can be found in the publication called the _____.

2. Cryotherapy causes _____.

3. In general, herbs tend to be less _____ than many drugs because the therapeutic substances are not as _____.

4. _____ is a protected term referring to the physical aspects of treating a disability or disorder, while rehabilitation may encompass lifestyle management.

5. The physiologic effects of acupuncture include both _____ and _____ effects, as the therapy stimulates both the central and peripheral nervous systems.

6. A _____ is used for muscle mass measurement.

7. _____ acupuncture points, which make up 67% of all points, are considered motor points.

8. _____ implantation provides long-term stimulation for chronic conditions.

9. Veterinary spinal manipulative therapy is similar to _____ in humans.

10. The hallmark, or "triad," of signs that occur with a subluxation includes _____, _____, and _____.

11. During hydrotherapy, _____ can be added with the use of jets.

12. _____ is particularly important for first-time VSMT patients because they are unsure about the process and may be nervous or frightened.

13. A(n) _____ is used to measure the range of motion (both flexion and extension) of all distal joints, including the carpus, elbow, shoulder, tarsus, stifle, and hip.

14. The goal of teaching patients to use the treadmill is to have them be comfortable getting on at one end and off at the other end when done, and _____ in between.

15. Sports massage can be classified into _____ massage and _____ maintenance massage.

16. _____ is a massage technique in which finger pressure is applied to acupuncture points.

17. _____ is the most commonly used massage stroke in animals.

18. The duration of a small animal massage is usually _____, and for a large animal it is approximately _____.

19. TENS is an acronym for _____ electrical nerve stimulation.

20. A voluntary muscle contraction involves slow-twitch, type _____ muscle fibers, whereas an electrically induced muscle contraction involves fast-twitch, type _____ fibers.

21. The technician's role in NMES is to shave and clean the skin with alcohol, apply gel, attach the pads, and use the NMES machine to obtain a strong, yet pain-free, _____.

22. TENS is the use of electric current to relieve _____ and _____.

23. LLLT decreases _____ by releasing beta-endorphins and serotonin and decreases _____ by inhibiting prostaglandin synthesis, thereby reducing inflammatory mediators.

24. To reach deeper tissue using LLLT, the laser should be set to a higher _____.

25. Strenth testing is measured on a scale of ___ to ___: Normal strength is ___/___.

26. PEMF is an acronym for _____.

27. The newest veterinary specialty recognized by the AVMA is _____.

28. Photobiomodulation is also known as _____.

EXERCISE 23.9 CASE STUDY #1: REHABILITATION AND COMPLEMENTARY MODALITIES

A Greyhound is being treated at your clinic for pain caused by trigger points. The veterinarian decides massage would be beneficial, and the owner has brought in her pet for its first massage session.

1. Explain to the owner the basic massage techniques that will be performed on her pet. _____

_____

_____

_____

EXERCISE 23.10 CASE STUDY #2: REHABILITATION AND COMPLEMENTARY MODALITIES

A 7-year-old, spayed, female Dachshund was diagnosed with intervertebral disc disease (IVDD) and underwent surgery to correct a compression at the lumbosacral junction.

1. What general types of complementary modalities might be used in the care of this patient, and what is the purpose of each modality?_____

_____

_____

EXERCISE 23.11 CASE STUDY #3: REHABILITATION AND COMPLEMENTARY MODALITIES

A 4-year-old, 65-pound German Shepherd is recovering from intervertebral disc disease (IVDD) and has minimal use of his hindlimbs. His owners are struggling with carrying him outside to urinate and defecate.

1. List two mobility aids that would benefit this patient, and discuss why each would be of benefit.

_____

_____

_____

EXERCISE 23.12 CASE STUDY #4: COMMONLY USED NUTRACEUTICALS AND CHONDROPROTECTANTS

The veterinary practice in which you work is interested in educating staff about supplements that can be used with dogs experiencing joint pain and dysfunction. The lead vet has requested that you provide a presentation on commonly used nutraceuticals and chondoprotectants.

1. Create a list with the names of supplements and their functions. Indicate which are not administered orally.

_____

_____

_____

EXERCISE 23.13 CASE STUDY #5: REHABILITATION AND COMPLEMENTARY MODALITIES

Bitsy, a 6-year-old mixed breed, has been adopted via a rescue group that found her in a hoarding situation. She is making very good progress in socialization and mental health and is improving her physical condition. However, she is still not used to being able to stretch and move at will, and is consequently not building muscle mass readily.

1. What treatments do you think the vet will suggest to address Bitsy's muscle atrophy?

_____

_____

_____

_____

24 Fluid Therapy and Transfusion Medicine

LEARNING OBJECTIVES

When you have completed this chapter, you will be able to:
1. Recognize, define, and apply all key terms in the chapter.
2. Explain the indications for fluid therapy and describe the body fluid compartments, including movement of fluids between these compartments.
3. Compare and contrast crystalloid and colloid fluids and describe the uses for and characteristics of each.
4. Do the following regarding the administration of fluids and fluid therapy additives:
   - Discuss the objectives of each phase of fluid therapy and the specific products and administration rates used during each phase.
   - Compare and contrast the indications for and techniques used to administer fluids by the intravenous, subcutaneous, intraosseous, and enteral routes.
   - Explain the indications for and techniques used to administer potassium chloride, dextrose, and sodium bicarbonate.
5. Do the following regarding monitoring and complications of fluid therapy:
   - Describe the methods used to monitor the effectiveness of fluid therapy.
   - Discuss common complications of fluid therapy, including appropriate interventions.
6. Do the following regarding transfusion medicine:
   - Describe the indications for blood, plasma, and blood component transfusion.
   - Discuss the selection and care of blood donors.
   - Explain pretransfusion testing, including blood typing, antibody screening, and cross-matching.
7. Do the following regarding collection techniques, blood products, and product administration:
   - Describe the techniques used to collect blood from dogs, cats, and horses.
   - List blood products, including the indications for and benefits provided by each.
   - Describe the technique used to administer blood products to a patient, including calculation of administration rates.
   - Discuss patient monitoring during blood transfusions and recognition and management of transfusion reactions.

EXERCISE 24.1 FILL-IN-THE-BLANK #1: TERMS AND DEFINITIONS

Instructions: Fill in each of the spaces provided with the missing word or words that complete the sentence.

1. Transfusion reactions from acute allergic _____ can include erythema, urticaria, and pruritus or anaphylaxis.

2. If DEA 1.1–positive blood is transfused to a dog with anti-DEA 1.1 antibodies, _____

   and _____ will result.

3. A solution composed of electrolytes and water is a _____ fluid.

4. Fluid resuscitation is aimed at restoration of vascular volume in an effort to reverse _____ and/or a shock state.

5. The _____ is the amount of fluid needed to fulfill the physiologic requirement for water.

6. Colloids may have the ability to move fluid from the interstitium into the vascular space by increasing the

_____ of blood.

7. The _____ is a large volume of fluid administered quickly.

8. Dehydration + Ongoing losses + Maintenance = _____.

9. Blood products that can be processed from whole blood include platelet-rich plasma, cryoprecipitate, and platelet

concentrate. Of these, _____ has a shelf life of one year.

10. Blood transfusion is likely to be necessary if _____ drops to below 20% to 25% during
an acute bleeding episode, though the decision should be based on the full clinical picture.

EXERCISE 24.2 MATCHING #1: BODY FLUID COMPARTMENTS

Instructions: Match each body fluid compartment term in column A with its corresponding statement in column B by writing the appropriate letter in the space provided.

Column A

1. _____ TBW

2. _____ Cell membrane

3. _____ ICF

4. _____ ECF

5. _____ Vascular endothelium

6. _____ ISF

7. _____ IVF

Column B

A. Separates the ISF and IVF

B. Approximately two-thirds of TBW

C. Approximately 60% of body weight

D. Approximately one-fourth of the ECF

E. Separates the ICF and ECF

F. Approximately three-fourths of ECF

G. Approximately one-third of TBW

EXERCISE 24.3 MATCHING #2: BODY TONICITY OF INTRAVENOUS FLUIDS

Instructions: Match each intravenous fluid in column A with its corresponding tonicity in column B by writing the appropriate letter in the space provided. (Note that responses may be used more than once.)

Column A

1. _____ Dextrose 5% in water

2. _____ 0.45% NaCl

3. _____ 7% NaCl

4. _____ Normosol M

5. _____ 0.9% Saline

6. _____ 0.45% Sodium chloride

7. _____ Lactated Ringer solution

8. _____ 3% NaCl

9. _____ Plasmalyte 148

10. _____ Plasmalyte 56

11. _____ Normosol R

Column B

A. Hypotonic

B. Isotonic

C. Hypertonic

EXERCISE 24.4 MATCHING #3: BLOOD GROUP FACTORS

Instructions: Match each species in column A with its corresponding blood group factors in column B by writing the appropriate letter in the space provided.

Column A

1. _____ Canine

2. _____ Equine

3. _____ Feline

4. _____ Cattle

Column B

A. Eight, including Aa, Ca, and Qa

B. More than 70; negative for factor J

C. Many, including DEA 1.1, 1.2, 3, 4, 5, and 7

D. A, B, and AB

EXERCISE 24.5 MATCHING #4: IDEAL AND UNIVERSAL BLOOD DONORS

Instructions: Match each species donor in column A with its corresponding description in column B by writing the appropriate letter in the space provided. (Note that not all responses will be used.)

Column A

1. _____ Universal canine donor

2. _____ Ideal equine donor

3. _____ Universal feline donor

4. _____ Ideal bovine donor

Column B

A. 3, 5, and 7 negative

B. No universal donor for this species

C. J negative

D. A negative

E. Ca and Pa negative

F. Positive for only the DEA 4 antigen

G. J, M, and R negative

H. Aa and Qa negative

EXERCISE 24.6 MATCHING #5: BLOOD PRODUCTS

Instructions: Match each blood product in column A with the corresponding primary indication for its use in column B by writing the appropriate letter in the space provided.

Column A

1. _____ Washed RBCs

2. _____ Packed RBCs

3. _____ Fresh plasma or fresh-frozen plasma

4. _____ Platelet-rich plasma or platelet concentrate

5. _____ Cryoprecipitate

6. _____ Hyperimmune plasma

Column B

A. Thrombocytopenia

B. Neonatal foals with failure of passive transfer

C. Anemia

D. Replace some coagulation factors

E. Neonatal isoerythrolysis

F. von Willebrand disease

Instructions: Read the following statements and write "T" for true or "F" for false in the blanks provided. If a statement is false, correct the statement to make it true.

1. _____ The circulating blood volume of a horse is approximately 40 to 60 mL/kg body weight.

2. _____ Both water and electrolytes are able to move freely across all fluid space barriers (the cell membrane and vascular endothelium) and so distribute throughout the total-body water.

3. _____ Colloids tend to remain in the vascular space.

4. _____ Dextrose 5% in water is an example of an isotonic fluid.

5. _____ Normosol R would be an appropriate fluid choice for a patient with severe acidemia.

6. _____ Administration of hypertonic saline IV will promote rapid and long-lasting expansion of the vascular volume.

7. _____ Routine cross-matching evaluates agglutination reactions but does not test for hemolytic reactions.

8. _____ Arterial blood pressure is an accurate indicator of response to fluid resuscitation.

9. _____ When calculating the ongoing losses so that the fluid administration rate can be increased appropriately, normal urinary losses should be included in this calculation.

10. _____ Pain or irritation when an IV catheter is flushed is a sign that the vein is inflamed.

11. _____ An advantage of subcutaneous fluid administration is that this route works well for resuscitation, replacement, or maintenance.

12. _____ Subcutaneous fluids can be given by a client at home.

13. _____ Only certain medications that are safe for IV administration can be given IO.

14. _____ Sodium bicarbonate is commonly used to treat a variety of conditions that lead to acidosis.

15. _____ Sodium bicarbonate can be used for severe cases of hyperkalemia to promote a shift of potassium into the cells.

16. _____ A normal blood pressure means everything is fine.

17. _____ If a patient has severe, acute hemorrhaging, the packed cell volume (PCV) will be decreased.

18. _____ The primary goal of blood transfusion is to improve oxygen delivery to the tissues.

19. _____ Dogs do not have naturally occurring antibodies to erythrocyte antigens, and so a reaction is less likely following a transfusion of red blood cells.

20. _____ Like dogs, cats do not have naturally occurring antibodies to erythrocyte antigens, so a reaction following a first transfusion is unlikely.

21. _____ Glass blood-collection bottles are preferred over bags because they preserve blood cells more effectively.

22. _____To achieve optimal RBC viability during blood storage, blood bags should be weighed to ensure adequate fill (blood-to-anticoagulant ratio).

23. _____Transfusion reactions will not occur as long as major and minor crossmatches indicate compatibility.

EXERCISE 24.8 MULTIPLE CHOICE: COMPREHENSIVE

Instructions: Circle the one correct answer to each of the following questions.

1. The circulating blood volume as a proportion of total body weight (mL/kg) is the lowest in a
   a. dog.
   b. horse.
   c. cow.
   d. cat.

2. When 0.9% saline solution is administered intravenously within a short time,_____ will remain in the vascular space.
   a. one-quarter.
   b. one-third.
   c. one-half.
   d. most of it.

3. Which of the following fluids is *not* a hypotonic fluid?
   a. 0.45% Saline.
   b. Normosol M.
   c. Plasmalyte 148.
   d. D5W.

4. Hypotonic fluids are used to treat
   a. shock.
   b. hypernatremia.
   c. hypokalemia.
   d. metabolic acidosis.

5. Which of the following fluids has an acidifying effect?
   a. LRS.
   b. 0.9% Saline.
   c. Normosol R.
   d. Plasmalyte 148.

6. Three percent or 7% hypertonic saline is used to treat
   a. heart failure.
   b. kidney failure.
   c. head trauma.
   d. hypernatremia.

7. Which of the following fluids would increase intravascular oncotic pressure in a patient with hypoproteinemia?
   a. Hetastarch.
   b. Normosol M.
   c. Plasmalyte 148.
   d. D5W.

8. The shock dose of isotonic crystalloid fluids in a cat is (in mL/kg body weight)
   a. 2 to 4.
   b. 10 to 15.
   c. 40 to 60.
   d. 80 to 90.

9. What is the correct catheter placement for a patient requiring multiple blood samples to be taken over a period of time or that needs multiple medications given by constant rate infusion?
   a. Cephalic.
   b. Central line.
   c. Butterfly.
   d. Peripheral.

10. Which of the following devices is often used to decrease the risk of fluid overload?
    a. Buretrol.
    b. Administration line filter.
    c. Carboy.
    d. 10 drops/mL drip set.

11. Fluids administered subcutaneously are usually absorbed in approximately
    a. 1 to 2 hours.
    b. 2 to 4 hours.
    c. 6 to 8 hours.
    d. 12 to 24 hours.

12. Even though it is isotonic, which of the following fluids can cause discomfort when given subcutaneously owing to its acidic pH?
    a. Lactated Ringer solution.
    b. Plasmalyte 148.
    c. Normosol R.
    d. Dextrose 5% in water.

13. Which of the following routes of fluid administration is used in neonates because it has essentially the same effect as IV administration but does not require catheterization of a vein?
    a. Intramuscular,
    b. Subcutaneous.
    c. Enteral (via stomach tube).
    d. Intraosseous.

14. Enteral fluids are often used to treat large-bowel impaction in
    a. cattle.
    b. cats.
    c. dogs.
    d. horses.

15. The combination of PU/PD, cardiac arrhythmias, and severe muscle weakness is very suggestive of
    a. hypokalemia.
    b. hypoglycemia.
    c. lactic acidosis.
    d. dehydration.

16. During the resuscitation phase of IV fluid therapy, arterial systolic blood pressure should be maintained at approximately
    a. 50 to 80 mm Hg.
    b. 80 to 110 mm Hg.
    c. 110 to 140 mm Hg.
    d. 140 to 170 mm Hg.

17. Given the decreased tolerance for sodium load in patients with heart and kidney disease, _____ may be more ideally suited to replace deficits or maintain hydration in these patients.
    a. hypotonic fluids.
    b. fresh plasma.
    c. isotonic fluids.
    d. hypertonic fluids.

18. A significant complication of fluid therapy is fluid overload. Of greatest concern in these patients is the possibility of
    a. coagulation abnormalities.
    b. cavitary effusion.
    c. pulmonary edema.
    d. peripheral edema.

19. During an acute bleeding episode, a blood transfusion is necessary if the PCV drops below
    a. 12% to 15%.
    b. 15% to 20%.
    c. 20% to 25%.
    d. 25% to 30%.

20. A blood plasma transfusion is not indicated for the treatment of
    a. low albumin.
    b. a blood-clotting disorder.
    c. failure of passive transfer of immunity in foals.
    d. anemia.

21. Canine blood-typing cards are used to detect
    a. DEA 1.1.
    b. DEA 1.2.
    c. DEA 4.
    d. DEA 7.

22. Which of the following statements regarding blood transfusions is most accurate?
    a. Transfusion of type A blood into a type B cat will result in decreased life span of transfused cells.
    b. Transfusion of type B blood into a type A cat is expected to cause a severe, potentially fatal hemolytic reaction.
    c. Transfusion of type B blood into a type AB cat is not expected to cause a reaction.
    d. Transfusion of type AB blood into any cat should not cause a reaction because this is the universal donor blood type in cats.

23. A "major crossmatch" detects
    a. reactions of a recipient's plasma with its own RBCs.
    b. reactions between donor RBCs and recipient plasma.
    c. reactions between donor plasma and recipient RBCs.
    d. reactions of a donor's plasma with its own RBCs.

24. The maximum recommended blood donation for dogs expressed as a percent of the blood volume is
    a. 5% to 10%.
    b. 10% to 15%.
    c. 15% to 20%.
    d. 20% to 25%.

25. Donor blood plasma is considered to be fresh plasma if used within _____ hours of collection.
    a. 4.
    b. 8.
    c. 12.
    d. 24.

26. When transfusing blood, it is usually given concurrently with isotonic crystalloid fluids. Which of the following fluids should not be used for this purpose because it can result in activation of the coagulation cascade?
    a. Normosol R.
    b. Plasmalyte 148.
    c. 0.9% Saline.
    d. Lactated Ringer solution.

27. Using the rule of thumb provided, if you want to raise the PCV of a 25-kg patient by 10%, you should give approximately
    a. 250 mL of whole blood or packed RBCs.
    b. 500 mL of whole blood or 250 mL of packed RBCs.
    c. 250 mL of whole blood or 500 mL of packed RBCs.
    d. 500 mL of whole blood or packed RBCs.

Instructions: Fill in each of the spaces provided with the missing word or words that complete the sentence.

1. The circulating blood volume of a dog is estimated to be approximately _____ to _____ mL/kg body weight.

2. The two main categories of fluids based on the size of their solute molecules are _____ and _____.

3. A 23% saline solution must be _____ before giving it IV to avoid osmotic injury to the tissues.

4. The product "VetStarch" is a synthetic _____ that has a decreased impact on blood coagulation than hetastarch.

5. The maintenance fluid administration rate includes losses from the following three sources: (a) the _____ system, (b) the _____, and (c) inappropriate _____ losses.

6. A route of fluid administration used in small animals but not usually in large animals is _____. A route of fluid administration used in large animals but not in small animals is via a(n) _____ tube.

7. Subcutaneously administered fluids should have an osmotic pressure that is approximately _____ to the extracellular fluid.

8. When tissues don't receive enough oxygen because of decreased tissue perfusion, the levels of _____ increase.

9. Volumes determined as "shock doses" for different fluids should be titrated based on _____.

10. Impaired blood coagulation is a possible side effect of administration of the synthetic colloid _____.

11. During severe, acute hemorrhage, the total protein (TP) will decrease before the packed cell volume (PCV) because of contraction of the _____.

12. The primary goal of blood transfusion is to increase the _____-carrying capacity of the blood.

13. The ideal equine blood donor is negative for factors _____ and _____.

14. The ideal bovine donor should be negative for factor _____.

15. If incompatible blood is given to a horse for a first transfusion, it takes approximately _____ to _____ days for RBC antibodies to form.

16. If a blood donation is taken from a dog in an amount equivalent to 20% of the blood volume, _____ to _____ mL/kg intravenous crystalloid fluids should be given to compensate for the fluid loss.

17. Concerning anticoagulants used for blood collection, if blood is going to be stored, either _____ or _____ anticoagulant should be used. If blood will be transfused immediately, _____ is acceptable. *(Note: The use of abbreviations is acceptable.)*

18. Donor blood plasma that is frozen within _____ hour(s) of collection and is less than _____ month(s) old is considered to be fresh-frozen plasma. Otherwise, it is considered to be frozen plasma.

19. When giving blood to hypothermic patients or those receiving large volumes of blood, refrigerated blood should be warmed to between _____ ° C and _____ ° C.

20. For patients with hemorrhage, the volume of blood to be transfused can be calculated based on the estimated blood _____, whereas for patients with chronic anemia, it can be calculated based on the _____.

EXERCISE 24.10 CASE STUDY #1: IV FLUID THERAPY

A 4-year-old, 50-pound, neutered male Basset Hound presents for anorexia and vomiting. He is estimated to be 6% dehydrated. The attending veterinarian orders a diagnostic workup, including blood work, urinalysis, and abdominal radiographs. She also orders intravenous lactated Ringer solution. She asks you to calculate the infusion and drip rates based on the sum of (a) the volume necessary to correct dehydration over the first 18 hours, (b) the standard maintenance rate, and (c) the amount necessary to replace ongoing losses.

1. Calculate the fluid deficit of this patient based on the estimated level of dehydration.

_____ mL

2. Calculate the fluid infusion rate in mL/hour for replacement of this deficit over 18 hours.

_____ mL/hour

3. Using the following formula, calculate the daily maintenance needs for this patient: 132*body weight (kg)(3/4)

(Note: This is accomplished on a multifunction calculator by taking the body weight in kg, multiplying it by itself twice (wt*wt*wt), then pressing the square root button twice, and, finally, multiplying the result by 132.)

_____ mL/day

4. Now calculate the hourly administration rate for maintenance.

_____ mL/hour

5. Calculate this patient's infusion rate (in mL/hour) necessary for replacement of the deficit and for maintenance.

_____ mL/hour

6. Calculate the drip rate in drops/second when using a drip set with a delivery rating of 10 drops/mL.

_____ gtt/second

7. During the first 6 hours, the patient vomited several times into two absorbent pads. The pads by themselves weighed 160 grams each; including the vomitus, the two pads weighed 580 grams. Approximately how much volume (mL) did this patient lose through vomiting?

_____ mL/hour

8. Adjust the infusion rate in mL/hour to replace this loss over the next 6 hours (as well as to replace the deficit and provide maintenance).

_____ mL/hour

9. Finally, calculate the drip rate in drops/second.

_____ gtt/second

EXERCISE 24.11 CASE STUDY #2: IV FLUID THERAPY AND TRANSFUSION THERAPY

A 2-year-old, neutered male mix-breed dog weighing 20 kg is presented after being hit by a car. He is estimated to have lost approximately 30% of his blood volume and is shocky. The doctor has ordered a variety of interventions, including IV fluid therapy and a transfusion of whole blood.

1. Calculate the estimated volume of blood lost (in mL) by this patient.

_____ mL

2. By this estimation, you determine that this patient needs about 1 unit of whole blood. During the first 10 to 20 minutes, there was no sign of a transfusion reaction. Based on this data, the doctor would like you to administer the whole blood at a rate of 20 mL/kg/hour. Calculate the infusion rate (in mL/hour) for this patient.

_____ mL/hour

3. Now calculate the drip rate in gtt/second. You are using a standard blood administration set rated at 10 gtt/mL.

_____ gtt/second

4. The donor dog at your clinic weighs 70 pounds. Calculate the maximum amount of blood you can collect from this donor using the rule of thumb in the text, and determine if this will be enough blood to meet this patient's needs.

_____ mL

Yes, it will be enough to meet this patient's needs. ❏

No, it will not be enough to meet this patient's needs. ❏

25 Emergency and Critical Care Nursing

LEARNING OBJECTIVES

When you have completed this chapter, you will be able to:

1. Pronounce, define, and spell all key terms in this chapter.
2. Triage a patient over the phone and upon arrival at the veterinary hospital.
3. Do the following regarding emergency and critical care assessment, initial diagnostics, and first aid:
   - Assess hydration and recognize hypovolemia in critical care patients.
   - Identify the diagnostic tests most commonly used in emergency and critical care settings.
   - Explain the principles of basic first aid.
   - Identify the ideal location for an emergency care station and/or resuscitation area and explain how to set up and stock a crash cart.
4. Compare and contrast the different types of shock, explain how each is treated, and identify and explain advanced emergency techniques most commonly performed on small animals.
5. Discuss disorders of the respiratory system seen in critically ill small animal patients.
6. Do the following regarding cardiopulmonary resuscitation:
   - List the common causes of cardiopulmonary arrest and explain the principles of cardiopulmonary resuscitation (CPR).
   - Describe the principles of basic and advanced life support in small animals and care of the post-arrest patient.
7. Describe methods used to monitor critically ill patients and the principles of effective patient monitoring.
8. Identify key aspects of recumbent patient care.
9. List common small animal emergencies and discuss appropriate patient stabilization and treatment.
10. Do the following regarding canine and feline electrocardiography:
    - List the indications for and discuss the principles of electrocardiography.
    - Explain the processes used to acquire, analyze, and interpret an electrocardiogram.
    - Identify and explain the significance of common cardiac arrhythmias.
11. Describe initial management, assessment, diagnostic, and treatment procedures for common equine emergencies.
12. Describe initial management, assessment, diagnostic, and treatment procedures for common food animal emergencies.

EXERCISE 25.1 FILL-IN-THE-BLANK #1: TERMS AND DEFINITIONS

1. Diagnosis of _____ is made when the patient meets physiologic criteria including tachycardia, tachypnea, fever, and marked increases or decreases in white blood cell count.

2. Cattle are at risk for _____, or inflammation of the uterus.

3. Clinical signs of _____ include gagging, retching, and excessive drooling.

4. _____ is often secondary to external trauma to the chest cavity that allows influx of air into the pleural space, which collapses the lung and prevents re-expansion.

5. _____ is complete cessation of all mechanical and electrical activity in the heart.

6. The term _____ refers to any condition that causes abdominal pain.

7. If gas fails to be expelled from the rumen, bloat, or _____, may occur.

8. _____ is the clinical term for a functional disorder of the small intestines in which motility is lost.

9. _____ is a rapid, irregularly irregular rhythm with supraventricular morphology QRS complexes, no identifiable P waves, and the presence of fibrillatory waves (f waves).

10. _____ results from excess acid in the blood caused by abnormal metabolism, excessive acid intake, renal retention, or excessive loss of bicarbonate.

11. If the SIRS response progresses to microvascular clotting, it can lead to permanent failure of the kidneys, liver, lungs, brain, and heart, a condition called _____.

12. The inflammatory response associated with _____ causes increased vasodilatation, which often presents as bright red mucous membranes and bounding pulses.

13. The clinical term for difficult birth is _____.

14. The pattern of concurrent thrombosis and bleeding is called _____, and is among the most serious complications of shock.

15. APCs are differentiated from _____ by their wide and bizarre QRS shape and by the presence or absence of a P wave.

16. A _____ is a device that uses obstetric wire to cut a dead fetus into smaller parts that can be extracted more easily.

17. Cyanotic (blue) membranes provide a tremendous amount of insight into a patient's degree of _____.

18. Ventricular fibrillation is often preceded by a rapid pulseless _____.

19. The clinical term for restriction of blood supply is _____.

20. During patient assessment, it is important to differentiate a dehydrated patient from a _____ patient, a condition marked by a loss of intravascular volume commonly occurring with shock, trauma, hemorrhage, or profuse vomiting and diarrhea.

21. Animals that cannot stand are referred to as _____.

22. Abnormal impulses originating from the atrial myocardium instead of the SA node are called _____.

23. If endotoxins are absorbed from septic secretions within the udder, endotoxemia can result, and the condition is termed _____.

24. Patients with _____ are suffering from a stomach that becomes twisted because it is full of gas. The animal presents with acute signs ranging from abdominal distention, agitation, repeated retching, lateral recumbency, and shock.

25. If the patient is in severe respiratory distress because of an upper airway obstruction, a temporary _____ should be performed immediately before the physical examination.

26. _____ anesthesia can be useful for reducing the pain associated with vaginal manipulation and for decreasing the force of uterine contractions so that vaginal manipulation of the fetus can be accomplished.

27. The condition of increased nitrogenous wastes in the blood is _____.

28. Urethral obstruction due to _____ (urinary calculi or stones) is common in male ruminants.

EXERCISE 25.2 DEFINITIONS: KEY TERMS

Instructions: Define each term in your own words.

1. Borborygmi: _____

   _____

2. Capillary refill time: _____

   _____

3. Eructation: _____

   _____

4. Stridor: _____

   _____

5. Syncope: _____

   _____

6. Tachycardia: _____

   _____

7. Tachypnea: _____

   _____

8. Tympany: _____

   _____

9. Toxin: _____

   _____

10. Urethral process: _____

    _____

11. Uterine prolapse: _____

    _____

12. Uterine torsion: _____

_____

13. Endometrial: _____

_____

14. Jugular vein: _____

_____

15. Perineal area: _____

16. _____

EXERCISE 25.3 MATCHING #1: TERMS AND DEFINITIONS RELATED TO PROCEDURES

Instructions: Match each term in column A with its corresponding definition in column B by writing the appropriate letter in the space provided.

Column A

1. _____ Abdominocentesis
2. _____ Cardiopulmonary resuscitation
3. _____ Chest tube
4. _____ Defibrillation
5. _____ Electrocardiogram
6. _____ Fetatome
7. _____ Fetotomy
8. _____ Primary survey
9. _____ Pulse oximeter
10. _____ Regional nerve block
11. _____ Rumenostomy
12. _____ Thoracocentesis
13. _____ Tracheostomy
14. _____ Tracheotomy
15. _____ Transfaunation
16. _____ Triage
17. _____ Tube cystostomy
18. _____ Urethrostomy

Column B

A. The transfer of beneficial microorganisms from the rumen of one individual to another

B. A procedure in which a relatively small amount of local anesthetic is injected near a nerve causing desensitization of a larger area of the body

C. A tube inserted into the pleural space

D. A device that is used to cut a fetus into smaller parts that can be extracted vaginally more easily

E. Aspiration of fluid by inserting a needle in the pleural space

F. Creation of a permanent opening from the skin into the urethra

G. A response to cardiac arrest

H. The brief, targeted exam performed to determine the most important aspects of the patient's condition

I. Creation of a permanent opening from the skin to the trachea

J. Aspiration of fluid by inserting a needle in the peritoneal cavity

K. Placement of a catheter through the abdominal wall and into the bladder

L. A procedure in which a dead fetus is cut into smaller pieces so that it can be extracted vaginally

M. The treatment for ventricular fibrillation

N. Sorting patients according to the severity of an injury

O. A visual representation of the electrical activity of the heart

P. Creation of a temporary opening from the skin to the trachea

Q. Creation of the permanent opening from the skin to the rumen

R. A monitor used to measure oxygen saturation of hemoglobin

EXERCISE 25.4 MATCHING #2: BREATHING PATTERNS

Instructions: Match each breathing pattern in column A with its corresponding description in column B by writing the appropriate letter in the space provided.

Column A

1. _____ Restrictive breathing

2. _____ Bradypnea

3. _____ Labored breathing

4. _____ Orthopnea

5. _____ Tachypnea

Column B

A. Condition of maintaining a specific posture to ease breathing

B. Decreased respiratory rate

C. Increased respiratory rate

D. Fast, short, and shallow breaths

E. Prolonged and deep respirations

EXERCISE 25.5 MATCHING #3: MENTATION

Instructions: Match each term used to describe mentation in column A with its corresponding description in column B by writing the appropriate letter in the space provided.

Column A

1. _____ Normal

2. _____ Dull

3. _____ Obtunded

4. _____ Stuporous

5. _____ Comatose

Column B

A. Only reacts to noxious stimuli

B. Not eager to interact with the environment

C. Interacts with the environment and is alert

D. Unresponsive to any stimuli

E. Reacts to stimuli more slowly than normal

EXERCISE 25.6 MATCHING #4: EVALUATION OF PUPILS AND POSTURE

Instructions: Match each pupillary assessment or postural finding in column A with its corresponding significance in column B by writing the appropriate letter in the space provided.

Column A

1. _____ Fixed and dilated pupils

2. _____ Rigid forelimbs and flexed hindlimbs with normal mentation

3. _____ Anisocoria

4. _____ Rigid forelimbs and flaccid hindlimbs when in lateral recumbency is typical

5. _____ Unresponsive midrange pupils

6. _____ Extreme rigidity of all four limbs with arching of the neck and back

Column B

A. A lack of connection between the forebrain and brainstem

B. Irreversible midbrain lesion

C. Schiff-Sherrington, associated with a T3 to L3 spinal lesion

D. Lesion in the medulla

E. Injury to the cerebellum

F. Injury of the cerebrum

EXERCISE 25.7 MATCHING #5: TYPES OF SHOCK

Instructions: Match each type of shock in column A with its corresponding cause in column B by writing the appropriate letter in the space provided.

Column A

1. _____ Septic shock

2. _____ Distributive shock

3. _____ Hypovolemic shock

4. _____ Cardiogenic shock

5. _____ Obstructive shock

Column B

A. Impaired venous return to the heart

B. Decreased circulating blood volume

C. Severe infection

D. Vasodilation and pooling of blood in the capillaries

E. Decreased cardiac output

EXERCISE 25.8 MATCHING #6: ABNORMAL RHYTHMS AND TREATMENTS

Instructions: Match each abnormal rhythm associated with cardiac arrest in column A with the drug(s) used to treat the abnormality in column B by writing the appropriate letter(s) in the space provided. (Note that there may be more than one correct response and that responses may be used more than once.)

Column A

1. _____ Ventricular tachycardia

2. _____ Asystole

3. _____ PEA

4. _____ Bradycardia

5. _____ Vagally mediated arrest or AV block

Column B

A. Epinephrine

B. Atropine

C. Vasopressin

D. Lidocaine

EXERCISE 25.9 MATCHING #7: DRUGS USED FOLLOWING CARDIOPULMONARY ARREST (CPA)

Instructions: Match each abnormality seen in patients that experience cardiac arrest in column A with the drug(s) used to treat the condition in column B by writing the appropriate letter(s) in the space provided. (Note that there may be more than one correct response.)

Column A

1. _____ Hypotension

2. _____ Pulmonary edema

3. _____ Cerebral edema

4. _____ Low cardiac output

5. _____ Hyperkalemia

Column B

A. Furosemide

B. Dobutamine

C. Mannitol

D. Vasopressin

E. Dopamine

F. Calcium gluconate

EXERCISE 25.10 MATCHING #8: ELECTROCARDIOGRAPHIC WAVEFORMS

Instructions: Match each waveform in column A with its corresponding significance in column B by writing the appropriate letter in the space provided.

Column A

1. _____ P wave

2. _____ PR interval

3. _____ QRS complex

4. _____ ST segment

5. _____ T wave

Column B

A. Time interval from ventricular depolarization to repolarization

B. Ventricular depolarization

C. Time it takes for the impulse to conduct through the AV node

D. Ventricular repolarization

E. Atrial depolarization

EXERCISE 25.11 PHOTO QUIZ: ECG TRACINGS

Instructions: Match each ECG tracing with the name corresponding to the cardiac rhythm by writing the name in the space provided. Then summarize the significance of each rhythm.

A. Normal sinus rhythm
B. Sinus arrhythmia
C. Atrial premature complexes (APCs)
D. Atrial tachycardia
E. Atrial fibrillation
F. Ventricular premature complexes (VPCs)
G. Ventricular tachycardia
H. Ventricular fibrillation
I. Atrial standstill
J. Second-degree AV block
K. Third-degree (complete) AV block

1. Name, reading summary, and significance of this rhythm: _____

_____

2. Name, reading summary, and significance of this rhythm:_____

_____

3. Name, reading summary, and significance of this rhythm:_____

_____

4. Name, reading summary, and significance of this rhythm:_____

_____

5. Name, reading summary, and significance of this rhythm:_____

_____

6. Name, reading summary, and significance of this rhythm:_____

_____

7. Name, reading summary, and significance of this rhythm:_____

_____

8. Name, reading summary, and significance of this rhythm:_____

_____

9. Name, reading summary, and significance of this rhythm:_____

_____

10. Name, reading summary, and significance of this rhythm:_____

_____

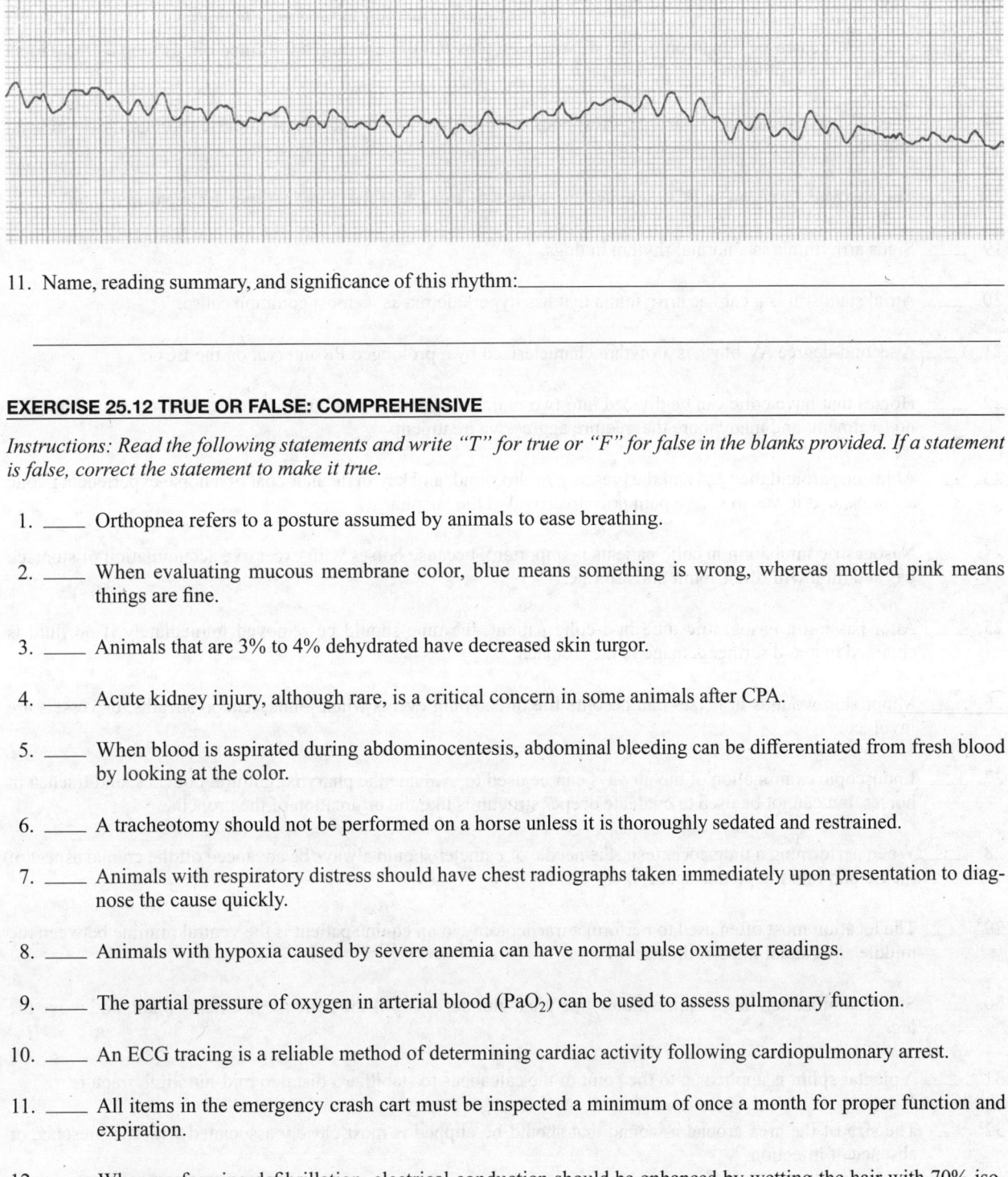

11. Name, reading summary, and significance of this rhythm:_____

_____

EXERCISE 25.12 TRUE OR FALSE: COMPREHENSIVE

Instructions: Read the following statements and write "T" for true or "F" for false in the blanks provided. If a statement is false, correct the statement to make it true.

1. ____ Orthopnea refers to a posture assumed by animals to ease breathing.

2. ____ When evaluating mucous membrane color, blue means something is wrong, whereas mottled pink means things are fine.

3. ____ Animals that are 3% to 4% dehydrated have decreased skin turgor.

4. ____ Acute kidney injury, although rare, is a critical concern in some animals after CPA.

5. ____ When blood is aspirated during abdominocentesis, abdominal bleeding can be differentiated from fresh blood by looking at the color.

6. ____ A tracheotomy should not be performed on a horse unless it is thoroughly sedated and restrained.

7. ____ Animals with respiratory distress should have chest radiographs taken immediately upon presentation to diagnose the cause quickly.

8. ____ Animals with hypoxia caused by severe anemia can have normal pulse oximeter readings.

9. ____ The partial pressure of oxygen in arterial blood (PaO_2) can be used to assess pulmonary function.

10. ____ An ECG tracing is a reliable method of determining cardiac activity following cardiopulmonary arrest.

11. ____ All items in the emergency crash cart must be inspected a minimum of once a month for proper function and expiration.

12. ____ When performing defibrillation, electrical conduction should be enhanced by wetting the hair with 70% isopropyl alcohol.

13. ____ The overall survival rate for all causes of witnessed in-hospital cardiopulmonary arrest patients is good, as long as treatment is initiated quickly.

14. ____ Thoracocentesis must be performed aseptically.

15. _____ Doppler blood pressure monitoring is only reliable for detecting systolic arterial blood pressure.

16. _____ The life-threatening condition gastric dilation volvulus (GDV) can be readily ruled out as long as the patient doesn't have visible abdominal distention.

17. _____ The "P" wave on an ECG tracing corresponds to propagation of the electrical impulse through the atrial heart muscle.

18. _____ The horizontal axis on an ECG tracing represents the strength of the electrical impulse measured in mV.

19. _____ Sinus arrhythmia is a normal rhythm in dogs.

20. _____ Atrial standstill is a cardiac arrhythmia that has hyperkalemia as its most common cause.

21. _____ A second-degree AV block is a rhythm characterized by a prolonged PR interval on the ECG.

22. _____ Horses that have colic can be divided into two main categories: a small number that resolve with minimal or no treatment, and many more that require aggressive treatment.

23. _____ Abrasions around the head and the presence of dirt, mud, and hay in the hair coat of a horse experiencing colic are signs that it was in severe pain prior to arrival at the hospital.

24. _____ Nasogastric intubation in colic patients is important, because horses with excessive accumulation of stomach gas and fluid will often vomit and aspirate.

25. _____ After passing a nasogastric tube in a colic patient, the tube should be removed immediately if no fluid is obtained to avoid further damage to the stomach.

26. _____ Minor skin wounds in horses can become life threatening events when joints, tendon sheaths, or vessels are involved.

27. _____ Endoscopic examination of the airways can be used to evaluate the pharynx, guttural pouches, and trachea in horses, but cannot be used to evaluate deeper structures like the bifurcation of the bronchi.

28. _____ When performing a thoracocentesis, the needle or catheter should always be advanced off the cranial aspect of the rib and into the pleural space.

29. _____ The location most often used to perform a tracheotomy in an equine patient is the ventral midline between the middle and caudal third of the neck.

30. _____ Splint stabilization of an equine elbow fracture is not necessary if the patient can extend, plant, and move the leg.

31. _____ A plantar splint is applied up to the point of the calcaneus to stabilize a distal to mid-hindlimb fracture.

32. _____ The size of the area around a wound that should be clipped is most closely associated with the presence or absence of infection.

33. _____ When checking a wound for joint involvement by tapping the joint, the needle should always be introduced at a site distant from the wound.

34. _____ Food animals seldom need emergency care because, with few exceptions, their value is seen as economic.

35. ____ Parasitism is the most common emergent condition treated in farm animals.

36. ____ Attacks on camelids, sheep, and goats can occur anywhere on the body but commonly occur around the groin, hindlimbs, and abdomen.

37. ____ The ruminal contents of a cow can be used to perform ruminal transfaunation of a goat.

38. ____ A veterinarian can usually diagnose urethral obstruction form a good history and physical examination.

39. ____ The rapidity with which joint luxation is treated is an important determinant of the likelihood of success.

40. ____ Sheep and goats that are targets of dog attacks often suffer puncture wounds, which, although potentially serious, usually involve only superficial structures.

41. ____ By using proper equipment, dystocias of food animals can usually be managed by the vet without additional help.

42. ____ When replacing a prolapsed uterus, a large plastic bag can be used to prevent further contamination and trauma of the prolapsed organ.

43. ____ When faced with a small ruminant with an inability to urinate, urethral stones can easily be ruled out by taking radiographs.

44. ____ General anesthesia is required to perform a urethrostomy in a goat.

EXERCISE 25.13 MULTIPLE CHOICE: COMPREHENSIVE

Instructions: Circle the one correct answer to each of the following questions.

1. Laryngeal paralysis and other extra-thoracic airway obstructions are characterized by
   a. fast, short, and shallow breaths.
   b. prolonged and deep breaths.
   c. long, slow inspirations and short exhalations.
   d. expiratory dyspnea with increased abdominal effort.

2. Increased bronchovesicular sounds indicate
   a. diaphragmatic hernia.
   b. pulmonary edema.
   c. pneumothorax.
   d. pleural effusion.

3. A weak, thready arterial pulse can indicate
   a. decompensated shock.
   b. anemia.
   c. compensated shock.
   d. aortic regurgitation.

4. A patient with pronounced loss of skin turgor, dry mucous membranes, tachycardia, weak pulses, and sunken eyes, but not in shock or comatose, is approximately _____ dehydrated.
   a. 5%
   b. 7%
   c. 10%
   d. > 10%

5. An elevated blood lactate indicates
   a. overhydration.
   b. brain injury.
   c. poor tissue perfusion.
   d. urinary blockage.

6. Radiographic evaluation of a wound provides the best assessment of
   a. infection.
   b. soft tissue injury.
   c. the source of the wound.
   d. bony structure involvement.

7. A complication of shock that is characterized by widespread inflammation of tissues resulting from lack of oxygen is known as
   a. MODS.
   b. DIC.
   c. BAR.
   d. SIRS.

8. When performing a thoracentesis to diagnose or treat pneumothorax, prepare the area around the
   a. fourth to fifth intercostal space between the top one-third and bottom two-thirds of the thorax.
   b. fourth to fifth intercostal space between the top two-thirds and bottom one-third of the thorax.
   c. seventh to ninth intercostal space between the top one-third and bottom two-thirds of the thorax.
   d. seventh to ninth intercostal space between the top two-thirds and bottom one-third of the thorax.

9. All animals in respiratory distress can die as a result of even small amounts of stress, but those most at risk are
   a. dogs.
   b. horses.
   c. camelids.
   d. cats.

10. Increased end-tidal carbon dioxide levels occur with
    a. hypoventilation.
    b. a leak in the anesthetic system.
    c. an incompletely inflated endotracheal tube cuff.
    d. decreased cardiac output.

11. PaO_2 is measured with
    a. end-tidal CO_2 monitoring.
    b. pulse oximetry.
    c. arterial blood-gas monitoring.
    d. oscillometry.

12. The first priority when performing CPR is considered by many critical care veterinarians to be
    a. providing breaths.
    b. chest compressions.
    c. placing an endotracheal tube.
    d. running an ECG tracing.

13. During cardiopulmonary arrest and subsequent CPR, which of the following end-tidal carbon dioxide monitor values indicate that chest compressions are adequate?
    a. 0 mm Hg
    b. 5 to 10 mm Hg
    c. 10 to 15 mm Hg
    d. 20 to 30 mm Hg

14. Which would be part of the secondary survey?
    a. Checking for fractures
    b. Checking for an open airway
    c. Digital palpation of pulse
    d. Assessment of mentation

15. During CPR, stimulation of the Governing Vessel 26 acupuncture point is used to
    a. stimulate the heart.
    b. increase tissue perfusion.
    c. increase blood oxygen.
    d. stimulate respirations.

16. The drug most commonly used to treat asystole during CPR is
    a. lidocaine.
    b. naloxone.
    c. epinephrine.
    d. calcium gluconate.

17. When administering advanced life support during CPR, some drugs may be given via the endotracheal tube. Which drug cannot be given this way?
    a. Naloxone
    b. Vasopressin
    c. Epinephrine
    d. Sodium bicarbonate

18. Asymmetry in pupil size is called
    a. strabismus.
    b. anisocoria.
    c. mydriasis.
    d. opisthotonus.

19. Hyperkalemia is often a feature of which emergency disease?
    a. Urethral obstruction
    b. Gastric dilatation volvulus
    c. Heart failure
    d. Respiratory distress

20. The ECG electrode that should be placed on the right rear limb is
    a. black.
    b. green.
    c. white.
    d. red.

21. Arrhythmias that originate from below the AV node are classified as
    a. tachyarrhythmias.
    b. supraventricular arrhythmias.
    c. bradyarrhythmias.
    d. ventricular arrhythmias.

22. A sinus arrhythmia is
    a. normal in the dog and cat.
    b. normal in the dog, but not the cat.
    c. normal in the cat, but not the dog.
    d. an abnormal rhythm in both cats and dogs.

23. Which of the following cardiac rhythms commonly occurs in normal animals as a response to pain, excitement, stress, or anxiety?
    a. Sinus arrhythmia
    b. Atrial fibrillation
    c. Sinus tachycardia
    d. Atrial tachycardia

24. Which of the following is a QRS complex that occurs too soon and is of identical or nearly identical shape as a normal QRS complex?
    a. Atrial premature complex
    b. Junctional escape beat
    c. Ventricular premature complex
    d. Ventricular escape beat

25. A cardiac arrhythmia that appears on an ECG tracing as a flat line is called
    a. atrial standstill.
    b. third-degree AV block.
    c. pulseless electrical activity.
    d. ventricular asystole.

26. In equine medicine, emergencies involving three major organ systems make up a large part of the caseload. Which organ system is typically not involved?
    a. Gastrointestinal system
    b. Genitourinary system
    c. Musculoskeletal system
    d. Respiratory system

27. The 10-cm × 10-cm location that should be clipped and surgically prepared prior to performing an abdominocentesis in colic patients is usually located
    a. 3 to 5 cm caudal to the umbilicus and 3 to 5 cm to the left of the midline.
    b. 3 to 5 cm caudal to the xiphoid and 3 to 5 cm to the left of the midline.
    c. 3 to 5 cm caudal to the umbilicus and 3 to 5 cm to the right of the midline.
    d. 3 to 5 cm caudal to the xiphoid and 3 to 5 cm to the right of the midline.

28. The most common reason for surgical intervention in a colic patient is to
    a. investigate a total absence of borborygmi.
    b. repair a rectal tear.
    c. investigate pain that is unresponsive to sedation.
    d. repair an intussusception.

29. An upper respiratory tract obstruction in an equine patient is generally characterized by
    a. rapid, shallow breathing and absent lung sounds.
    b. severe distress and inspiratory stridor.
    c. abnormal lung sounds, including crackles and wheezes.
    d. rapid, shallow breathing with abnormal lung sounds.

30. Effective treatment of equine pneumonia may require a bacterial culture and cytologic evaluation of respiratory secretions. Samples for these tests are best obtained by
    a. thoracocentesis.
    b. lower airway endoscopy.
    c. transtracheal wash.
    d. tracheotomy.

31. A bandage designed to stabilize a fracture of the proximal metacarpus of the horse must extend from the coronary band to the
    a. highest point of the elbow.
    b. top of the metacarpus.
    c. top of the carpus.
    d. highest point of the shoulder.

32. Equine patients with _____ should always be assessed for blood loss, which is commonly associated with this condition.
    a. colic
    b. an upper respiratory obstruction
    c. a wound
    d. heaves

33. A nonviable segment of bone that acts as a foreign body and frequently prevents full wound healing until it is removed is called a(n)
    a. osteoblast.
    b. chondrocyte.
    c. bone fragment.
    d. sequestrum.

34. A cow in hypovolemic shock should receive a rapid 1-L IV infusion of
    a. normal (0.9%) saline.
    b. lactated Ringer solution.
    c. hypertonic (7%) saline.
    d. Ringer solution.

35. The area that must be prepared prior to abdominal surgery in cattle to correct GI abnormalities such as an abomasal volvulus or cecal volvulus is typically
    a. the right paralumbar fossa.
    b. the left paralumbar fossa.
    c. the ventral midline.
    d. the paramedian region.

36. A large-bore tube used to remove ingesta, liquid, and gas from the rumen of a cow is called a(n)
    a. nasoesophageal tube.
    b. Kingman tube.
    c. rumenostomy tube.
    d. urethrostomy tube.

37. The term *down animal* or *downer* is typically used to describe
    a. animals that need to be removed from the herd.
    b. animals in a downward posture as the result of an infection.
    c. animals that cannot stand.
    d. animals experiencing gastrointestinal distress in the evening.

38. The best option for supporting cows that can't stand for long periods of time is
    a. hydroflotation.
    b. slings.
    c. hip lifters.
    d. water beds.

39. A Krey hook is a device used to
    a. support downer cows.
    b. correct a uterine torsion.
    c. retrieve foreign objects.
    d. perform a fetotomy.

40. A "breech" presentation of a fetus during parturition is one in which
    a. the head presents first.
    b. the front legs present first.
    c. the rump presents first.
    d. the hind legs present first.

41. The "plank-in-the-flank" method is a technique used to correct a(n)
    a. uterine torsion in a cow.
    b. cecal impaction in a horse.
    c. uterine prolapse in a ewe.
    d. dystocia in a camel.

42. Urolithiasis is a condition most often seen in
    a. cows.
    b. bulls.
    c. male sheep and goats.
    d. female sheep and goats.

43. The most common place for a urinary stone to lodge in a goat is the
    a. sigmoid flexure of the urethra.
    b. neck of the bladder.
    c. prostatic urethra.
    d. urethral process.

44. Holter monitoring is used to
    a. diagnose suspected arrhythmia.
    b. evaluate suspected airway obstruction.
    c. resolve suspected arrhythmias.
    d. A and B

45. To minimize the likelihood of development of urolithiasis in goats, it is important to
    a. decrease salt intake.
    b. limit hay intake.
    c. alkalinize the urine.
    d. eliminate grain from the diet.

EXERCISE 25.14 FILL-IN-THE-BLANK #2: COMPREHENSIVE

Instructions: Fill in each of the spaces provided with the missing word or words that complete the sentence.

1. During an initial triage examination, the _____, _____, and _____ organ systems should be systematically and carefully evaluated.

2. The term _____ refers to sudden onset of abdominal pain that is often severe and of unknown cause.

3. A nonpalpable dorsal metatarsal arterial pulse in a dog indicates a mean arterial pressure (MAP) lower than _____ mm Hg, whereas a nonpalpable femoral pulse in a dog or cat indicates a MAP lower than _____ mm Hg.

4. The clip-like probe of a pulse oximeter is designed to attach to a(n)_____, sparsely haired area.

5. Shock occurs as a result of altered blood flow, and ultimately impaired delivery of _____ to the tissues.

6. Normal arterial blood pressure values for dogs and cats are in the range of _____ _____ mmHG systolic and _____ _____ mmHg (diastolic).

7. The heart, lungs, brain, _____, and _____ are the organs most often affected by MODS.

8. A pulse oximeter measures the percentage of hemoglobin that is saturated with _____.

9. During CPR, when performing chest compressions and interposed abdominal compressions, the abdomen is compressed during the _____ phase of the chest compression.

10. A pulse that is _____ has a very large pulse pressure with an extremely rapid rise and fall, often occurring with anemia, patent ductus arteriosus, or severe aortic regurgitation.

11. Once the respiratory, cardiovascular, and neurologic systems have been initially assessed, a quick abdominal _____ to check for pain, tympany, or a fluid wave is conducted.

12. Cats in shock often present with _____, rather than with _____, as is seen in dogs with shock.

13. A blood pressure cuff is properly sized if the _____ of the cuff is approximately 40% of the _____ of the limb.

14. Patients with emergency respiratory disease are often treated with particular drugs related to the primary problem. For instance, patients in respiratory distress benefit from sedation with an opioid drug such as _____, cats suspected to have asthma should receive the drug _____ by inhalation, and patients suspected to be in heart failure should receive _____.

15. The most commonly used electrocardiographic leads are I, II, III, aVR, aVL, and aVF. I, II, and III are known as _____ leads, and aVR, aVL, and aVF are known as _____ leads.

16. When acquiring an ECG, the tracing should be recorded at a paper speed of _____ or _____ mm/sec, and a calibration of _____ mm/mV.

17. A(n) _____ should be placed to remove large amounts of fluid if more than two thoracocenteses are needed within a few hours.

18. When a QRS complex is normal in shape, this suggests that it is _____ in origin, but if it is wide and bizarre in shape, this suggests that it is _____ in origin.

19. In a patient with a sinus arrhythmia, the HR typically increases during _____ and decreases during _____.

20. Ventricular premature complexes (VPCs) may occur in groups of two, three, four, or more, and may occur in patterns. A group of two sequential VPCs is called a(n)_____, and a group of three sequential VPCs is called a(n)_____. A(n)_____ is a rhythm in which every other beat is a VPC, and a(n)_____ is a rhythm in which every third beat is a VPC.

21. Nasogastric intubation is typically performed in colic patients to remove excess gas and fluid from the stomach. This excess fluid is called _____ _____.

22. On physical examination, mucous membrane color is an important indicator of various conditions. For instance, an animal that presents with blue mucous membranes, also known as _____, should immediately be provided with _____.

23. In horses, thoracic problems, such as diaphragmatic hernia and pneumothorax, can lead to signs of respiratory distress or _____ (a disease of the gastrointestinal system).

24. _____ supplementation is required in patients with respiratory distress when the PaO_2 is less than 100 mm Hg.

25. When supplementing oxygen to an adult equine patient, a flow rate of at least _____ L/min should be used, whereas foals and miniature horses may require as little as _____ L/min.

26. Bovine patients with bloat may have respiratory compromise because the rumen becomes distended and cranially pushes on the _____.

27. Microbial function of the ruminal contents can be determined by a methylene blue reduction test. If rumen flora is normal, the ruminal contents will change from a(n)_____ color to a(n) _____ color within 5 minutes.

28. In a ruminant, the incision for a C-section is usually made in the _____ _____ with the animal awake.

29. Cattle with metritis and mastitis can develop endotoxemia and may present with signs of _____, which include tachycardia and tachypnea.

30. Animals with urinary obstructions frequently have serious electrolyte abnormalities. The most dangerous of these is _____ because it may lead to fatal _____.

31. The surgical procedure performed to create an opening in the urethra proximal to an obstruction is called a(n) _____.

EXERCISE 25.15 CASE STUDY: MANAGEMENT OF RECUMBENT PATIENTS

Leslie, a 10-year-old, spayed female Shepherd mix is presented for management of recumbency caused by paralysis secondary to a rupture of an intervertebral disc. She has not been eating well and has disturbed fluid balance. She is also in pain secondary to the disc rupture and has developed several open ulcers over her elbows and other bony prominences. Because she is panting a lot, she has dry oral mucous membranes, and she also has red and irritated skin around her rear quarters because she is often lying in a pool of her own urine. In addition to these problems, if her recumbency is prolonged, she will be prone to loss of muscle mass, and contracture and edema of her limbs.

Recumbent patients may also require placement of an endotracheal tube or tracheostomy tube and/or may be on mechanical ventilation. For the problems Leslie is facing, as well as the additional problems common to recumbent patients, indicate the reasons that each occurs and then summarize the care that must be provided to manage each problem appropriately and effectively.

1. Inadequate nutritional intake

   Reasons: _____

   _____

   Management: _____

   _____

   _____

   _____

   _____

   _____

2. Pain

   Reasons: _____

   Management: _____

   _____

   _____

   _____

   _____

   _____

3. Dry oral mucous membranes and other oral problems

Reasons: _____

Management: _____

_____

_____

_____

_____

4. Peripheral edema, muscle wasting, and contracture

Reasons: _____

Management: _____

_____

_____

_____

_____

_____

5. Urine scald

Reasons: _____

Management: _____

_____

_____

_____

_____

_____

_____

6. Placement of an endotracheal tube or tracheostomy tube and/or mechanical ventilation

Reasons: _____

Management: _____

_____

_____

_____

_____

_____

_____

26 Toxicology

When you have completed this chapter, you will be able to:

1. Pronounce, spell, and define all the key terms in this chapter.
2. Assess and stabilize a patient presenting with a toxicologic emergency.
3. Use appropriate decontamination techniques for ocular, dermal, and oral toxin exposure to prevent absorption and/or remove the toxin from the body.
4. Provide supportive care to a patient being treated for toxicosis.
5. Do the following regarding common household hazards, including dangerous food items, household cleaning agents, and miscellaneous household items:
   - Identify the toxic component of the item or product.
   - Describe clinical signs expected with toxicosis.
   - Describe specific decontamination techniques used to prevent absorption and/or remove the toxin from the body.
6. Do the following regarding dangerous plants, including *Rhododendron* species, cardiac glycoside–containing plants, castor beans, cycad palms, lilies, and insoluble calcium oxalate crystal containing plants:
   - Identify the toxic component of the item or product.
   - Describe clinical signs expected with toxicosis.
   - Describe specific decontamination techniques used to prevent absorption and/or remove the toxin from the body.
7. Do the following regarding pesticides, including ant and roach baits, flea/tick products, methomyl, molluscicides, and rodenticides:
   - Identify the toxic component of the item or product.
   - Describe clinical signs expected with toxicosis.
   - Describe specific decontamination techniques used to prevent absorption and/or remove the toxin from the body.
8. Do the following regarding antifreeze products, including methanol, propylene glycol, and ethylene glycol:
   - Identify the toxic component of the item or product.
   - Describe clinical signs expected with toxicosis.
   - Describe specific decontamination techniques used to prevent absorption and/or remove the toxin from the body.
9. Do the following regarding human medications, including acetaminophen, nonsteroidal anti-inflammatory drugs, aspirin, pseudoephedrine, amphetamines, isoniazid, calcipotriene, and 5-fluorouracil:
   - Identify the toxic component of the item or product.
   - Describe clinical signs expected with toxicosis.
   - Describe specific decontamination techniques used to prevent absorption and/or remove the toxin from the body.
10. Do the following regarding drugs of abuse, including marijuana, cocaine, ethanol, and methamphetamine:
    - Identify the toxic component of the item or product.
    - Describe clinical signs expected with toxicosis.
    - Describe specific decontamination techniques used to prevent absorption and/or remove the toxin from the body.

EXERCISE 26.1 MATCHING #1: KEY TERMS—INFECTIOUS AGENTS

Instructions: Match each term in column A with its corresponding definition in column B by writing the appropriate letter in the space provided.

Column A

1. _____ Alkalis
2. _____ Anionic detergent
3. _____ Toxin
4. _____ Cationic detergents
5. _____ Decontamination
6. _____ Acids
7. _____ Toxicosis

Column B

A. Any disease of toxic origin
B. A poisonous substance
C. Neutralization of injurious agents
D. Produce(s) an initially nonpainful, deep, and penetrating wound
E. Produce(s) an initially painful wound
F. Found in shampoos
G. Found in fabric softeners

EXERCISE 26.2 MATCHING #2: CLASSIFICATION OF TOXINS

Instructions: Match each toxic substance in column A with its corresponding toxin category in column B by writing the appropriate letter in the space provided. (Note that responses may be used more than once.)

Column A

1. _____ St. John's wort
2. _____ Tobacco
3. _____ Yew
4. _____ Lantana
5. _____ Raisins
6. _____ Marijuana
7. _____ Cocklebur
8. _____ Avocado
9. _____ White and yellow sweet clover
10. _____ Bermuda grass
11. _____ Cotton
12. _____ Milkweed
13. _____ Buckwheat
14. _____ Shamrock
15. _____ Agave
16. _____ Fescue
17. _____ Rhubarb
18. _____ Common juniper
19. _____ Queen Anne's lace
20. _____ Amanita mushrooms

Column B

A. Neurotoxic
B. Hepatotoxic
C. Nephrotoxic
D. Dermal
E. Fungal
F. Reproduction
G. Cardiotoxic

EXERCISE 26.3 COMPLETING TREATMENT OPTIONS: ORALLY INGESTED TOXINS

Instructions: Complete the chart by supplying the missing information for each treatment/agent identified.

Treatment/Agent	Indication	Dose	Contraindications/Exceptions
Dilution—Milk or water			
Emesis—Hydrogen peroxide			
Activated Charcoal			
Enemas—Plain warm or soapy water			
Gastric Lavage			
Enterogastric Lavage			

EXERCISE 26.4 FILL-IN-THE-BLANK: COMPREHENSIVE

Instructions: Fill in each of the spaces provided with the missing word or words that complete the sentence.

1. Toxicity is dependent upon the _____ and _____ dose, as well as the _____, _____, and _____ of the animal.

2. The general rule of toxicology is to _____.

3. _____ is the preferred emetic agent for dogs.

4. Sedation that can result from the use of apomorphine hydrochloride can be reversed with _____.

5. _____ or _____ should never be used as an emetic.

6. _____ % solution of hydrogen peroxide has been shown to be an effective emetic for dogs, ferrets, and _____.

7. As a general rule, the _____ and more _____ the chocolate, the more toxic it likely is.

8. Members of the *Allium* family that can be harmful to all animals include onions, _____, _____, _____, and _____.

9. _____ is recommended in patients with hemoglobinuria.

10. Grapes and raisins have been shown to cause _____ in some dogs when eaten.

11. _____ is the only toxin that will cause intermittent seizures.

12. _____ and _____ are effective chelating agents that can be administered in the case of lead poisoning.

13. Signs of nicotine poisoning usually occur within _____ to _____ minutes of ingestion.

14. _____ is commonly found in snail or slug bait and is highly toxic.

15. Anticoagulant rodenticides act by competitive inhibition of vitamin _____.

16. _____ _____ is the most dangerous type of antifreeze.

17. _____ are more sensitive to acetaminophen than dogs.

18. Initial signs of marijuana toxicity in dogs include _____ and _____ that can progress into _____.

19. An ataxic animal dribbling urine is considered to be intoxicated by _____ until proven otherwise.

20. Ingestion of members of the *Rhododendron* family can lead to _____.

EXERCISE 26.5 TRUE OR FALSE: COMPREHENSIVE

Instructions: Read the following statements and write "T" for true or "F" for false in the blanks provided. If a statement is false, correct the statement to make it true.

1. _____ The best way to prevent serious problems from toxicosis is to have emetics and activated charcoal on hand.

2. _____ Taking a good history will be critical for preparation for the toxicologic emergency.

3. _____ The general rule of toxicology is to "treat the patient, not the poison."

4. _____ Decontamination is performed to prevent other animals from similar ingestion.

5. _____ With any ocular exposure, the eyes should be flushed repeatedly with tepid water or saline solution for a minimum of 20 to 30 minutes.

6. _____ To remove sticky substances from birds, work a small amount of vegetable oil, mineral oil, mayonnaise, or peanut butter through the rest of the substance until it breaks down into "gummy balls."

7. _____ Hypothermia is not a concern when treating a patient for toxicosis.

8. _____ Emesis is contraindicated in rodents, rabbits, birds, horses, and ruminants.

9. _____ Emesis is more likely to be productive if the animal is fed a large, moist meal before inducing vomiting.

10. _____ Food-grade hydrogen peroxide is an acceptable grade for animal use.

11. ____ Salt water should be administered within 10 minutes of arrival to the clinic when ingestion of a caustic agent is suspected.

12. ____ Chocolate contains theobromine and caffeine, which are both classified as methylxanthines.

13. ____ If ingested by dogs, macadamia nuts may cause weakness, depression, vomiting, ataxia, tremors, and hyperthermia.

14. ____ Grapes and raisins, when eaten, cause cardiovascular episodes in cats.

15. ____ Alkali burns are initially nonpainful.

16. ____ Acid and alkali burns are treated the same.

17. ____ Bathing and dilution are the cornerstones in treating contact with bleach.

18. ____ The treatment for zinc ingestion is dilution.

19. ____ Lead must be in an acidic environment to be absorbed into the bloodstream.

20. ____ Toxicity risks for the ingestion of dangerous plants are similar for all plant types.

21. ____ One of the most potent plant toxins is contained in the castor bean, for which there is no anecdote.

22. ____ Delaying treatment for the ingestion of an Easter lily in a cat beyond 18 hours frequently results in death.

23. ____ Outdoor plants contain calcium oxalate crystals; common houseplants do not.

24. ____ Cats are extremely sensitive to concentrated permethrin.

25. ____ The first step in treating symptomatic cats exposed to permethrin compounds is emesis.

26. ____ Cats are very sensitive to bromethalin; dogs are more resistant.

27. ____ Vitamin B12 increases the absorption of calcium, stimulates bone resorption, and enhances kidney reabsorption of calcium.

28. ____ The smell of rotten fish in the air could signal a phosphine gas, dangerous to both humans and animals.

29. ____ Large ingestions of methanol require monitoring for acidosis.

30. ____ The ingestion of ethylene glycol can cause acute renal failure.

31. ____ Apomorphine and ropinirole work well on cats and dogs to stimulate vomiting.

32. ____ The toxin in grapes, raisins, and Zante currants is tartaric acid.

EXERCISE 26.6 SHORT ANSWER: COMPREHENSIVE

Instructions: Each of the following is a TRUE statement. In the space provided, please provide a short answer as to WHY the statement is true.

1. Apples and cherries can cause problems in grazing animals.

   _____

2. The ingestion of certain grasses (Dallis, Perennial ryegrass, Bermuda, Phalaris) can cause grass staggers and tremors.

   _____

3. Aspiration is a concern with the ingestion of ethanol.

_____

4. In treating cocaine ingestion, emesis should only be induced within 15 minutes of ingestion.

_____

5. Aspirin can be used therapeutically in both dogs and cats but must be used cautiously in cats.

_____

6. In cats, 10 mg/kg of acetaminophen has produced signs of toxicity.

_____

7. The test kit for EG poisoning must be used very carefully with consultation of the package insert and directions.

_____

8. When managing a zinc phosphide case, if any staff develop a headache or shortness of breath, they should seek medical attention.

_____

9. Guinea pigs are not affected by bromethalin.

_____

10. A drooling cat should be evaluated for ingestion of topical insecticides or sprays.

_____

11. Clinical signs associated with the ingestion of calcium oxalate-containing plants include oral irritation; intense burning and irritation of the mouth, lips, and tongue; excessive drooling; vomiting; and difficulty in swallowing.

_____

12. Ingestion of raw yeast bread dough can be life-threatening to dogs.

_____

13. Onions and other members of the *Allium* family can be harmful to all animals.

_____

14. Cats are considered to be at higher risk for onion toxicity.

_____

15. The veterinary staff should take extra steps to keep the bladder empty, either through catheterization or frequent walking in a patient who has ingested chocolate.

_____

16. As a general rule, the darker and more bitter the chocolate, the more toxic it likely is.

_____

17. Samples collected should always be kept and properly labeled.

_____

18. It is extremely important to maintain nutritional requirements in a cat undergoing treatment.

_____

19. A 3% hydrogen peroxide solution has been shown to be an effective emetic for dogs, ferrets, and pigs.

_____

20. The use of hydrogen peroxide as an emetic in the cat is not recommended.

_____

21. Emesis should be induced on a hard surface where the vomitus can be examined.

_____

22. It is especially important to make sure young animals are kept warm after a bath.

_____

23. When dealing with sticky substances (e.g., gum, glue traps, tar), the use of solvents should be avoided.

_____

24. For birds, do not follow all the same instructions for the removal of sticky substances as for other animals.

_____

Wound Management and Bandaging

LEARNING OBJECTIVES

When you have completed this chapter, you will be able to:
1. Pronounce, define, and spell all key terms in the chapter.
2. Identify the phases of wound healing and describe patient, wound, and treatment factors that adversely affect wound healing.
3. Do the following regarding wound management in the small animal:
   - Describe the objectives and principles of immediate wound care, including wound lavage.
   - Describe the goals and methods of wound debridement.
   - Differentiate among primary, delayed primary, and secondary wound closure and among primary, second, and third intention healing.
   - Compare methods of managing wound drainage and wound infection.
   - Explain the nature and appearance of abrasions, lacerations, degloving injuries, penetrating wounds, burns, decubitus ulcers, and pressure sores and discuss the methods used to treat each.
4. Identify the principles of bandaging and discuss the purpose of the primary, secondary, and tertiary layers of a bandage, including the specific materials used for each.
5. Discuss the uses for and characteristics of the following external coaptation methods in small animals and their application technique:
   - Robert Jones bandage and modified Robert Jones bandage
   - Casts and splints
   - Ehmer, 90/90 flexion, Velpeau, and carpal flexion sling, hobbles
   - Bandages for the head, chest, abdomen, tail, and areas that are difficult to bandage, such as the pelvis and the axilla
6. Explain aftercare of bandages, splints, casts, and slings, including complications that may occur.
7. Discuss the principles of equine wound care, including treatment of exuberant granulation tissue.
8. Do the following regarding application of bandages, splints, and casts in horses:
   - Discuss uses for, characteristics of, and the technique used to place a lower limb wound bandage or a support bandage on an equine limb.
   - Discuss uses for and characteristics of equine casts and splints and techniques used to place a cast or a splint on an equine limb.
   - Describe the technique used to remove a cast.
9. Discuss uses for and characteristics of bandages, splints, and casts used for cattle and describe technique used to place a claw block and a modified Thomas splint on a ruminant limb.

Across

4 A wound dressing that is a primary layer impermeable to moisture
8 Wound caused by pressure on skin over bony prominences (2 words)
9 Cells recruited into a wound during the proliferative phase that help form granulation tissue
10 Sharp cut or tear of skin
12 Having an affinity for water
14 Wound healing involving treatment that does not allow the wound to dry out
15 A primary wound dressing that allows air and moisture to move through
17 Closure of a wound by apposing the skin over healthy granulation tissue
18 Healing of a wound across a surgically closed incision. (2 words)
20 The opposite side
22 Vascularized fibrous tissue that covers a wound if left to heal by second intention
23 Tissue also known as proud flesh (2 words)
24 Healing of a wound by granulation tissue formation, epithelialization and contraction (2 words)
25 Pertaining to the groin area
26 Type of injury that features a large section of skin torn off the underlying tissue in a glove-like fashion

Down

1 Having an osmotic pressure equivalent to that of blood plasma
2 Having an osmotic pressure greater than that of blood plasma.
3 Surgical closure of a wound
5 Meshwork-like substance in a wound, attached to the outer cell surface that provides support and anchorage (2 words)
6 Space between tissues allowing accumulation of fluid (2 words)
7 A cell with contractile properties that is responsible for wound contraction
8 Removal of foreign matter and dead tissue from a wound.
11 The process in which skin cells advance in a single layer across the wound
13 Wound healing by secondary closure after allowing granulation tissue to form (2 words)
16 A Teflon pad is one example of this type of wound dressing
19 Deposited into a wound by fibroblasts during the proliferative phase of healing
21 An area of skin that has been superficially scraped

Chapter **27** **Wound Management and Bandaging**

EXERCISE 27.2 MATCHING #1: WOUND CLASSIFICATIONS

Instructions: Match each wound type in column A with its corresponding classification in column B by writing the appropriate letter in the space provided. (Note that responses may be used more than once.)

Column A

1. _____ A wound with a high bacterial count

2. _____ Surgical wound that enters the GI tract

3. _____ Surgical wound

4. _____ An open traumatic wound

5. _____ An old traumatic wound

6. _____ A surgical wound with a minor break in sterile technique

7. _____ A surgical wound into the respiratory tract

8. _____ A natural wound with minor contamination

9. _____ A surgical wound with a major break in sterile technique

Column B

A. Clean wound

B. Clean-contaminated wound

C. Contaminated wound

D. Dirty and infected wound

EXERCISE 27.3 MATCHING #2: BANDAGES, SLINGS, SPLINTS, AND CASTS

Instructions: Match each device in column A with its corresponding description in column B by writing the appropriate letter in the space provided.

Column A

1. _____ Carpal flexion sling

2. _____ Cast

3. _____ Ehmer sling

4. _____ Modified Thomas splint

5. _____ Modified Robert Jones bandage

6. _____ Robert Jones bandage

7. _____ Schroeder-Thomas splint

8. _____ Spica splint

9. _____ Velpeau sling

10. _____ 90/90 Flexion sling

11. _____ Hobbles

Column B

A. A traction splint constructed of rods used for stabilizing long bone fractures in large animals

B. Maintains the limb in extension; includes a lateral splint that reaches over the shoulder or hip

C. Prevents abduction of the pelvic limbs; primarily used after reduction of ventral hip luxations

D. Used for the forelimb in any situation where weight-bearing should be avoided, but some movement of the elbow and shoulder joints is acceptable

E. A very bulky bandage used to immobilize a limb distal to the elbow or stifle joint

F. A device that prevents weight-bearing of the pelvic limb; frequently used after closed reduction of craniodorsal hip luxations

G. A device that prevents weight-bearing of the thoracic limb; primarily used after reduction of medial shoulder luxations

H. A device used to immobilize fractures that is most often made of fiberglass material

I. Used in puppies after repair of distal femoral fractures to prevent quadriceps tie-down or contracture

J. The most commonly used distal limb bandage in small animals; also known as a soft-padded bandage

K. An immobilization device with a rigid metal frame (no longer recommended)

EXERCISE 27.4 MATCHING #3: WOUND CLOSURE AND HEALING

Instructions: Match each statement in column A with the corresponding type of healing that will follow in column B by writing the appropriate response in the space provided.

Column A

1. No closure of a wound will lead to ____.

2. Primary closure of a wound will lead to ____.

3. Secondary closure of a wound will lead to ____.

Column B

A. primary intention wound healing

B. third intention wound healing

C. second intention wound healing

EXERCISE 27.5 MATCHING #4: BURNS

Instructions: Match each type of burn in column A with its corresponding description in column B by writing the appropriate letter in the space provided.

Column A

1. ____ First-degree burn

2. ____ Second-degree burn

3. ____ Third-degree burn

4. ____ Fourth-degree burn

Column B

A. Skin that is thick, leathery, and often black

B. The skin may appear yellow-white, black, or charred

C. A burn that involves tissues deep into the skin

D. Skin is red and painful

Instructions: Match each bandage material in column A with its corresponding characteristics in column B by writing the appropriate letter in the space provided. (Note that responses may be used more than once.)

Column A

1. _____ Elastikon elastic adhesive tape (Johnson & Johnson Medical, Arlington, TX)

2. _____ Curagel hydrogel (Kendall/Covidien, Mansfield, MA)

3. _____ Cotton sheets

4. _____ NU-GEL hydrogel (Johnson & Johnson Medical, Arlington, TX)

5. _____ Cast padding (3M Skin and Wound Care, St. Paul, MN)

6. _____ 20% sodium chloride dressing

7. _____ Vetrap elastic bandage (3M Animal Care Products, St. Paul, MN)

8. _____ Hydrosorb Plus Foam (Kendall/Covidien, Mansfield, MA)

9. _____ Military field bandage

10. _____ Petrolatum-impregnated gauze

11. _____ Ultec hydrocolloid dressing (Kendall/Covidien, Mansfield, MA)

12. _____ Flannel track wrap

13. _____ Kling conforming gauze (Johnson & Johnson Medical, Arlington, TX)

14. _____ Honey

15. _____ Bioclusive polyurethane film (Johnson & Johnson Medical, Arlington, TX)

16. _____ Rolled cotton (Johnson & Johnson Medical, Arlington, TX)

17. _____ Teflon pads

18. _____ Tegaderm transparent dressing (3M Skin and Wound Care, St. Paul, MN)

19. _____ Quilted leg wraps

20. _____ Sterile wide-mesh gauze

21. _____ Tegaderm hydrocolloid (3M Skin and Wound Care, St. Paul, MN)

22. _____ Ace bandage

23. _____ Granulated sugar

Column B

A. Primary layer adherent

B. Primary layer nonadherent, nonocclusive

C. Primary layer nonadherent semiocclusive

D. Primary layer nonadherent occlusive

E. Primary layer hypertonic or hyperosmolar

F. Secondary layer

G. Tertiary layer

Instructions: Match each bandage, cast, or sling with its corresponding photo by writing the name in the space provided. Then list the primary indication(s) for each bandage, cast, or sling.

1. Hobbles

2. Modified Robert Jones bandage

3. Robert Jones bandage

4. Fiberglass cast

5. Velpeau sling

6. Carpal flexion sling

7. Ehmer sling

1. Name and primary indication(s):_____

_____

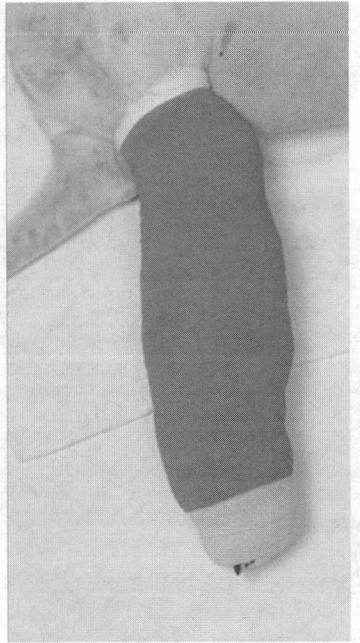

2. Name and primary indication(s):_____

_____

A

B

C

3. Name and primary indication(s):_____

_____

4. Name and primary indication(s):_____

_____

5. Name and primary indication(s):_____

_____

A

B

6. Name and primary indication(s):_____

_____

7. Name and primary indication(s):_____

_____

EXERCISE 27.8 ORDERING: APPLYING A CAST TO A HORSE'S LIMB

A cast is the external coaptation most frequently used to manage various orthopedic injuries or problems in horses when maximum support and immobilization are required. Collecting all necessary materials is the first step when applying a cast. A number of other specific steps must be performed in the correct order to apply the cast properly.

Instructions: Place the steps of applying a cast to a horse's limb in the proper order from first to last by writing the appropriate number (2 through 16) in the space provided. The first step has already been completed.

A. __1__ Collect all necessary materials.

B. _____ Place wire traction loops, if using, through the hoof.

C. _____ Apply two to three layers of 4- to 5-inch fiberglass material.

D. _____ Induce general anesthesia.

E. _____ Cover the limb with a double layer of stockinette.

F. _____ Clean the sole, remove the shoe, and trim the hoof.

G. _____ Place a wooden wedge underneath the heel.

H. _____ Dry the skin and powder it with talcum or boric acid.

I. _____ Apply two layers of 3-inch plaster material.

J. _____ Cut off the excess stockinette, leaving about 4 cm, and incorporate this into the last layer of the cast.

K. _____ Protect the bottom of the cast with hard acrylic.

L. _____ Apply orthopedic felt at points of pressure.

M. _____ Cut the traction wires, if used, and have an assistant support the leg.

N. _____ Apply support foam.

O. _____ Apply fiberglass material by overlapping one-third to one-half of its width as it's applied.

P. _____ Place adhesive tape around the top of the cast and attach it to the skin.

EXERCISE 27.9 TRUE OR FALSE: COMPREHENSIVE

Instructions: Read the following statements and write "T" for true or "F" for false in the blanks provided. If a statement is false, correct the statement to make it true.

1. _____ During the maturation phase of wound healing, the tissue regains normal strength.

2. _____ Corticosteroids delay all phases of wound healing.

3. _____ When lavaging a highly contaminated wound for the initial removal of debris and contamination, the type of fluid is more important than the amount you use.

4. _____ Fluid drainage from a wound is a reliable sign of infection and warrants antimicrobial therapy.

5. _____ Healthy granulation tissue is naturally resistant to infection and, therefore, does not require routine antimicrobial therapy.

6. ＿＿ Bite wounds are usually relatively easy to assess because the extent of the damage is visually apparent.

7. ＿＿ Bite wounds should always be considered contaminated.

8. ＿＿ Most burns in domestic animals are a result of accidental or deliberate injury from things like barn fires, car mufflers, electrical cords, or hot liquids.

9. ＿＿ The best treatment for pressure sores arising from splints or casts is the use of occlusive, nonadherent dressings.

10. ＿＿ The wet-to-dry bandage technique has largely been replaced by the nonadherent dressing.

11. ＿＿ The Robert Jones bandage is a frequently used bandage for small animal patients.

12. ＿＿ Cattle are notorious for their inability to tolerate bandages and casts, and other forms of wound care or immobilization are preferred.

13. ＿＿ As long as the device has been applied correctly, dogs with bandages, slings, and casts can be permitted to play in a fenced-in yard.

14. ＿＿ To keep a bandage dry, it should be covered with a plastic bag or an empty fluid IV bag at all times.

15. ＿＿ Basic wound management in horses is very similar to that of small companion animals.

16. ＿＿ Horses with open wounds on a limb below the carpus or tarsus are at risk for the development of exuberant granulation tissue.

17. ＿＿ Full limb casts can easily be applied to a horse under standing sedation.

18. ＿＿ Fiberglass casting tape is the preferred material to use due to its rigid, lightweight properties.

19. ＿＿ Stall confinement is mandatory after equine cast application.

20. ＿＿ The management of lameness in cattle is aided by the number of weight-bearing digits on each foot.

21. ＿＿ Platelet Rich Plasma and Tilapia skin grafts can be successful options in treating animal burns.

22. ＿＿ 1% Silver Sulfadiazine (SSD) cream has not proven successful in veterinary medicine for the treatment of burns.

EXERCISE 27.10 MULTIPLE CHOICE: COMPREHENSIVE

Instructions: Circle the one correct answer to each of the following questions.

1. The inflammatory phase of wound healing is also known as the
   a. lag phase.
   b. second phase.
   c. final phase.
   d. contraction phase.

2. All of the following treatments but one negatively impact wound healing. Which one does not negatively affect wound healing?
   a. Chemotherapy
   b. Corticosteroids
   c. Antimicrobials
   d. Radiation

3. The preferred antiseptic for wound lavage is
   a. 1:40 (0.05%) dilution of chlorhexidine solution and water.
   b. warm isotonic crystalloid fluid.
   c. 1% povidone-iodine solution.
   d. 2% chlorhexidine gluconate surgical scrub.

4. Wound debridement by use of a wet-to-dry bandage causes debridement that is classified as
   a. debridement en bloc.
   b. selective biologic debridement.
   c. staged selective surgical debridement.
   d. nonselective debridement.

5. Surgical wounds closed by direct apposition heal by
   a. moist wound healing.
   b. primary intention healing.
   c. second intention healing.
   d. third intention healing.

6. Wound drains should be removed when the amount of fluid decreases. This is often after approximately
   a. 1 to 2 days.
   b. 3 to 5 days.
   c. 5 to 7 days.
   d. 7 to 10 days.

7. Patients with a severely infected wound and systemic signs (such as lethargy, pain, and decreased appetite) often require that antimicrobials be given
   a. topically.
   b. orally.
   c. intramuscularly.
   d. intravenously.

8. Burn wounds are classified based on
   a. the depth and size.
   b. the size and duration.
   c. the duration and location.
   d. the location and depth.

9. A partial-thickness burn that is characterized by blisters and discoloration would be classified as
   a. first-degree.
   b. second-degree.
   c. third-degree.
   d. fourth-degree.

10. A full-thickness burn that is characterized by tough, discolored skin, but without involvement of deep tissues, would be classified as
    a. first-degree.
    b. second-degree.
    c. third-degree.
    d. fourth-degree.

11. Splints, casts, and slings can be used only to immobilize injuries below the
    a. metacarpus and metatarsus.
    b. carpus and tarsus.
    c. elbow and stifle.
    d. hip and shoulder.

12. There is a risk of complications from tightening the tertiary layer of a
    a. modified Robert Jones bandage.
    b. chest bandage.
    c. head bandage.
    d. Robert Jones bandage.

13. In small animals, the most commonly used device for treatment of the distal limb is the
    a. modified Robert-Jones bandage.
    b. fiberglass cast.
    c. Schroeder-Thomas splint.
    d. Robert-Jones bandage.

14. When applying cast padding and conforming gauze that comes on a roll, often it should be overlapped by approximately
    a. 30%.
    b. 50%.
    c. 70%.
    d. 0%; it should not be overlapped.

15. Most forelimb splints should be applied to the
    a. cranial surface.
    b. lateral surface.
    c. medial surface.
    d. caudal surface.

16. Most rear limb splints (with the exception of metatarsal and foot splints) should be applied to the
    a. cranial surface.
    b. lateral surface.
    c. medial surface.
    d. caudal surface.

17. Non–weight-bearing slings, like the Ehmer and the Velpeau, should not be maintained for more than
    a. 7 to 10 days.
    b. 1 to 2 weeks.
    c. 2 to 3 weeks.
    d. 4 to 6 weeks.

18. The toes of an animal with a distal limb bandage must be monitored for complications daily. An increased distance between the toenails of a foot is a sign of
    a. decreased viability.
    b. nothing; it is normal.
    c. swelling.
    d. skin maceration.

19. Horses can get proud flesh in wounds on the distal limb. The term *proud flesh* refers to
    a. an infected wound.
    b. excessive granulation tissue.
    c. a healthy-looking wound bed.
    d. a nonhealing open wound.

20. Casting material used in horses may include
    a. polyvinyl chloride (PVC) pipe.
    b. wooden slats.
    c. metal bars.
    d. all of the above.

21. When applying a cast to a limb, for optimal effectiveness, the cast must immobilize
    a. the joints proximal and distal to the injury.
    b. all the joints of the limb.
    c. only the joint proximal to the injury.
    d. only the bone that is fractured.

22. Application of excessive padding under a cast will
    a. cause it to get wet.
    b. cause pressure necrosis of the skin.
    c. result in cast sores.
    d. prevent cast sores.

23. When removing an equine distal limb cast, it should be split on
    a. the medial and lateral surfaces.
    b. the cranial and caudal surfaces.
    c. the diagonal surfaces.
    d. all four surfaces.

24. The best method for controlling proud flesh in horses is usually
    a. cryotherapy.
    b. electrocautery.
    c. topical treatment.
    d. surgical removal.

25. Despite advances in external and internal skeletal fixation, modified Thomas splints are still often used in
    a. horses.
    b. dogs.
    c. cattle.
    d. cats.

26. A "beehive" and aluminum rod are used to construct a
    a. coaptation splint.
    b. fiberglass cast.
    c. Modified Thomas splint.
    d. Robert Jones bandage.

27. The term for a partial or total separation of previously approximated wound edges is
    a. lag phase.
    b. dehiscence.
    c. primary healing.
    d. primary closure.

EXERCISE 27.11 FILL-IN-THE-BLANK: COMPREHENSIVE

Instructions: Fill in each of the spaces provided with the missing word or words that complete the sentence.

1. Wound strength is lowest during the _____ phase of healing.

2. Concerning the proliferative phase of wound healing, granulation tissue begins to form approximately _____ to _____ days after the injury; epithelialization begins approximately _____ to _____ days after the injury; and contraction of the wound begins approximately _____ days after the injury.

3. Healthy granulation tissue is _____ in color. If it is unhealthy, it is _____ in color.

4. When caring for a wound in a patient first presented for treatment, the first objective is always to prevent further _____ of the wound.

5. _____ intention healing is often used on the distal limb in situations where there is little available skin.

6. When treating patients with wound infections, antimicrobials are often chosen _____ (i.e., based on experience or observation). If the correct medication was chosen, the infection should generally resolve within _____ to _____ days of initiation of treatment.

7. Gunshot wounds and wounds caused by sticks are often treated in a similar manner to _____ wounds.

8. You might know that a pressure sore is starting to form if you see _____ of the skin with _____.

9. When treating wounds, once granulation tissue has formed and epithelialization begins, a(n) _____ primary layer must be used to promote second intention healing.

10. A cast that has been cut on both sides to create a top and bottom half is said to have been _____.

11. A properly applied Ehmer sling will internally _____ and _____ the femur, thereby forcing the _____ into the _____ and maintaining reduction.

12. After placing a tail bandage, a(n) _____ should be used to provide additional protection for the tip of the tail.

13. Bandages covering wounds with a lot of exudate should be replaced _____ times a day, whereas support bandages should be changed about every _____ days to check for complications.

14. A lower limb wound bandage on a horse is defined as a bandage distal to the _____ or the _____.

15. When applying an equine cast to the forelimb, _____ must be placed over pressure points.

EXERCISE 27.12 CASE STUDY: WOUND CARE

Signalment: Mindy, a 2-year-old, female, spaniel mix

History: The owner reported that Mindy jumped over the fence and disappeared from the yard 2 days ago. This morning, they found her lying on the front porch. She was covered with burs and had a large laceration on her left forelimb. The owner is not sure what happened, but it appears that she may have gotten caught on the fence and torn her skin as she jumped over.

Physical examination: Other than the laceration and mats and burs in her hair, Mindy appears normal. The wound is approximately 10 cm long; there is a 1 to 2 cm gap between the edges of the wound; and the wound is visibly dirty, appears to have some dead tissue around the edges, and is covered with a thick discharge. It appears that some skin was torn away, and it does not appear that there will be enough skin to completely cover the wound. After talking with the doctor, the owner elected to treat it as an open wound and let it heal by second intention. Answer the following questions regarding the management of this case.

1. What type of bandage could be used to nonselectively debride this wound?

_____

   a. Summarize the steps used to apply this bandage.

_____

_____

_____

_____

_____

_____

_____

b. Briefly explain how this bandage works to debride the wound.

_____

_____

_____

_____

c. What precautions must you take when using this type of bandage?

_____

_____

_____

_____

_____

_____

_____

2. What type of primary layer is often preferred to prevent destruction of granulation tissue and other healthy tissue? Give a few examples of the specific types of materials that can be used for this alternative type of primary layer.

_____

_____

_____

_____

_____

_____

3. Mindy was kept for the day while the wound was treated and the bandage was applied. The attending veterinarian has now asked you to discharge Mindy from the hospital and speak with her owner about the care of the bandage until they return the next day.

a. What instructions would you need to give Mindy's owner regarding the care of this bandage?

_____

_____

_____

_____

_____

_____

b. What signs should Mindy's owner watch for that would alert her of a complication that would need to be addressed?

_____

_____

_____

_____

_____

_____

28 | Pharmacology and Pharmacy

LEARNING OBJECTIVES

When you have completed this chapter, you will be able to:

1. Pronounce, define, and spell all key terms in this chapter.
2. Do the following related to types of drugs:
   - List approval categories of drugs and compare and contrast prescription drugs and over-the-counter drugs.
   - Explain the concept of a valid veterinarian–client–patient relationship and explain how it affects the use of prescription drugs.
   - Discuss laws affecting the use of controlled substances and list commonly used drugs that are classified as controlled substances.
3. List the dosage forms of medications, the routes by which medications may be administered, and factors that affect route selection, and discuss dosage terminology.
4. Do the following related to pharmacokinetics and pharmacodynamics:
   - Describe the principles of basic pharmacokinetics, including drug absorption, distribution, metabolism, and elimination.
   - Describe the principles of basic pharmacodynamics, including mechanism of action, side effects, and adverse drug reactions.
   - Discuss the impact of disease (specifically cardiovascular, kidney, and liver diseases) on drug pharmacokinetics.
   - Discuss aging and drug pharmacokinetics.
5. Do the following regarding drug nomenclature and the systemic approach to drug classification:
   - Discuss the different ways drugs can be identified.
   - List the main drug classes used to treat major animal diseases and give examples of drugs in each class, including their mechanism of action and common side effects.
6. Do the following regarding regulatory pharmacology:
   - List state and federal agencies regulating drug use and explain how they work together to ensure that available drugs are safe and effective and are used appropriately to treat and prevent animal diseases.
   - Define extra-label drug use and discuss circumstances under which drugs may or may not be used in this manner, including special restrictions on extra-label drug use in food-producing animals.
   - Discuss the significance of drug residues in food-producing animals and the importance of observing withdrawal times to keep the human food supply safe.
   - Define drug compounding and explain legal issues related to the compounding of medications.
7. Describe regulatory issues related to the procurement, storage, and disposal of pharmacologic agents.
8. Do the following regarding prescribing and dispensing drugs:
   - Correctly describe how to write a prescription and explain the parts of a prescription label.
   - Perform dosage calculations required to dispense drugs and administer drugs to patients.

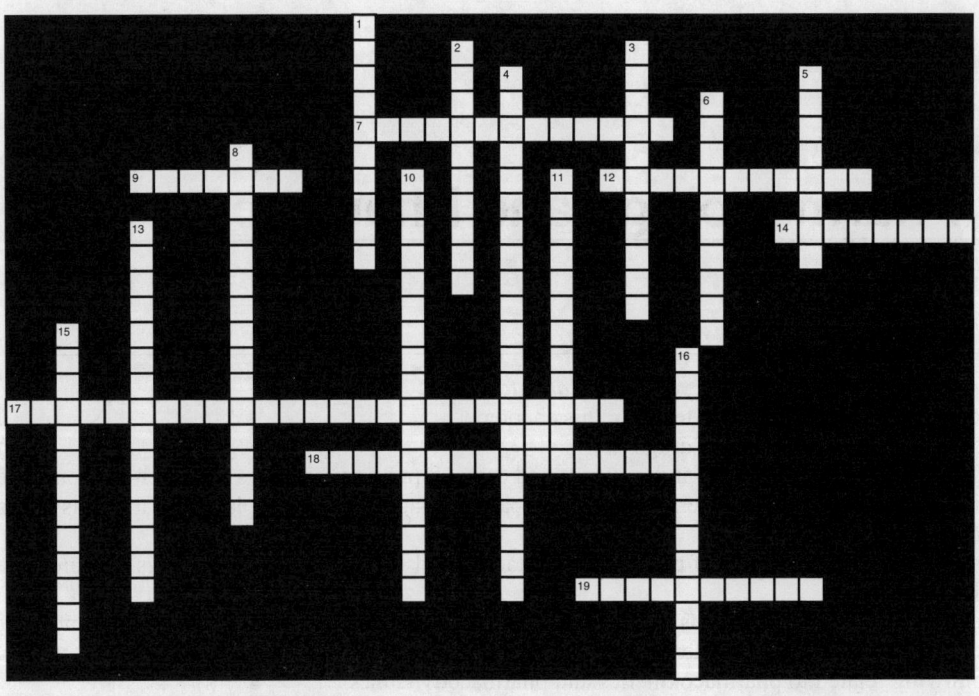

Across

7   A nondrug substance administered orally to provide substances required for normal body structure and function

9   A drug that activates a receptor, producing the same action as an endogenous substrate

12 Soluble in water

14 A drug's capacity, once bound to its receptor, to produce an effect

17 The periodic measurement of the amount of a drug in the blood (3 words)

18 A term summarized by the phrase "what the drug does to the body"

19 Use of a formulation of human insulin to treat type I diabetes in a dog is an example of this drug use (2 words)

Down

1   The term for administration of a drug by injection

2   Naloxone is one of these within the opioid family of drugs

3   When the amount of drug administered equals the amount of drug eliminated, the blood level is said to have reached _____ (2 words)

4   A drug will be expected to have the desired effect when the concentration in the bloodstream is within this level (3 words)

5   The time required for the amount of a drug in the body to decrease by 50%; used to estimate the dosing interval (2 words)

6   Absorption across cell membranes is more efficient for these drugs, than for hydrophilic drugs

8   A measure of the percentage of a drug dose that reaches the bloodstream

10 The chemical modification of a drug by the body

11 Another name for an Rx drug

13 Preparation of a flavored suspension of metronidazole to facilitate accurate oral dosing in a cat is a form of this (2 words)

15 A predictable reaction to a drug, the likelihood of which increases as the drug dose increases (2 words)

16 An unpredictable reaction to a drug that does not occur immediately, but after several days of treatment, and that is often associated with an immune system response

EXERCISE 28.2 MATCHING #1: TERMS RELATED TO REGULATORY ISSUES

Instructions: Match each term related to regulatory issues in column A with its corresponding definition in column B by writing the appropriate letter in the space provided.

Column A

1. _____ Animal Medicinal Drug Use Clarification Act (AMDUCA)

2. _____ Center for Veterinary Medicine (CVM)

3. _____ Drug Enforcement Agency (DEA)

4. _____ Environmental Protection Agency (EPA)

5. _____ Federal Food, Drug, and Cosmetic Act (FFD&C Act)

6. _____ U.S. Department of Agriculture (USDA)

7. _____ U.S. Pharmacopoeia (USP)—National Formulary (NF)

8. _____ Veterinarian–client–patient relationship (VCPR)

9. _____ Compendium of Veterinary Products (CVP)

Column B

A. A set of requirements that must be met in order for a veterinarian to prescribe a drug for a patient

B. The federal law that required manufacturers to provide evidence of safety under conditions prescribed on the label

C. The governing body that regulates the manufacture and distribution of drugs, food additives, and medical devices used in veterinary species

D. The government agency that regulates veterinary biologics

E. An amendment of the FFD&C Act that allows extra-label drug use for the treatment of veterinary species, provided specific conditions are met

F. A compilation of information about veterinary drugs and biologics

G. The government agency charged with overseeing and regulating pesticides

H. The official legal drug compendium for the United States; a compilation of all drug substances and products focused on providing active ingredients

I. The agency that categorizes controlled substances into five schedules (I, II, III, IV, and V) based on their potential for abuse

Instructions: Match each drug class or group in column A with its corresponding primary indication in column B by writing the appropriate letter in the space provided.

Column A

1. _____ Antiemetics
2. _____ Mitotane or trilostane
3. _____ Immunosuppressive drugs
4. _____ Decongestants
5. _____ Antibiotics
6. _____ Fludrocortisone
7. _____ Methimazole or radioactive iodide
8. _____ Anticoagulants
9. _____ Antitussives
10. _____ Insulin
11. _____ Antihypertensive
12. _____ Anticonvulsants
13. _____ Antiparasitics
14. _____ NSAIDs
15. _____ Diuretics
16. _____ L-thyroxine
17. _____ Antifungal drugs
18. _____ Inotropic agents
19. _____ Diazepam
20. _____ Antiarrhythmics

Column B

A. Diabetes mellitus
B. Hyperadrenocorticism
C. Prevent life-threatening thrombi
D. Immune-mediated diseases
E. Dermatophyte infections
F. Hypoadrenocorticism
G. Vomiting
H. Hyperthyroidism
I. High blood pressure
J. Coughing
K. Cluster seizures and status epilepticus
L. Inflammation
M. Edema
N. GI nematode and arthropod infestations
O. Hypothyroidism
P. Swelling and congestion of the nasal passages
Q. Improved contractility of cardiac muscle
R. Control heart rhythm abnormalities
S. Epilepsy
T. Bacterial infections

EXERCISE 28.4 MATCHING #3: ADVERSE DRUG REACTIONS

Instructions: Column A lists characteristics that apply to drug reactions. Indicate whether each characteristic applies to dose-dependent reactions, idiosyncratic reactions, or both by writing an "A," "B," or "C" in the space provided. (Note that responses will be used more than once.)

Column A

1. _____ Associated with an immune-system response
2. _____ Occur at standard and inappropriate doses
3. _____ Unpredictable
4. _____ Treatment requires drug avoidance
5. _____ May be prevented by therapeutic drug monitoring
6. _____ Affect all members of a species
7. _____ Not dose-dependent
8. _____ Not related to the action of the drug
9. _____ Predictable
10. _____ May cause adverse T-cell sensitization
11. _____ Therapeutic drug monitoring will not prevent them
12. _____ Often affects multiple species
13. _____ Occur after several days of treatment
14. _____ May or may not affect multiple species
15. _____ More severe at higher doses
16. _____ Often respond to dose reduction
17. _____ Affect a small portion of treated animals

Column B

A. Dose-dependent drug reactions

B. Idiosyncratic drug reactions

C. Both dose-dependent and idiosyncratic drug reactions

EXERCISE 28.5 MATCHING #4: ANTIBACTERIAL DRUGS

Instructions: Match each antibacterial drug in column A with the corresponding class to which it belongs in column B by writing the appropriate letter in the space provided. (Note that responses may be used more than once.)

Column A

1. _____ Cephalexin
2. _____ Marbofloxacin
3. _____ Oxytetracycline
4. _____ Amikacin
5. _____ Sulfamethoxazole
6. _____ Ampicillin
7. _____ Metronidazole
8. _____ Tilmicosin
9. _____ Florfenicol
10. _____ Gentamicin
11. _____ Amoxicillin
12. _____ Cefpodoxime
13. _____ Tylosin
14. _____ Enrofloxacin
15. _____ Erythromycin
16. _____ Trimethoprim
17. _____ Azithromycin
18. _____ Lincomycin
19. _____ Clindamycin
20. _____ Doxycycline

Column B

A. Cephalosporins
B. Aminoglycosides
C. Sulfonamides
D. Potentiated sulfonamides
E. Fluoroquinolones
F. Amphenicols
G. Macrolides
H. Lincosamides
I. Tetracyclines
J. Nitroimidazoles
K. Aminopenicillins

EXERCISE 28.6 MATCHING #5: MECHANISM OF ACTION

Instructions: Match each commonly used drug in column A with its mechanism of action in column B by writing the appropriate letter in the space provided. (Note that responses may be used more than once.)

Column A

1. ____ Benazepril
2. ____ NSAIDs
3. ____ Digoxin
4. ____ Tetrahydropyrimidines
5. ____ Apomorphine
6. ____ Sulfadiazine
7. ____ Furosemide
8. ____ Quinidine
9. ____ Famotidine
10. ____ Heparin
11. ____ Aspirin
12. ____ Enalapril
13. ____ Omeprazole
14. ____ Neomycin
15. ____ Diphenhydramine
16. ____ Lidocaine

Column B

A. Histamine antagonist

B. Inhibits bacterial production of folic acid

C. Suppresses prostaglandin synthesis by inhibiting cyclooxygenase

D. Inhibits angiotensin-converting enzyme

E. Binds to histamine receptors

F. Agonist at parasitic nicotinic acetylcholine receptors

G. Blockade of fast sodium channels (slow action potential conduction)

H. Produces sedation as a dopamine receptor agonist

I. Inhibits sodium/potassium/chloride (Na +/K +/2Cl −) reabsorption in the loop of Henle

J. Increases the strength of heart muscle contraction by increasing the calcium concentration in cardiac muscle cells

K. Inhibits bacterial ribosomal protein production

L. Proton pump inhibitor

M. Interferes with clot formation by inhibiting the conversion of prothrombin to thrombin

EXERCISE 28.7 MATCHING #6: DRUGS USED TO TREAT GASTROINTESTINAL DISEASE

Instructions: Match each drug or group of drugs used to treat gastrointestinal disease in column A with the corresponding mechanism of action to which it belongs in column B by writing the appropriate letter in the space provided. (Note that responses may be used more than once.)

Column A

1. ____ Famotidine and ranitidine
2. ____ Maropitant citrate
3. ____ Prochlorperazine and chlorpromazine
4. ____ Cisapride
5. ____ Omeprazole
6. ____ Pancrelipase
7. ____ Cyproheptadine
8. ____ Sucralfate
9. ____ Docusate potassium
10. ____ Loperamide
11. ____ Dronabinol
12. ____ Metoclopramide
13. ____ Xylazine

Column B

A. Serotonin receptor agonist

B. Histamine antagonist

C. Promotes gastric ulcer healing

D. Reduces water absorption from the colon

E. Neurokinin 1 receptor antagonist

F. Dopamine receptor, histamine receptor, cholinergic receptor, and adrenergic receptor antagonist

G. Increase segmental contractions

H. Digestive enzyme supplement

I. Proton pump inhibitor

J. Serotonin receptor antagonist

K. Dopamine antagonist

L. Affects cannabinoid receptors in the vomiting receptor

M. Alpha$_2$ receptor agonist

EXERCISE 28.8 MATCHING #7: DRUGS USED TO TREAT CARDIOVASCULAR DISEASE

Instructions: Match each drug or group of drugs used to treat cardiovascular disease in column A with the corresponding class to which it belongs in column B by writing the appropriate letter in the space provided. More than one selection from Column B is possible.

Column A

1. _____ Atenolol and propranolol
2. _____ Pimobendan
3. _____ Diltiazem
4. _____ Furosemide and spironolactone
5. _____ Lidocaine and quinidine
6. _____ Benazepril and enalapril
7. _____ Hydralazine
8. _____ Amlodipine
9. _____ Digoxin
10. _____ Sotalol
11. _____ Sildenafil

Column B

A. Diuretic

B. ACE inhibitor (antihypertensive)

C. Positive inotrope

D. Calcium channel blocker (class IV antiarrhythmic)

E. β-adrenergic blocker (class II antiarrhythmic)

F. Phosphodiesterase V inhibitor (antihypertensive)

G. Fast sodium channel blocker (class I antiarrhythmic)

H. Alters calcium metabolism of vascular smooth muscle cells (antihypertensive)

I. Calcium channel blocker (antihypertensive)

J. Phosphodiesterase III inhibitor (balanced vasodilator/positive inotrope)

K. Potassium channel blocker (class III antiarrhythmic)

EXERCISE 28.9 MATCHING #8: DRUGS PROHIBITED FOR USE IN FOOD-PRODUCING ANIMALS

Instructions: Match each drug or drug class in column A with the reason that it is banned in food-producing animals in column B by writing the appropriate letter in the space provided. (Note that responses may be used more than once.)

Column A

1. _____ Fluoroquinolones
2. _____ Clenbuterol
3. _____ Chloramphenicol
4. _____ Glycopeptides (vancomycin)
5. _____ Adamantanes
6. _____ Nitrofurans
7. _____ Sulfonamides
8. _____ Nitroimidazoles

Column B

A. Microbial drug resistance in humans

B. Used for treating or preventing influenza A

C. Carcinogenicity

D. Toxicity and death associated with human consumption of edible tissues

E. Carcinogenicity and mutagenicity

F. Idiosyncratic bone marrow toxicosis in humans

Instructions: Read the following statements and write "T" for true or "F" for false in the blanks provided. If a statement is false, correct the statement to make it true.

1. ____ To achieve therapeutic blood levels, hydrophilic drugs must be administered by injection.

2. ____ Drugs leave the vascular space by the process of adsorption.

3. ____ Biotransformation tends to make most drugs more hydrophilic prior to elimination in the urine or bile.

4. ____ Drug metabolism most often occurs in the kidney.

5. ____ Drug side effects are commonly related to the drug's mechanism of action.

6. ____ Glucocorticoids are classified according to the receptor they bind to.

7. ____ The term antibacterial is used in reference to substances that kill or inhibit the growth of bacteria.

8. ____ The most common side effects of antimicrobial drugs are vomiting and diarrhea.

9. ____ When treating disseminated fungal infections, most systemic antifungal drugs are given for approximately 10 days to 2 weeks.

10. ____ Feline hyperthyroidism is generally treated with levothyroxine.

11. ____ Mitotane kills the cells in the adrenal gland that produce cortisol, whereas trilostane does not.

12. ____ The molecular structure of insulin varies widely among the common domestic species.

13. ____ Because insulin is usually given in very small doses, a tuberculin syringe should be used to administer it.

14. ____ Glargine insulin has a bioactivity of 40 U/mL.

15. ____ Therapeutic strategies used in the treatment of gastrointestinal (GI) disease include nonspecific supportive therapies and targeted therapies based on the primary underlying disease process.

16. ____ Treatment of congestive heart failure is one of the main indications for diuretics such as furosemide.

17. ____ The class I antiarrhythmic lidocaine is administered orally to treat ventricular tachycardia.

18. ____ Potassium bromide may be used as an alternative to phenobarbital to control seizures in dogs with liver disease.

19. ____ Macrocyclic lactones, such as ivermectin and milbemycin oxime, have a prolonged effect because they are packaged in a slow-release form.

20. ____ Collies and related breeds have a genetic predisposition for CNS toxicity to milbemycins and avermectins.

21. ____ State laws cover drug distribution within the state, whereas federal laws cover drug manufacturing.

22. ____ Regulation of online pharmacies is primarily in the hands of the FDA.

23. ____ The single most important rule in successfully performing drug calculations is to keep track of the units.

24. ____ Dose-dependent drug reactions are unpredictable and do not respond to dose reduction or drug withdrawal.

25. _____ Drug compounding is a form of extra-label drug use.

26. _____ Vitamins, minerals, and herbs are considered to be dietary supplements, whereas nutraceuticals are classified as drugs.

27. _____ Internet companies are uniformly reliable sources of high-quality drugs and information about those drugs.

28. _____ A reverse distribution company (RDC) will dispose of expired drugs, including controlled substances.

29. _____ The units used to express most drug dosages are gm/unit body weight (lb).

EXERCISE 28.11 MULTIPLE CHOICE: COMPREHENSIVE

Instructions: Circle the one correct answer to each of the following questions.

1. A drug's pharmacokinetics are not used to determine its
   a. dose.
   b. withdrawal time.
   c. dosing regimen.
   d. action.

2. A drug will be 100% bioavailable when it is given
   a. SC.
   b. orally.
   c. IV.
   d. IM.

3. Because of a genetic mutation, Collies and a few other dog breeds have a nonfunctional p-glycoprotein pump. This abnormality makes these breeds more sensitive to the drug ivermectin because it
   a. decreases protein binding of the drug.
   b. decreases the action of the blood–brain barrier.
   c. increases its lipid solubility.
   d. increases tissue binding of the drug.

4. One example of a drug that is metabolized by the body into a toxic metabolite is
   a. acetaminophen.
   b. digoxin.
   c. Enalapril.
   d. selamectin.

5. Aspirin can be used in cats to prevent thrombus formation, but it must be used with caution because of
   a. the short half-life.
   b. the slow metabolism in the cat.
   c. the gastrointestinal side effects (bleeding).
   d. secondary infection.

6. The half-life of a drug is used to determine the
   a. dose.
   b. prescription duration.
   c. dose interval.
   d. potency.

7. A drug's pharmacokinetics are least likely to be affected by
   a. kidney disease.
   b. liver disease.
   c. heart disease.
   d. CNS disease.

8. Blood flow to the kidneys is negatively impacted by
   a. NSAID-class drugs.
   b. penicillin-class drugs.
   c. benzodiazepine-class drugs.
   d. tetracycline-class drugs.

9. Respiratory drugs include
   a. bronchodilators and barbiturates.
   b. neuraminidase inhibitors.
   c. expectorants and mucolytics.
   d. nutraceuticals.

10. "Dry eye" (a deficiency of the tear film) is a known dose-dependent adverse drug reaction to which class of antibacterial drugs?
    a. Potentiated sulfonamides
    b. Amphenicols
    c. Aminoglycosides
    d. Fluoroquinolones

11. Which of the following attributes is not associated with long-acting glucocorticoids?
    a. Doses cannot be effectively tapered.
    b. They stay in the body until they are naturally eliminated.
    c. They are available in oral, injectable, optical, otic, and ophthalmic forms.
    d. Their use increases the production of natural glucocorticoids.

12. The glucocorticoid _____ has a long duration of action.
    a. prednisone
    b. betamethasone
    c. hydrocortisone
    d. triamcinolone

13. Which of the following immunosuppressive drugs causes a wide variety of adverse effects, including polyphagia, polydipsia, polyuria, and delayed wound healing?
    a. Azathioprine
    b. Cyclosporine A
    c. Prednisolone
    d. Chlorambucil

14. The penicillin-class drug or combination that has activity against beta-lactamase is
    a. ampicillin.
    b. penicillin G.
    c. amoxicillin.
    d. amoxicillin and clavulanate.

15. Which class of antibacterial drugs is known for causing kidney toxicity?
    a. β-Lactams
    b. Tetracyclines
    c. Aminoglycosides
    d. All of the above

16. The cephalosporin-class antibacterials are classified according to
    a. the duration of action.
    b. the subclass.
    c. generation (first, second, third, etc.).
    d. strength.

17. Which two classes of antibacterial drugs have efficacy against protozoa?
    a. Sulfonamides and nitroimidazoles
    b. Penicillins and cephalosporins
    c. Tetracyclines and amphenicols
    d. Aminoglycosides and lincosamides

18. Which class of antibacterials is known to damage cartilage in young animals and cause blindness in cats as a part of its adverse effect profile?
    a. Amphenicols
    b. Macrolides
    c. Fluoroquinolones
    d. Sulfonamides

19. Which two antibacterial drugs and/or drug classes are banned in food-producing animals?
    a. β-Lactams and enrofloxacin
    b. Tetracycline and the macrolides
    c. Chloramphenicol and nitroimidazoles
    d. Aminoglycosides and lincosamides

20. Which of the following drugs is an imidazole-class antifungal used to treat disseminated fungal infections?
    a. Trilostane
    b. Amphotericin B
    c. Clotrimazole
    d. Ketoconazole

21. Since multiple manufacturers may produce the same drug, the drug may be known by multiple
    a. trade names.
    b. generic names.
    c. chemical names.
    d. capitalized names.

22. Hyperthyroidism is a condition that is seen most frequently in
    a. cats.
    b. horses.
    c. dogs.
    d. cattle.

23. Insulin is a hormone produced in the beta cells of the pancreas and is responsible for cellular uptake of
    a. glucose.
    b. phosphate.
    c. potassium.
    d. All of the above.

24. Which of the following types of insulin can be given intravenously?
    a. NPH
    b. PZIR
    c. Glargine
    d. Regular

25. NPH insulin is an example of
    a. intermediate-acting insulin.
    b. long-acting insulin.
    c. fast-acting insulin.
    d. short-acting insulin.

26. The phrase "first-pass effect" refers to which organ?
    a. Heart
    b. Kidney
    c. Liver
    d. Brain

27. Which of the changes associated with aging has the most clinically significant impact on drug elimination?
    a. Increased fatty tissue
    b. Decreased hepatic metabolism
    c. Reduced kidney function
    d. Decreased cardiac output

28. Amlodipine is most commonly used to treat
    a. canine pulmonary hypertension.
    b. hypertension in cats and dogs.
    c. congestive heart failure.
    d. CHF secondary to mitral insufficiency.

29. Which of the following antiarrhythmics is a β-adrenergic blocker?
    a. Lidocaine
    b. Sotalol
    c. Diltiazem
    d. Quinidine

30. The abbreviation "bid" on a written prescription means
    a. before meals.
    b. after meals.
    c. two times a day.
    d. once a day.

31. Which of the following antiparasitics is effective against cestodes?
    a. Pyrantel
    b. Fenbendazole
    c. Netobimin
    d. Praziquantel

32. Ectoparasite agents are most commonly given
    a. subcutaneously.
    b. orally.
    c. topically.
    d. intramuscularly.

33. Which of the following ectoparasiticides targets the parasite's growth and development by inhibiting development of the parasite's exoskeleton?
    a. Imidacloprid
    b. Lufenuron
    c. Fipronil
    d. Carbamate

34. Which agency regulates the manufacture and distribution of veterinary drugs and food additives?
    a. Environmental Protection Agency (EPA)
    b. Drug Enforcement Agency (DEA)
    c. U.S. Department of Agriculture (USDA)
    d. FDA's Center for Veterinary Medicine

35. The Drug Enforcement Agency (DEA) categorizes controlled drugs
    a. as Schedule I, II, III, IV, or V.
    b. as Rx or non-Rx.
    c. based on their chemical structure.
    d. based on the severity of their side effects.

36. Schedule II controlled substances have a high abuse potential and require the completion of a special form when ordering them. Which of the following controlled substances is classified as a Schedule II substance?
    a. Codeine
    b. Phenobarbital
    c. Fentanyl
    d. Ketamine

37. Nutraceuticals
    a. are subject to safety evaluations by the FDA.
    b. are made using a standardized manufacturing process.
    c. are classified as over-the-counter drugs.
    d. may be administered without medical supervision.

38. Which of the following abbreviations used in prescription writing is not universally understood by human medical professionals?
    a. s.i.d.
    b. p.r.n.
    c. t.i.d.
    d. q.o.d.

39. The FDA requires standard expiration dates on all approved drug products except
    a. antiparasitics.
    b. rodenticides.
    c. benzimidazoles.
    d. The FDA requires standard expiration dates on all approved drugs without exception.

40. Which of the following is not true of the online pharmacy?
    a. Regulated by the FDA and the NABP
    b. Requires a valid hard copy provided directly from the prescriber
    c. Offers a toll-free phone number and street address
    d. Allows direct contact with its pharmacists for consultation

41. Percent solutions may be expressed as volume/volume ratio. For instance, a 5% solution contains
    a. 5 mL in 1 mL of solution.
    b. 5 mL in 1 L of solution.
    c. 5 mL in 100 mL of solution.
    d. 5 mL in 100 L of solution.

42. Which of the following metric system weight conversions is correct?
    a. 1 kg = 100 g
    b. 1 mcg = 1000 mg
    c. 10 ng = 1 mcg
    d. 1000 mg = 1 g

43. Which of the following metric system volume conversions is correct?
    a. 100 mL = 1 dL
    b. 100 mL = 1 L
    c. 1 mcL = 1000 mL
    d. 1000 mcL = 1 L

EXERCISE 28.12 FILL-IN-THE-BLANK: COMPREHENSIVE

Instructions: Fill in each of the spaces provided with the missing word or words that complete the sentence.

1. The study of drugs used in the diagnosis, treatment, or prevention of disease is known as _____.

2. The relationship between the amount of drug in the _____ and the concentration in the _____ is measured by the volume of distribution (Vd).

3. The protein that protects the brain from exposure to various drugs and substances by actively pumping them out of the cells is referred to as the _____.

4. Most drugs are eliminated from the body by the _____ into the _____.

5. It takes approximately _____ half-lives for a drug to reach a steady state after it is first administered.

6. Whereas the antiseizure drug _____ is known to cause a dose-dependent adverse drug reaction involving the liver in dogs, the antiseizure drug _____ is known to cause an idiosyncratic adverse drug reaction involving the liver in cats.

7. Immunosuppressive drugs are used to treat _____ diseases.

8. The use of glucocorticoids concurrently with _____ _____ drugs (NSAIDs) is contraindicated because of the increased risk of gastrointestinal bleeding, _____, or perforation.

9. The method of choosing a specific antibacterial based on observation and experience is called _____ antibacterial therapy.

10. The two specific classes of drugs that are part of the larger β-lactam class are the _____ and _____.

11. The adverse effects of antifungal drugs result from targeting the _____ in the cell membranes of the treated patient.

12. _____ and _____ are two topical antifungal drugs used to treat yeast otitis.

13. Medical therapies for feline hyperthyroidism include the drug _____ and radioactive _____ therapy.

14. One cause of hyperadrenocorticism is overproduction of ACTH in the brain (called _____ -dependent hyperadrenocorticism), and the other cause is overproduction of cortisol by a(n) _____ tumor.

15. The concentration of insulin is expressed in _____ of activity per mL.

16. Congestive heart failure will result in an accumulation of fluid in the _____, _____ _____, and _____.

17. Drugs used to treat patients with heart failure include _____, _____, _____, and _____.

18. Diuretics eliminate fluid buildup by inhibiting the _____ of sodium at different parts of the _____.

19. The goal of therapy with lactulose in patients with hepatic encephalopathy is to make the stool _____, but not to produce _____.

20. Diuretic medications are intended to increase excretion of _____ and _____.

21. Digoxin has a narrow _____ _____ (a low ratio between the therapeutic plasma levels and toxic plasma levels).

22. The drugs enalapril and benazepril work by inhibiting _____ converting enzyme (ACE).

23. Whereas arrhythmias that originate from the atria are referred to as _____, arrhythmias that originate from the ventricles are referred to as _____.

24. The anticonvulsant of choice in cats is _____, because potassium bromide causes _____ symptoms in 40% of treated cats.

25. Endoparasites include three classes: (a) _____, (b) _____, and (c) _____.

26. Although used to control flies, ticks, mites, and mosquitoes, pyrethrins are not safe for use in _____.

27. The Animal Medicinal Drug Use Clarification Act (AMDUCA) enables veterinarians to use and prescribe animal and human drugs for _____ use under defined conditions.

28. The time interval between the last administered drug dose to a food-producing animal and the time that the animal can be slaughtered or animal products such as eggs or milk can be used is known as the _____ _____.

29. The presence of a drug or its metabolite in cells, tissues, organs, or other edible products of an animal is referred to as a(n) _____.

30. An enteric coating is designed to prevent exposure of an oral medication to the acid environment of the _____ and delay absorption until it reaches the higher pH of the _____.

31. Some injectable drugs are able to cross the oral mucous membranes of some species. An example of a drug that is absorbed transmucosally in cats is the opioid analgesic _____.

32. No expiration date is required on the label of drugs regulated by the _____ (an acronym).

EXERCISE 28.13 DOSAGE CALCULATIONS: COMPREHENSIVE

Perform each of the following dosage calculations according to guidelines A through D.

A. When performing calculations involving administration of oral tablets, express answers that are less than 1 tablet as a fraction (e.g., "½ tablet" instead of "0.5 tablet").

B. When performing calculations involving administration of injectable medications, express fractions of a milliliter (mL) as a decimal (e.g., "2.5 mL" instead of "2½ mL").

C. When writing instructions for the client, write it as you would on the label (e.g., "Give 1 tablet by mouth twice daily for 10 days" instead of "1 tab. P.O. BID × 10 d").

D. When writing instructions for the client, only limit the duration of administration (e.g., "Give 1 tablet once daily for 10 days" or "Give 1 tablet once daily until gone") if the medication is being given for a limited time. If the medication is ongoing, and the client will need to come in for a refill, do not include either of these phrases.

1. **Order:** 22 mg/kg amoxicillin P.O. The patient weighs 25 lb. The tablet strength is 100 mg, and the tablets are scored. How many tablets will you give? (Note: You may round your answer down to the nearest ½ tablet.)

   _____ tablet(s)

2. **Order:** 0.25 mg/lb butorphanol P.O. The patient weighs 30 lb. The tablet strength is 5 mg, and the tablets are scored. How many tablets will you give? (Note: You may round your answer down to the nearest ½ tablet.)

   _____ tablet(s)

3. **Order:** 0.01 mg/lb fludrocortisone P.O. The patient weighs 60 lb. The tablet strength is 0.1 mg. How many tablets will you give?

   _____ tablet(s)

4. **Order:** 0.5 mg/kg prednisolone. The patient weighs 66 lb. The tablet strength is 5 mg. How many tablets will you give?

_____ tablet(s)

5. **Order:** 62.5 mg sulfasalazine. The tablet strength is 500 mg. How many tablets will you give?

_____ tablet(s)

6. **Order:** 0.01 mg/lb soloxine q 24 hr. *(Note that this drug will be given for the remainder of the patient's life.)* The patient weighs 34 lb. The tablet strengths available are 0.1 mg, 0.2 mg, and 0.6 mg. The pills are scored. Determine the patient's total dose in mg, the most convenient pill size to dispense to achieve this dose (you may round down to the nearest size), how many tablets the owner will need to give each dose, the number of tablets you will dispense to supply this patient for 30 days, and instructions to the client.

This patient's total dose in mg (each time the drug is administered): _____

Pill size you would dispense: _____

Number of tablets the owner will give each dose: _____

The number of tablets to dispense: _____

Your instructions to the client: _____

_____

_____

7. **Order:** 5 mg/kg amoxitabs BID for 10 days. *(This medication will not be ongoing.)* The patient weighs 25 lb. The tablet strengths available are 50 mg, 100 mg, 200 mg, and 400 mg. The pills are *not* scored. Determine the patient's total dose in mg, the most convenient pill size to dispense to achieve this dose (you may round down to the nearest size), how many tablets the owner will need to give each dose, the number of tablets you will dispense, and the instructions to the client.

This patient's total dose in mg (each time the drug is administered): _____

Pill size you would dispense: _____

Number of tablets the owner will give each dose: _____

The number of tablets to dispense: _____

Your instructions to the client: _____

_____

_____

_____

8. **Order:** 15 mg prednisolone BID for 2 weeks, then 15 mg q 24 hr × 2 weeks; then 15 mg QOD for 2 weeks. *(This medication will not be ongoing.)* The tablet strength available is 5 mg only. The pills are scored. Determine how many tablets the owner will need to give each dose, the number of tablets you will dispense, and the instructions to the client.

   Number of tablets the owner will give each dose: _____

   The number of tablets to dispense: _____

   Your instructions to the client: _____

   _____

   _____

   _____

9. **Order:** 36 mg prednisolone injectable SQ. The prednisolone injection strength is 10 mg/mL. What volume will you administer expressed in mL?

   _____ mL

10. **Order:** 14 mEq of potassium chloride is to be added to a 1 L bag of fluids. The KCl solution strength is 20 mEq/10 mL. How many mL will you add to the bag of fluids?

    _____ mL

11. **Order:** 5 mg/kg sodium dexamethasone phosphate injectable IV. The patient weighs 35 lb. The solution strength is 4 mg/mL. Determine the total dose for this patient (mg) and how many mL you will give.

    Total dose for the patient in mg: _____

    How many mL you will give: _____

12. **Order:** 1 mg/lb lidocaine IV. The patient weighs 50 lb. The solution strength is 2%. How many mL do you give? Determine the total dose for this patient (mg) and how many mL you will give.

    Total dose for the patient in mg: _____

    How many mL you will give: _____

EXERCISE 28.14 CASE STUDY #1: VETERINARIAN–CLIENT–PATIENT RELATIONSHIP

An acquaintance asks that you request a prescription for heartworm medication for her dog from the veterinarian who owns the practice where you work. You ask her to schedule an appointment for her dog to be seen by your vet. She asks why you can't just get the prescription without her dog being seen by the vet. What do you say?

_____

_____

_____

_____

_____

_____

_____

_____

_____

EXERCISE 28.15 CASE STUDY #2: DISPENSING MEDICATIONS

Annie, a 4-year-old, spayed female, black Labrador Retriever, is presented for treatment of inhalant allergies. This is a recurrent problem in the fall, and allergy testing has indicated a sensitivity to several allergens, including ragweed pollen. At the height of the season, she often gets so itchy that she must be given both antihistamines and glucocorticoids to control it, or she will develop dermatitis with hair loss and a secondary pyoderma. At this point, Annie has no skin lesions but is very pruritic. The doctor wants to prescribe antihistamines and prednisolone now so that the itching can be brought under control before she develops skin lesions.

1. Consider the following written prescription:

   a. Use your knowledge of abbreviations used in prescription writing to interpret this order by writing the prescription out in longhand.

   _____

   _____

   _____

b. Now prepare a label to be affixed to the bottle with all the required information for a noncontrolled substance.

Disp. #30, 5 mg, prednisolone; Sig: Give 1 tab PO q 12 h × 2d, then 1 tab q.o.d. until gone.

St. Francis Veterinary Associates
10000 Main Ave.
Anywhere, USA 98765
987-000-1234

29 Pain Management

LEARNING OBJECTIVES

When you have completed this chapter, you will be able to:

1. Pronounce, define, and spell all key terms in the chapter.
2. Explain how the technician can use effective communication, observation, and interpretation skills to advocate for the patient and help provide effective and appropriate analgesia.
3. List common causes and physiologic and behavioral signs of pain in small animals, including the negative effects of untreated pain.
4. Describe the physiologic aspects of pain, including the phases of nociception in mammals, and compare acute, chronic, inflammatory, neuropathic, somatic, and visceral pain and explain the significance of the "wind-up phenomenon."
5. Do the following regarding the treatment of pain in small animals:
   - Describe the basic principles of effective analgesia protocol design and pain management, including preemptive and multimodal analgesia concepts.
   - Compare and contrast agents used to treat pain in small animals, including nonsteroidal anti-inflammatory drugs (NSAIDs), local anesthetics, opioids, and alpha$_2$ agonists.
   - List the analgesics commonly given by constant rate infusion (CRI) and perform the calculations required to administer a drug by CRI.
   - List the "adjunctive analgesics" and nonpharmacologic treatment options for pain control and describe the uses and benefits of each.
6. Do the following regarding the treatment of pain in large animals:
   - List causes and signs of pain in large animals and explain why large animals often are undertreated for pain.
   - Compare and contrast agents used to treat pain in large animals, including NSAIDs, opioids, alpha$_2$ agonists, and local anesthetics.
   - Discuss the role of joint supplements, chondroprotective agents, miscellaneous agents, alternative and complementary therapy, and good husbandry in the treatment of pain in large animals.
7. Describe analgesic agents and techniques commonly used in horses, cattle, sheep, goats, camelids, and pigs, and explain how economics and drug residues influence the decision to treat pain in food animals.

Instructions: Match each term in column A with its corresponding definition in column B by writing the appropriate letter in the space provided.

Column A

1. _____ Transduction
2. _____ Antagonist
3. _____ Agonist
4. _____ Nociception
5. _____ Breakthrough pain
6. _____ Transmission
7. _____ Agonist-antagonist
8. _____ Dysphoria
9. _____ Wind-up phenomenon
10. _____ Allodynia
11. _____ Neurotransmitters
12. _____ Hyperalgesia
13. _____ Multimodal analgesia
14. _____ Preemptive analgesia
15. _____ Partial agonist
16. _____ Modulation

Column B

A. A drug that blocks receptors

B. Pain management administered before any trauma occurs to prevent expected pain

C. Movement of a nerve impulse along peripheral nerves to the spinal cord

D. A situation in which less and less stimulation is required to initiate pain

E. A drug that stimulates some receptors and blocks others

F. The combination of allodynia and hyperalgesia

G. Transmission of pain impulses by fibers that normally carry pleasant or neutral impulses

H. Conversion of mechanical, chemical, and thermal energy into electrical impulses

I. Pain exceeding the usual protocol

J. The process by which pain is detected by the nervous system

K. Amplifying or dampening of a nerve impulse in the CNS

L. The use of two or more analgesic drugs to alter more than one phase of the pain pathway

M. An emotional state characterized by anxiety, depression, or unease

N. A drug that causes partial stimulation of receptor sites

O. A drug that simulates receptors

P. Chemicals that transmit nerve impulses between nerve cells

EXERCISE 29.2 MATCHING #2: EXPECTED LEVEL OF PAIN ASSOCIATED WITH COMMON CONDITIONS AND PROCEDURES

Instructions: Match each condition or procedure in column A with its corresponding expected level of pain in column B by writing the appropriate letter in the space provided. (Note that responses may be used more than once.)

Column A

1. _____ Cervical disc herniation
2. _____ Laparotomy
3. _____ Castration
4. _____ Limb amputation
5. _____ Mass removal
6. _____ Declawing
7. _____ Fracture repair
8. _____ Dental procedures
9. _____ Ear canal ablation

Column B

A. Mild to moderate pain

B. Severe pain

EXERCISE 29.3 MATCHING #3: ANALGESICS AND ANALGESIC CLASSES

Instructions: Match each analgesic in column A with the corresponding class to which it belongs in column B by writing the appropriate letter in the space provided. (Note that responses may be used more than once.)

Column A

1. _____ Phenylbutazone
2. _____ Morphine
3. _____ Ketamine
4. _____ Naloxone hydrochloride
5. _____ Lidocaine
6. _____ Romifidine
7. _____ Buprenorphine
8. _____ Carprofen
9. _____ Xylazine
10. _____ Flunixin meglumine
11. _____ Butorphanol
12. _____ Mepivacaine
13. _____ Atipamezole
14. _____ Sodium hyaluronate
15. _____ Ketoprofen
16. _____ Dexmedetomidine
17. _____ Fentanyl
18. _____ Firocoxib
19. _____ Hydromorphone
20. _____ Aspirin
21. _____ Bupivacaine
22. _____ Detomidine
23. _____ Polysulfated GAGs
24. _____ Meloxicam

Column B

A. NSAID
B. α_2 Agonist
C. α_2 Antagonist
D. Local anesthetic
E. NMDA-receptor antagonist
F. Joint supplement and chondroprotective agent
G. Pure opioid agonist
H. Partial opioid agonist
I. Opioid agonist-antagonist
J. Opioid antagonist

EXERCISE 29.4 TRUE OR FALSE: COMPREHENSIVE

Instructions: Read the following statements and write "T" for true or "F" for false in the blanks provided. If a statement is false, correct the statement to make it true.

1. _____ Like people, domestic animals tend to readily show that they are in pain.

2. _____ Pain tolerance varies widely between species and individuals within a species.

3. _____ In animals, pain is usually easy to differentiate from normal postoperative behaviors.

4. _____ Although pain has many negative physiologic effects, these effects are confined to the nervous system.

5. _____ Nociceptors are specialized nerve fibers that carry pain information but not pleasant or neutral sensations.

6. _____ Allodynia is the phase of wind-up in which less and less stimulation is required to initiate pain.

7. _____ Administering analgesics after pain occurs is often just as effective as giving them before it occurs.

8. _____ Lower doses of individual analgesics can be used when an analgesic protocol includes agents from multiple classes that attack more than one phase of the pain pathway.

9. _____ Even though pain has many damaging consequences, it can also be beneficial by limiting activity.

10. _____ Even though multiple analgesics are often given concurrently, it is recommended that no more than one NSAID be given to a patient at a time.

11. _____ Lidocaine with epinephrine is helpful for feline declaw blocks because it reduces bleeding.

12. _____ Lidocaine, bupivacaine, or tetracaine can be used topically to reduce pain associated with minor procedures such as urethral catheterization.

13. _____ For oral mass removal, the entire muzzle can be anesthetized by blocking the infraorbital and mandibular foramen.

14. _____ Opioids classified as partial agonists have a decreased effect but very similar side effects to pure agonists.

15. _____ Giving butorphanol with a fentanyl patch will maximize the analgesic effects of the patch.

16. _____ Diazepam does not provide pain relief.

17. _____ Because it can cause heart toxicity, lidocaine is not recommended for use in cats.

18. _____ Analgesics are generally used more often in large animals than in small animals.

19. _____ Large animals do not experience pain in the same way as small domestic animals and people.

20. _____ GI ulceration is the primary side effect of NSAIDs in large animals.

EXERCISE 29.5 MULTIPLE CHOICE: COMPREHENSIVE

Instructions: Circle the one correct answer to each of the following questions.

1. Signs of pain can be classified as physiological or behavioral. Examples of behavioral signs of pain are
   a. tachycardia, dilated pupils, and howling.
   b. biting, hiding, and hypertension.
   c. tachypnea, reluctance to move, and failure to groom.
   d. whimpering, escaping, and tucking the abdomen.

2. During which phase of nociception does the mechanical, chemical, or thermal energy that causes tissue damage get turned into electrical impulses by the nerve endings?
   a. Transduction
   b. Transmission
   b. Modulation
   d. Perception

3. The drug gabapentin has particular efficacy for
   a. acute pain.
   b. deep pain.
   c. neuropathic pain.
   d. abdominal pain.

4. NMDA-receptor antagonists such as ketamine have a particular place in preventing and treating
   a. chronic pain.
   b. wind-up pain.
   c. neuropathic pain.
   d. preexisting pain.

5. Drugs that provide analgesia by modifying inflammation are
   a. opioids.
   b. α_2 agonists.
   c. NSAIDs.
   d. local anesthetics.

6. The analgesics of choice for the treatment of osteoarthritis are
   a. NSAIDs.
   b. opioids.
   c. local anesthetics.
   d. α_2 agonists.

7. Because of potential side effects of NSAIDs, patients should not receive them if they have
   a. bleeding abnormalities.
   b. hypertension.
   c. parasites.
   d. Any of the above

8. Dogs receiving NSAIDs are particularly prone to adverse effects relating to the GI system, whereas cats are particularly prone to adverse effects relating to the
   a. liver.
   b. CNS.
   c. kidneys.
   d. blood.

9. Cats can be given NSAIDs when indicated but should never be given
   a. meloxicam.
   b. carprofen.
   c. acetaminophen.
   d. aspirin.

10. Local anesthetics work by
    a. decreasing inflammation.
    b. blocking mu receptors.
    c. inhibiting norepinephrine release.
    d. disrupting neural transmission.

11. A circumferential ring block for declawing requires an SQ injection of 0.5% bupivacaine at a dose of
    a. mL/10 lb body weight.
    b. mL/10 kg body weight.
    c. mL per cat.
    a. mL/10 lb body weight.

12. An epidural injection of lidocaine or morphine will provide analgesia to the
    a. pelvis only.
    b. caudal abdomen only.
    c. tail only.
    d. caudal half of the body.

13. The stinging sensation caused by injection of local anesthetics can be reduced by adding 0.1 mL of
    _____ to 10 mL of the local agent.
    a. bupivacaine
    b. epinephrine
    c. sodium bicarbonate
    d. saline

14. The class of opioids with the most severe side effects are the
    a. pure agonists.
    b. partial agonists.
    c. mixed agonist-antagonists.
    d. antagonists.

15. One of the following species is more sensitive to morphine and, therefore, requires lower doses of this pure agonist. Which one is it?
    a. Dog
    b. Cat
    c. Cow
    d. Horse

16. An opioid that has a significantly longer duration of action than most is
    a. morphine.
    b. hydromorphone.
    c. butorphanol.
    d. buprenorphine.

17. Vomiting is a common side effect of morphine, occurring more frequently
    a. when the drug is administered to young animals.
    b. when the drug is administered via CRI.
    c. when the drug is administered as a premedication.
    d. when the drug is administered with butorphanol.

18. The drug romifidine is an α_2 agonist analgesic. Which of the drugs listed below is also in this class?
    a. Ketamine
    b. Acepromazine
    c. Dexmedetomidine
    d. Morphine

19. This class of analgesics works by inhibiting the release of the neurotransmitter norepinephrine.
    a. NMDA inhibitors
    b. α_2 agonists
    c. NSAIDs
    d. Anticonvulsants

20. Which of the following drug combinations is representative of the anesthetic protocol known as "kitty magic"?
   a. Morphine, acepromazine, and ketamine
   b. Fentanyl, ketoprofen, and ketamine
   c. Buprenorphine, meloxicam, and dexmedetomidine
   d. Buprenorphine, dexmedetomidine, and ketamine

21. As compared with morphine, the main advantages of fentanyl are
   a. shorter half-life and faster onset of action.
   b. faster onset of action and longer half-life.
   c. longer half-life and slower onset of action.
   d. slower onset of action and shorter half-life.

22. Which of the following drugs is safe for use in patients with GI disturbances and thus is a good choice for dogs with gastric dilatation-volvulus (GDV), unlike many analgesics?
   a. Carprofen
   b. Hydromorphone
   c. Lidocaine
   d. Dexmedetomidine

23. An NMDA receptor antagonist used to prevent wind-up phenomena is
   a. gabapentin.
   b. xylazine.
   c. acepromazine.
   d. ketamine.

24. In view of the efficacy gabapentin has in treating neuropathic pain, which of the following conditions would it be used to treat?
   a. Resistance to being touched at a location with no tissue damage
   b. Pain secondary to a severe infection
   c. Postsurgical incisional pain
   d. Limb pain resulting from trauma

25. The most commonly used NSAIDs in large animals are
   a. flunixin meglumine and carprofen.
   b. carprofen and ketoprofen.
   c. ketoprofen and phenylbutazone.
   d. phenylbutazone and flunixin meglumine.

26. The opioid most commonly used in large animals is
   a. morphine.
   b. butorphanol.
   c. fentanyl.
   d. buprenorphine.

27. Which of the following analgesic adjuncts is a nutraceutical and consequently is not regulated by the FDA?
   a. Gabapentin
   b. Tramadol
   c. Chondroitin sulfate
   d. Phenylbutazone

28. The analgesic class most commonly used in horses is
   a. opioids.
   b. α_2 agonists.
   c. NSAIDs.
   d. local anesthetics.

29. The analgesic class most commonly used in ruminants is
   a. opioids.
   b. α_2 agonists.
   c. NSAIDs.
   d. local anesthetics.

EXERCISE 29.6 FILL-IN-THE-BLANK: COMPREHENSIVE

Instructions: Fill in each of the spaces provided with the missing word or words that complete the sentence.

1. Signs of pain in animals can be categorized according to whether they are _____ (e.g., tachycardia or hypertension) or _____ (e.g., biting or guarding an incision).

2. Pain is now considered by some to be the fifth vital sign. The other four vital signs are _____, _____, _____, and _____.

3. Tissue damage results in inflammation. The classic signs of inflammation are localized _____, _____, and _____.

4. The phase of the pain pathway in which there is the awareness that something hurts is called

   _____.

5. Pain is subdivided into two categories based on the duration. The sensation experienced with each category differs. _____ pain is characterized by a sharp, stabbing sensation, whereas _____ pain is characterized by a dull, throbbing sensation.

6. An extreme form of pain sometimes occurs when the CNS is bombarded by persistent pain impulses. This extreme form is called "central sensitization" or _____.

7. The four main categories of analgesic drugs are_____, _____, _____, and _____.

8. To prevent adverse effects on kidney function, patients that are receiving NSAIDs should always have _____ monitored intraoperatively.

9. Adding the drug _____ to lidocaine at a 1:200,000 dilution will increase its duration of action.

10. Most cases of local anesthetic toxicity are a result of accidental _____ or _____ administration.

11. A correctly performed declaw block using bupivacaine will provide analgesia for up to_____ hours after surgery.

12. Morphine can be injected intra-articularly to provide analgesia of the joint. The use of this technique results in the maintenance of a smooth plane of anesthesia when the joint capsule is incised. When this technique is not used, an

    increase in the _____ is often observed as the joint capsule is entered.

13. Analgesia can be provided to patients following thoracotomy by injecting bupivacaine in the pleural space. When

    using this technique, the drug is thought to work by directly blocking the _____ nerves.

14. The specific effects that a particular opioid will have are dependent on the specific _____ in the CNS that it binds to.

15. Analgesia provided by opioids is primarily a result of the binding of the drug to the _____ receptors in the CNS.

16. Hydromorphone has similar analgesic effects as morphine but is less likely to cause_____

    or _____ (two adverse effects).

17. The injectable opioid _____ is readily absorbed across mucous membranes in cats as a

    result of the unique _____ in this species and can consequently be given orally.

18. Analgesics in the class _____ work synergistically with opioids to _____ the intensity and duration of pain relief beyond what can be accounted for by the separate action of each drug.

19. The drug used to reverse the effects of the α_2 agonist dexmedetomidine is _____.

20. After being given any sedative, the patient should be placed in a quiet environment for_____ minutes to allow the drug(s) to take effect.

21. Different large animal species have different sensitivities to α_2 agonists. _____ are most resistant, _____ are moderately sensitive, and _____ are the most sensitive.

22. _____ pain has a rapid onset and serves to warn that something is wrong with the body; _____ pain persists over time and serves no purpose.

23. A RUMM block, which stands for _____, _____, _____, and _____, is used to block the _____.

EXERCISE 29.7 CASE STUDY: ADMINISTERING ANALGESICS BY CONSTANT RATE INFUSION

Signalment: 4-year-old, 110-pound, neutered, male Bull Mastiff

History: This patient came up lame on the left rear limb while playing in the backyard 3 days ago. He has no history of previous medical problems.

Physical examination: On presentation, the patient was three-legged lame, and physical findings were compatible with an anterior cruciate ligament rupture. All other findings were normal.

Preoperative workup: Results of routine preoperative blood work were normal.

Treatment plan: This patient was admitted to the hospital for surgical management of the anterior cruciate ligament rupture. The doctor has asked you to give this patient a 5 mcg/kg loading dose of fentanyl, followed by a 12 mcg/kg/hr (or 0.2 mcg/kg/min) CRI intraoperatively. The patient will be receiving lactated Ringer solution in a 1 L bag at a rate of 10 mL/kg/hr. You are asked to calculate both the loading dose and the constant rate infusion for this patient.

1. Calculate the loading dose by following these steps:

    a. Calculate this patient's body weight in kg.

       Patient's body weight: _____ kg

    b. Calculate the loading dose of fentanyl in mL. The concentration of fentanyl is 0.05 mg/mL. Set this problem up by multiplying the body weight and the dose and divide the product by the drug concentration.

       Loading dose of fentanyl: _____ mL

2. Now calculate the constant rate infusion by following the steps below.

    a. Calculate the fluid infusion rate for this patient in mL/hr. Set this problem up by multiplying the body weight and the prescribed fluid administration dosage.

       Fluid infusion rate during surgery: _____ mL/hr

    b. Calculate the number of hours the bag of lactated Ringer solution will last. Set this problem up by converting the fluid bag size to mL and then dividing by the figure from the previous step.

       Number of hours the bag will last: _____ hours

344

c. Calculate the number of minutes the bag of lactated Ringer solution will last. Set this problem up by converting the figure from the previous step into minutes.

Number of minutes the bag will last: _____ minutes

d. Calculate the total number of micrograms of fentanyl to add to the bag. Set this problem up by multiplying the patient weight by both the prescribed dose in mcg/kg/min and the figure from the previous step.

Number of micrograms to add to the bag: _____ micrograms

e. Convert this value to milligrams. Set this problem up by converting the figure from the previous step into milligrams.

Number of milligrams to add to the bag: _____ milligrams

f. Calculate the drug volume to add to the bag. Set this problem up by dividing the figure from the previous step by the drug concentration.

Drug volume to add to the bag: _____ mL

You will next add this volume of fentanyl to the bag after removing an equivalent volume of fluids from the bag. Then, you will run the fluids for the duration of the surgery at the rate calculated in part 2a above using a controlled rate infusion pump.

30 Veterinary Anesthesia

LEARNING OBJECTIVES

When you have completed this chapter, you will be able to:

1. Pronounce, define, and spell all key terms in the chapter.
2. Differentiate general anesthesia, sedation, tranquilization, neuroleptanalgesia, and local anesthesia; differentiate among the periods of general anesthesia (premedication, induction, maintenance); and list the objectives of anesthesia and techniques used to achieve these objectives, including the concept of balanced anesthesia.
3. Discuss each aspect of patient preparation for anesthesia, including fasting, gathering historical information, physical assessment, stabilization, and physical status classification.
4. Do the following regarding injectable anesthetic agents:
   - Describe the ways anesthetic agents are classified, and differentiate among agonists, partial agonists, agonist–antagonists, and antagonists.
   - Describe the effects, adverse effects, properties, and uses of anticholinergics, phenothiazine and benzodiazepine tranquilizers, alpha$_2$ adrenergic agents, opioids, propofol, alfaxalone, dissociatives, etomidate, and guaifenesin.
5. Explain how vapor pressure, blood–gas partition coefficient, and minimum alveolar concentration influence the way inhalant anesthetics are used and describe the effects, adverse effects, properties, and uses of halogenated inhalant anesthetics.
6. Do the following regarding the use of anesthetic equipment:
   - Discuss the characteristics, uses, and maintenance of endotracheal tubes, laryngoscopes, and anesthesia masks and chambers.
   - Describe the characteristics of an anesthesia machine, including the four general machine systems.
   - Explain how to assemble an anesthesia machine, check for leaks, and set the pop-off valve before use.
   - Describe the structure, function, and use of each component of the carrier gas supply, including compressed gas cylinder, pressure gauge, pressure-reducing valve, flowmeter, and oxygen flush valve.
   - List and calculate the oxygen flow rates used for various species, systems, and periods of the anesthetic procedure.
   - Describe the structure, function, and uses of precision and non-precision vaporizers.
   - Discuss rebreathing and non-rebreathing systems and explain the criteria used to choose an appropriate breathing system for any given patient.
   - Describe the structure, function, and use of each component of the breathing system, including unidirectional flow valves, reservoir bag, pop-off valve, carbon dioxide absorber canister, pressure manometer, negative pressure relief valve, and breathing tubes.
   - Discuss the function and uses of passive and active scavenging systems.
   - Describe the procedures used to maintain anesthesia machines.
7. Do the following regarding endotracheal intubation:
   - Discuss the principles of endotracheal intubation, including the equipment needed to place an endotracheal tube and the criteria used to select and prepare an appropriate endotracheal tube for any given patient.
   - Describe placement of an endotracheal tube in a small animal (SA), horse, adult ruminant, and small ruminant; how to check an endotracheal tube for proper placement; and how to inflate the cuff.
   - Discuss laryngospasm and other complications of intubation, including causes and methods of prevention.
   - Compare and contrast supraglottic airway devices and endotracheal tubes.
8. Do the following regarding anesthetic monitoring:
   - Explain the principles of anesthetic monitoring and how monitoring parameters can be used to identify the classic stages and planes of anesthesia.
   - Identify physical monitoring indicators of circulation, oxygenation, and ventilation.
   - Discuss the methods used to assess vital signs, including normal values, and common causes of abnormal values.
   - Describe methods used to assess reflexes and other monitoring indicators and explain how they are used to determine anesthetic depth.
   - Discuss the function, setup, and limitations of monitoring equipment used to assess circulation, oxygenation, and ventilation, and interpretation of data generated by these instruments.

9. Do the following regarding SA anesthesia:
   - Describe the sequence of events required to take an SA patient from consciousness to surgical anesthesia and back to consciousness.
   - Describe agents and methods commonly used to induce anesthesia in an SA patient through intramuscular or intravenous injection, mask, or chamber.
   - Describe agents and methods used to maintain anesthesia in an SA patient and considerations for patient positioning, comfort, safety, and recovery.
10. Explain the sequence of events in an anesthetic event in a horse, including ways in which the anesthetic procedure for equines differs from that for an SA patient.
11. Explain the sequence of events in an anesthetic event in a ruminant, including ways in which the anesthetic procedure for ruminants differs from that for an SA patient.
12. List the common problems and emergencies, associated causes, and interventions in relation to anesthesia.

EXERCISE 30.1 CROSSWORD PUZZLE: TERMS AND DEFINITIONS

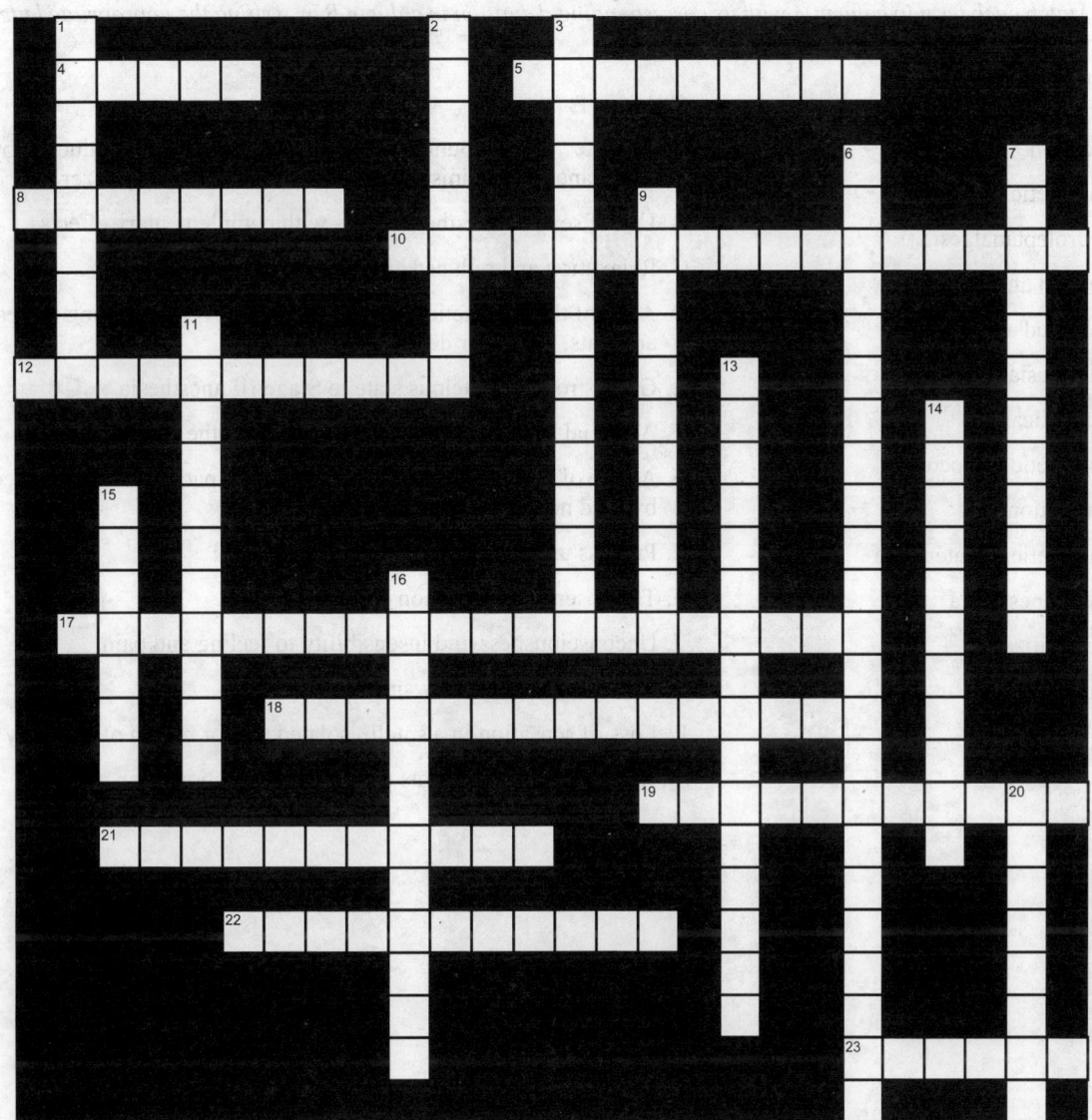

Across

4 A respiratory rate of 0 breaths/min
5 The opposite of miosis
8 A drug that induces sleep
10 Also known as a circle system (2 words)
12 Increased heart rate
17 An anesthetic machine configuration used for patients weighing less than 2.5 kg (2 words)
18 Decreased respiratory rate and/or tidal volume
19 Mapleson E nonrebreathing circuit (2 words)
21 The volume of air breathed in during each breath (2 words)
22 A body temperature of 97° F in a cat
23 Constricted pupils

Down

1 Increased respiratory rate
2 Lack of pain sensation
3 Decreased RR and/or VT
6 The product of respiratory rate and tidal volume (3 words)
7 Air in the chest cavity
9 Collapse of a portion of the lung
11 Elevated blood CO2
13 The percentage of binding sites on the hemoglobin molecules occupied by oxygen (2 words)
14 Modified Mapleson D circuit (2 words)
15 Reduced oxygen in the tissues
16 A side effect of acepromazine that leads to hypotension
20 A physical indicator of hypoxemia

Instructions: Match each term in column A with its corresponding definition in column B by writing the appropriate letter in the space provided.

Column A

1. _____ Sedation

2. _____ Anesthetic induction

3. _____ Neuroleptanalgesia

4. _____ General anesthesia

5. _____ Balanced anesthesia

6. _____ Anesthesia

7. _____ Premedication

8. _____ Anesthetic protocol

9. _____ Ventilation

10. _____ Anesthetic maintenance

11. _____ Local anesthesia

12. _____ Tranquilization

13. _____ Narcosis

Column B

A. A state of profound sedation and analgesia produced by simultaneous administration of an opioid and tranquilizer

B. Use of several anesthetic drugs with complementary effects

C. Relaxation and reduced anxiety

D. A list of the anesthetic drugs that will be given, including routes, amounts, and other details

E. Going from a conscious state to Stage III anesthesia

F. Artificial delivery of anesthetic gases into the patient's lungs

G. A state of profound sedation, from which a patient can be aroused by loud noises or other stimulation

H. Process used to keep a patient anesthetized

I. The absence of sensation

J. Unconsciousness and insensibility to feeling and pain

K. A state of calm or drowsiness

L. Loss of sensation in a small, isolated part or region of the body

M. Administration of agents prior to the induction of anesthesia

Instructions: Match each anesthetic machine part in column A with its corresponding description in column B by writing the appropriate letter in the space provided.

Column A

1. _____ Pressure manometer

2. _____ Oxygen cylinder

3. _____ Oxygen flush valve

4. _____ Line pressure gauge

5. _____ Pressure-reducing valve

6. _____ Vaporizer inlet port

7. _____ Carbon dioxide absorber canister

8. _____ Reservoir bag

9. _____ Yoke

10. _____ Negative pressure relief valve

11. _____ Tank pressure gauge

12. _____ Flowmeter

13. _____ Pop-off valve

14. _____ Exhalation unidirectional valve

Column B

A. This part reduces the pressure of the gas from 40 to 50 psi to approximately 15 psi.

B. This is the point where oxygen and other carrier gases enter the vaporizer from the flowmeter.

C. This part is most commonly used when preparing a patient for recovery or when a crisis has arisen.

D. This part provides the patient an adequate volume of anesthetic gases during inspiration to fill the lungs.

E. This part prevents rebreathing of carbon dioxide.

F. This part reduces the pressure of the gas exiting the compressed gas cylinder to 40 to 50 psi.

G. This part indicates the pressure in a compressed gas cylinder.

H. This part measures pressure in the breathing circuit and in the patient's lungs.

I. This part should be emptied and refilled after 6 to 8 hours of machine use.

J. This part indicates pressure in the line connecting the pressure-reducing valve and the flowmeter(s).

K. This part (also referred to as an adjustable pressure-limiting or APL valve) allows excess gases to exit the breathing circuit.

L. When the oxygen pressure inside this part is 500 psi, it should be changed.

M. This part prevents asphyxiation when the bag is empty.

N. This part holds the oxygen tank onto the anesthesia machine.

Instructions: Match each complication of endotracheal intubation in column A with its corresponding cause or causes in column B by writing the appropriate letter in the space provided. (Note that responses may be used more than once.)

Column A

1. _____ Aspiration of foreign material and fluid during dental cleaning

2. _____ Dyspnea and hypoxia

3. _____ Damage to the tube from chewing

4. _____ Necrosis of the tracheal mucosa

5. _____ Intubation of only one main stem bronchus, leading to hypoxia and difficulty in keeping the patient anesthetized

6. _____ Changes in patient position may dislodge the tube from the glottis

7. _____ Trauma or tracheal rupture resulting in pneumomediastinum and/or pneumothorax

8. _____ Pollution of the workspace with anesthetic gas

9. _____ Increased resistance to breathing with increased respiratory effort

10. _____ Transmission of infectious agents leading to tracheitis, bronchitis, or pneumonia

Column B

A. Tube too short

B. Cuff overinflated/tube diameter too large

C. Tube kinked or obstructed

D. Tube not cleaned and disinfected

E. Tube too long

F. Cuff not inflated/underinflated or tube diameter too small

G. Tube not removed before return to consciousness

H. Overzealous intubation

I. Tube diameter too small

Instructions: Match each monitoring device in column A with the corresponding parameter or parameters it detects in column B by writing the appropriate letter in the space provided.

Column A

1. _____ Esophageal stethoscope

2. _____ Electrocardiograph

3. _____ Ultrasonic Doppler monitor

4. _____ Oscillometric monitor

5. _____ Pulse oximeter

6. _____ Apnea monitor

7. _____ Capnograph

Column B

A. Oxygen saturation and HR

B. Relative HR and irregularity in heart sounds

C. Carbon dioxide in inspired and expired air and RR

D. Relative HR and systolic blood pressure

E. Relative RR only

F. Blood pressure and HR

G. HR and rhythm

EXERCISE 30.6 PHOTO QUIZ: ENDOTRACHEAL TUBE PARTS

Instructions: Match each endotracheal tube part with its corresponding name by writing the appropriate letter in the space provided.

Part Names

1. _____ Connector

2. _____ Cuff

3. _____ Pilot balloon

4. _____ Valve

5. _____ Patient end

6. _____ Measurement of the internal diameter

7. _____ Murphy eye

8. _____ Machine end

9. _____ Tie

10. _____ Measurement of tube length

EXERCISE 30.7 TRUE OR FALSE: COMPREHENSIVE

Instructions: Read the following statements and write "T" for true or "F" for false in the blanks provided. If a statement is false, correct the statement to make it true.

1. _____ Anticholinergics are expected to increase tear and salivary secretions because of their parasympathetic nervous system blockade.

2. _____ Adverse effects of the phenothiazine tranquilizer acepromazine include vomiting and cardiac arrhythmias.

3. _____ The benzodiazepine diazepam should not be given IM because of pain when given by this route and erratic absorption from this site.

4. _____ As a result of significant adverse cardiovascular effects, benzodiazepines should be given with caution in old, young, or ill patients.

5. _____ Ruminants are very sensitive to the drug xylazine, and therefore need only approximately one-tenth of the dose used for horses.

6. _____ An advantage of using the antagonist yohimbine to reverse the effects of xylazine is that dangerous adverse effects will be reversed, but the analgesic effects will persist.

7. _____ In addition to providing analgesia, opioid agonists produce cough suppression, respiratory depression, bradycardia, and hypotension.

8. _____ Most opioid agonists have a relatively long duration of action and must be administered only 2 to 3 times a day.

9. _____ Rapid IV administration of the ultra–short-acting anesthetic propofol can cause apnea, which may be severe.

10. _____ Guaifenesin is the only barbiturate-class general anesthetic still in regular use in the United States.

11. _____ The intravenous, injectable anesthetic etomidate is not commonly used because of its relatively higher cost and adverse effects.

12. _____ As a rule, drugs that are milky in appearance should not be administered intravenously, and propofol is not an exception to this rule.

13. _____ An inhalant anesthetic with a high blood-gas partition coefficient produces faster inductions than one with a low blood-gas partition coefficient.

14. _____ The halogenated inhalant anesthetic sevoflurane induces a more significant dose-dependent hypotension than isoflurane and so must be used with caution.

15. _____ Anesthetic masks may be used to induce but not to maintain general anesthesia.

16. _____ Oxygen is the carrier gas used during all anesthetic procedures.

17. _____ Oxygen flowmeters have an indicator that is shaped either like a ball or like a rotor. When setting oxygen flow, read the top of the ball or center of the rotor indicator.

18. _____ Precision vaporizers are located in the breathing circuit so that the patient's respiratory drive is able to move the carrier gas through the vaporizer as the patient breathes.

19. _____ A semi-closed rebreathing system is a safe, practical system to use with all patients greater than or equal to 2.5 kg in body weight.

20. _____ Closed rebreathing systems are a practical and economical alternative for both small and large animal patients.

21. _____ When in use, a reservoir bag should be approximately one-quarter full at peak expiration.

22. _____ When using a semi-closed rebreathing system, the pop-off valve should be kept partially open except when providing manual ventilation.

23. _____ An endotracheal tube should extend from the tip of the nose to the larynx.

24. _____ Under the traditional system of stages and planes of anesthesia, there are four stages, and stage IV is divided into four planes.

25. _____ Physical status class ASA I patients should be monitored every 5 minutes at a minimum.

26. _____ In general, vital signs are only loosely correlated with depth of anesthesia.

27. ____ Cyanotic mucous membranes are an early indicator of hypoxemia.

28. ____ Abdominal breathing is a breathing pattern in which there is a long pause after inhalation and a short pause after exhalation.

29. ____ The corneal reflex is not reliable in small animals but is useful to determine if a large animal patient is too deep.

30. ____ The electrocardiogram is an accurate indicator concerning whether or not the heart is beating.

31. ____ When administering injectable anesthetics by the intramuscular route, generally they are given "to effect."

32. ____ When turning a patient from side to side, the endotracheal tube should be temporarily disconnected from the breathing circuit.

33. ____ As soon as the patient is in the recovery area, most of the danger has passed and the frequency of anesthetic monitoring can be decreased.

34. ____ Horses naturally can breathe only through their noses and will become distressed and compromised if they are unable to.

35. ____ Many ruminants are difficult to handle and require heavy sedation, along with physical restraint prior to and during anesthetic induction.

36. ____ During surgery, all ruminants should have the head positioned higher than the body.

37. ____ During anesthetic recovery, once a ruminant is in sternal recumbency, does not require support, and is in no danger of bloating, it can be left unattended for short periods of time (15 to 20 minutes).

38. ____ Hypoventilation is an uncommon complication during equine anesthetic procedures.

EXERCISE 30.8 MULTIPLE CHOICE: COMPREHENSIVE

Instructions: Circle the one correct answer to each of the following questions.

1. Which of the following general fasting recommendations is incorrect?
   a. Dogs: No food × 8 to 12 hours
   b. Adult cattle: No food × 24 to 48 hours
   c. Adult equine: No food × 8 to 12 hours
   d. Pediatric patients: No food × 2 to 4 hours

2. A patient that has a life-threatening disease such as a ruptured bladder should be put in which of the following ASA physical status classifications?
   a. ASA I
   b. ASA II
   c. ASA III
   d. ASA IV
   e. ASA V

3. Anticholinergics are expected to
   a. decrease the heart rate in dogs.
   b. thicken the airway mucous in cats.
   c. constrict the bronchi in any species.
   d. protect against cardiac arrhythmias in cats.

4. Which of the following drugs is commonly given in doses that are significantly lower than the doses listed on the label?
   a. Diazepam
   b. Dexmedetomidine
   c. Acepromazine
   d. Glycopyrrolate

5. Young, healthy dogs are resistant to the tranquilizing effects of
   a. diazepam.
   b. acepromazine.
   c. xylazine.
   d. butorphanol.

6. Which of the following agents often causes vomiting in cats?
   a. Acepromazine
   b. Xylazine
   c. Atropine
   d. Midazolam

355

7. α_2 agonists have significant cardiovascular system effects. These drugs cause all of the following effects with the exception of
   a. high heart rate.
   b. decreased cardiac output.
   c. decreased blood pressure.
   d. heart block.

8. All of the following are examples of pure opioid agonists except
   a. fentanyl.
   b. hydromorphone.
   c. morphine.
   d. buprenorphine.

9. This mixed opioid agonist-antagonist is used to treat mild to moderate pain, and as an antitussive.
   a. Hydromorphone
   b. Buprenorphine
   c. Butorphanol
   d. Fentanyl

10. The antagonist used to reverse the effects of opioid agonists such as morphine is
   a. yohimbine.
   b. naloxone.
   c. tolazoline.
   d. flumazenil.

11. Which of the following injectable drugs is *not* a controlled substance?
   a. Propofol
   b. Thiopental sodium
   c. Diazepam
   d. Methohexital

12. Which of the following drugs does not provide significant analgesia?
   a. Morphine
   b. Dexmedetomidine
   c. Fentanyl
   d. Propofol

13. Dissociatives should not be given to patients with seizure disorders for which of the following reasons?
   a. Increases salivation
   b. May induce seizure-like activity during recovery
   c. Causes thickened mucous production and choking
   d. Creates corneal dryness

14. The use of barbiturates as anesthetics has gradually declined over the past several decades due to the availability of ultra-short-acting injectable drugs such as
   a. methohexital and pentobarbital.
   b. phenobarbital and methohexital.
   c. thiopental sodium.
   d. alfaxalone and propofol.

15. Which of the following barbiturate drugs is still regularly used for induction of general anesthesia in laboratory animals by intraperitoneal injection?
   a. Methohexital
   b. Pentobarbital sodium
   c. Phenobarbital
   d. Thiopental sodium

16. Which of the following injectable anesthetics is most appropriate to use as an induction agent in patients with severe heart disease because it has little effect on cardiovascular function?
   a. Methohexital
   b. Propofol
   c. Thiopental sodium
   d. Etomidate

17. Which of the following properties of inhalant anesthetics reveals information regarding the type of vaporizer used to administer it?
   a. Minimum alveolar concentration (MAC)
   b. Vapor pressure
   c. Blood-gas partition coefficient
   d. Boiling point

18. Which of the following is incorrect regarding oxygen administration during anesthesia?
   a. Oxygen carries the anesthetic.
   b. Oxygen compensates for diminished RR.
   c. Oxygen compensates for diminished VT.
   d. Oxygen should only be used during induction, not maintenance, of anesthesia.

19. What specific type of endotracheal tube is designed specifically for birds and other animals that do not have an expandable trachea?
   a. Murphy tube
   b. Silicone tube
   c. Cuffed tube
   d. Cole tube

20. Laryngoscopes are most often used in
   a. dogs, cats, and horses.
   b. pigs, small ruminants, and camelids.
   c. horses, pigs, and adult ruminants.
   d. cats, adult ruminants, and camelids.

21. The force that moves the gases around a rebreathing circuit is
   a. the pressure in the oxygen tank.
   b. the unidirectional valves.
   c. the patient's lungs.
   d. the flowmeter.

22. Which of the following is not the name of a nonre-breathing circuit?
    a. Lack
    b. Bain
    c. Murphy
    d. Jackson-Rees

23. Carbon dioxide absorbent granules should be changed at all of the following times except
    a. when they are soft and can be crushed with the fingers.
    b. when they have turned violet or blue.
    c. when they turn from white to off-white.
    d. after 6 to 8 hours of use.

24. An activated charcoal cartridge removes halogenated anesthetic from waste gases. It should be changed
    a. after 6 to 8 hours of use.
    b. when it gains 50 g of weight.
    c. when it changes color.
    d. after 6 to 8 uses.

25. Using the guidelines listed in the text, a _____ mm endotracheal tube should be prepared for a 30-kg dog.
    a. 9.5 to 10
    b. 10.5 to 11
    c. 11.5 to 12
    d. 12.5 to 13

26. Which of the following is an indicator that the endotracheal tube is in the esophagus instead of the trachea?
    a. Only one firm tube-like structure is palpable in the neck.
    b. The patient whines or cries following placement.
    c. The reservoir bag expands and contracts with respiratory movements.
    d. The patient coughs during placement.

27. Laryngospasm is most commonly encountered in
    a. dogs, cats, and horses.
    b. horses, pigs, and adult ruminants.
    c. cats, adult ruminants, and dogs.
    d. pigs, small ruminants, and cats.

28. The stage of anesthesia during which the patient loses voluntary control but has involuntary reactions such as vocalizing, reflex struggling, and paddling, and during which reflexes are present and muscle tone is marked, is
    a. Stage I.
    b. Stage II.
    c. Stage III.
    d. Stage IV.

29. Decreased or absent palpebral reflex, present corneal reflex, heart rate showing no or mild increase in response to surgical stimulation, moderate muscle tone, and absent pedal and swallowing reflexes indicate which of the following depths of anesthesia in a patient?
    a. Inadequate depth
    b. Surgical anesthesia
    c. Excessive depth
    d. Preanesthesia depth

30. During anesthesia, a variety of heart rhythms may be seen, depending on the species. Sinus arrhythmia is normal in
    a. dogs and camelids.
    b. cats.
    c. cats and dogs.
    d. dogs and horses.

31. Which equipment can be used to monitor blood pressure indirectly?
    a. Pulse oximeter and Doppler monitor
    b. Oscillometric monitor and capnograph
    c. Doppler monitor and oscillometric monitor
    d. Capnograph and pulse oximeter

32. Malignant hyperthermia is a complication of general anesthesia that is most commonly seen in
    a. pigs.
    b. dogs.
    c. cats.
    d. horses.

33. Which of the following is not a typical location for placement of an ultrasonic Doppler probe?
    a. The ventral surface of the forepaw proximal to the metacarpal pad
    b. The lateral surface of the tail
    c. The dorsomedial surface of the hock
    d. The ventral surface of the hind paw proximal to the metatarsal pad

34. Which of the following is not a usual location for placement of a blood pressure cuff?
    a. Around the foreleg
    b. Around the metatarsus
    c. Around the tail base
    d. Around the upper front limb (humerus)

35. Sensors from which of the following monitoring equipment increase mechanical dead space?
    a. Pulse oximeter and apnea monitor
    b. Apnea monitor and capnograph
    c. Capnograph and Doppler monitor
    d. Doppler monitor and pulse oximeter

36. If excessive depth of anesthesia is detected, what is NOT a required action?
    a. The veterinarian should be informed immediately.
    b. The patient should be extubated.
    c. The administration of all anesthetics should be stopped.
    d. The flow of oxygen should be increased.

37. All of the drugs listed below must be given intravenous (IV) except one, which can be given either IV or intramuscular (IM). Which drug can be given IM?
    a. Ketamine
    b. Etomidate
    c. Propofol
    d. Methohexital

38. During anesthetic recovery, the oxygen flow rate should be turned to
    a. 5 to 10 mL/kg/min.
    b. 20 to 40 mL/kg/min.
    c. 50 to 100 mL/kg/min.
    d. 200 to 300 mL/kg/min.

39. Which of the following is not a sign of normal recovery?
    a. Vocalization
    b. Excitement
    c. Hyperventilation
    d. Seizures

40. In contrast to most other domestic animals, many surgical procedures can be done using local or regional anesthetic techniques in this species.
    a. Feline
    b. Canine
    c. Ruminant
    d. Equine

41. Anesthetic agents used in veterinary patients may be classified in a number of ways, including all but which of the following?
    a. Manufacturer
    b. Route of delivery
    c. Chemistry
    d. Primary use

42. Animals of which species often breathe rapidly and shallowly, somewhat like a panting dog, during general anesthesia?
    a. Horse
    b. Cow
    c. Pig
    d. Cat

43. To prevent atelectasis during general anesthesia, healthy small animal patients should be bagged approximately every
    a. 1 to 2 minutes.
    b. 2 to 5 minutes.
    c. 5 to 10 minutes.
    d. 20 to 30 minutes.

44. When anesthetizing a dog, to prevent regurgitation of stomach contents, you should
    a. position the head level with or slightly higher than the body.
    b. position the head lower than the body.
    c. pack gauze into the throat.
    d. position the patient in lateral recumbency.

EXERCISE 30.9 FILL-IN-THE-BLANK: COMPREHENSIVE

Instructions: Fill in each of the spaces provided with the missing word or words that complete the sentence.

1. Neuroleptanalgesia is a state of profound sedation and analgesia produced by simultaneous administration of a(n) _____ and a(n) _____.

2. The use of _____ prior to induction increases body oxygen storage and tolerance to apnea.

3. Drugs classified as agonists bind to receptors and exert one or more effects. Drugs classified as _____ exert a decreased effect at the receptors, those classified as mixed _____ partially reverse the effects of pure agonists, and those classified as _____ completely block the action of the corresponding agonist.

4. The preanesthetic medications used to counteract bradycardia and excess salivation are called _____. The drugs _____ and _____ are examples of these agents.

5. The main adverse effect on the cardiovascular system caused by acepromazine is _____.

6. The two drugs contained in the combination telazol are the benzodiazepine _____ and the dissociative _____.

7. The reversal agent _____ can be given after either formulation of dexdomitor to awaken patients undergoing minor procedures.

8. Opioid drugs work by stimulating specific receptors in the brain and spinal cord. The effect of each opioid depends on its affinity for the various receptors. For instance, opioid agonists primarily stimulate the _____ receptors.

9. The dissociative anesthetics most commonly used in veterinary patients are _____ and _____.

10. Dissociative anesthetics cause a unique state called _____, in which the patient appears to be awake but is immobile and does not respond to its surroundings.

11. A combination of diazepam and ketamine is often used to induce general anesthesia in small animals. To do this, these drugs are mixed in a(n) _____:_____ ratio by volume, and given at a dosage of about 1 mL of the mixture for every _____ pounds of body weight. So, a 50-pound dog would need about _____ mL of this mixture for induction.

12. The drug combination "TKX" contains the drugs _____, _____, and _____.

13. _____, a drug used as an induction agent in healthy dogs and cats, may cause hyperthermia, especially in dogs.

14. A drug used as a muscle relaxant and sedative in large animals is _____ (also known as "GG" or glyceryl guaiacolate).

15. The anesthetic combination of xylazine, ketamine, and guaifenesin, used to maintain general anesthesia in horses, is commonly called "_____."

16. To produce surgical anesthesia in the average patient, you must select a vaporizer dial setting of approximately _____ times the minimum alveolar concentration (MAC).

17. The inhalant anesthetic _____ induces more rapid inductions and recoveries than any other halogenated agent.

18. When checking a nonrebreathing system for leaks, the inflated reservoir bag should remain inflated for at least _____ seconds if no leaks are present.

19. When checking a rebreathing system for leaks, the reservoir bag should be inflated to a pressure of _____ cm of water. No leaks are present if the pressure decreases to no less than _____ cm of water over 10 seconds, or if an oxygen flow of no more than _____ mL/min is necessary to maintain pressure.

20. When setting the pop-off valve of a rebreathing system, the oxygen should be turned on to the maximum rate you anticipate will be needed for the procedure. The pop-off valve should then be opened until the pressure manometer indicates a pressure of _____ to _____ cm of water.

21. When turning on any dial or valve on an anesthetic machine, the dial or valve should be turned in a _____ direction.

22. An E-size oxygen cylinder with a pressure of 500 psi contains approximately _____ L of oxygen. At a flow rate of 2 L/min, the oxygen will last approximately _____ minutes.

23. An H-size oxygen cylinder with a pressure of 500 psi contains approximately _____ L of oxygen, which will last approximately _____ hours at a flow rate of 2 L/min.

24. To avoid confusion, an isoflurane vaporizer is identified by the color _____, and a sevo-flurane vaporizer is identified by the color _____.

25. A nonrebreathing circuit is recommended for patients weighing less than _____ kg of body weight but is mandatory for patients weighing less than _____ kg of body weight.

26. If a rebreathing system is used for a 5-kg patient, it should be fitted with _____ breathing tubes.

27. A 45-pound patient requires use of a(n) _____ L rebreathing bag.

28. The pressure manometer should read no more than _____ cm of water when providing manual or mechanical ventilation to small animals, and should read no more than _____ cm of water when providing manual or mechanical ventilation to large animals, unless the chest cavity is open.

29. The primary benefit of pediatric breathing tubes is that they decrease mechanical _____.

30. The anesthetic machine should be professionally serviced at least _____.

31. When inflating the cuff of the endotracheal tube, compress the reservoir bag and inflate the cuff until the leak just ceases at a pressure of _____ cm of water.

32. Anesthetized patients often experience decreased respiratory rate, and approximately a(n) _____% decrease in VT. These patients often require periodic manual ventilation about every _____ to _____ minutes during anesthesia to prevent this complication.

33. Eye position is _____ during light anesthesia, gradually shifts to _____ position, and finally shifts back to _____.

34. The width of a blood pressure cuff should be _____% to _____% of the circumference of the extremity.

35. Oxygen saturation of hemoglobin greater than _____% is normal; between _____% and _____% indicates desaturation; less than _____% indicates hypoxemia; and less than _____% for longer than 30 seconds is a medical emergency.

36. In a normal anesthetized patient, the carbon dioxide level as measured with a capnograph should be _____ mm Hg during inspiration, and _____ to _____ mm Hg at the end of expiration.

37. When giving an injectable anesthetic IM, the onset of action will be _____ and the duration of action will be _____ than if the same drug were given IV.

38. When inducing a patient by chamber, use an oxygen flow rate of _____ L/min, and _____% to _____% isoflurane or _____% to _____% sevoflurane.

39. Hypotension in a horse is defined as a mean arterial blood pressure of less than _____ mm Hg.

40. Ruminants normally _____ gas to expel it from the rumen. Because this does not happen during anesthesia, _____ can occur.

41. Regurgitation of stomach contents is very common in ruminants during anesthesia, especially when the anesthetic depth is _____ or _____.

42. A laryngoscope visualizes the _____.

43. _____ animals may have a "stiff" jaw that is related to arthritis rather than an indication of inadequate anesthetic depth.

EXERCISE 30.10 CASE STUDY: COMPREHENSIVE

You are serving as an anesthetist for a 6-month-old, 48-pound female mixed-breed dog scheduled for an ovariohysterectomy. The doctor has prescribed the following anesthetic protocol:

Preanesthetic medications: Hydromorphone 0.1 mg/kg IM

Dexmedetomidine 0.005 mg/kg IM

Anesthetic induction: Propofol 4 mg/kg IV to effect

Anesthetic maintenance: Isoflurane 1.5% to 2.5% via endotracheal tube

You are expected to premedicate, induce, and maintain this patient, and to monitor her throughout the anesthetic event until fully recovered. Answer the following questions regarding anesthetic management of this case.

1. First you must prepare and administer the prescribed preanesthetic medications for this patient.

   a. Calculate the volume of each preanesthetic medication you will administer to this patient. (The concentration of hydromorphone is 2 mg/mL. The concentration of dexmedetomidine is 0.5 mg/mL.)

   Volume of hydromorphone you will administer (mL): _____

   Volume of dexmedetomidine you will administer (mL): _____

b. What general effects would be expected from these premedications?

Hydromorphone:_____

_____

Dexmedetomidine:_____

_____

c. The patient should be placed in a quiet location while the preanesthetic medications take effect. Why is this necessary?_____

_____

_____

d. How much time should you allow for the medications to take effect before proceeding?

_____

2. Next, you must prepare the anesthetic machine and associated equipment including the equipment required for endotracheal intubation.

a. Using the rule-of-thumb regarding selection of an endotracheal tube, what tube size (internal diameter in mm) would you prepare for this patient? _____ **mm**

b. What other equipment would you prepare for endotracheal intubation?

_____

_____

_____

c. Would you select a rebreathing or a nonrebreathing circuit for this patient? Why?

_____

_____

_____

d. What size rebreathing bag would you prepare for this patient? _____ **L bag**

e. When using a semi-closed rebreathing system, what are the steps for setting the pop-off valve?

_____

_____

_____

f. Calculate the oxygen flow rate for this patient following IV induction, during any change in anesthetic depth, or during recovery in L/min.

_____ **L/min**

g. Now calculate the oxygen flow rate for this patient during anesthetic maintenance.

_____ **L/min**

h. You are using a machine with size E oxygen tanks. The tank pressure gauge shows 1200 psi. Approximately how many liters of oxygen are left in the tank?

_____ **L**

i. At an oxygen flow rate of 2 L/min, approximately how long (in hours) would this oxygen supply last?

_____ **hours**

3. Now you must induce this patient with propofol.

a. Calculate the volume (in mL) of propofol you will draw up for this patient. The concentration of propofol is 10 mg/mL.

_____ **mL**

b. Will you administer the entire calculated dose to this patient? Why or why not?

_____

_____

_____

c. Describe the specific technique you will use to administer the propofol.

_____

_____

_____

_____

_____

_____

d. What general effects do you expect from this agent?

_____

_____

_____

_____

_____

e. What adverse effects may occur if the propofol is injected too rapidly?

_____

_____

4. During anesthetic maintenance, you will be monitoring this patient to be sure that it is safe, and to determine anesthetic depth.

a. Summarize the findings regarding vital signs and machine parameters you would expect to see during Stage III, general anesthesia (medium surgical anesthesia).

Vital Signs:

Heart rate/rhythm	
Respiratory rate	
Respiratory character	
Body temperature	
Mucous membrane color	
Capillary refill time	
Pulse quality	

Machine Monitoring Parameters:

Oxygen saturation	
Systolic arterial blood pressure	
Diastolic arterial blood pressure	
Mean arterial blood pressure	
Minimally acceptable mean during anesthesia	

b. Which of these vital signs and machine parameters are indicators of circulation, which are indicators of oxygenation, and which are indicators of ventilation?

Indicators of circulation:_____

_____

Indicators of oxygenation:_____

_____

Indicators of ventilation:_____

_____

c. Now summarize the findings regarding reflexes, ocular signs, and other indicators that would indicate that your patient is in Stage III general anesthesia (medium surgical anesthesia).

_____

Reflexes, Ocular Signs, and Other Indicators

Palpebral reflex	
Pedal reflex	
Swallowing reflex	
Corneal reflex	
Pupillary light reflex	
Pupil size	
Eyeball position	
Muscle tone	
Lacrimation	
Response to surgical stimulation	

5. The surgery was completed without incident, and the patient is ready for recovery.

   a. Indicate how you would prepare your patient for recovery, including the appropriate oxygen flow rate for this patient.

_____

_____

_____

_____

_____

_____

_____

_____

   b. Discuss steps you would take to hasten recovery.

_____

_____

_____

   c. What signs would tell you that the recovery is progressing normally?

_____

_____

_____

   d. How do you know when you can remove the endotracheal tube?

_____

31 Surgical Instruments and Aseptic Technique

LEARNING OBJECTIVES

When you have completed this chapter, you will be able to:
1. Pronounce, define, and spell all key terms in this chapter.
2. Do the following regarding general surgery instruments and stapling equipment:
   - Name and describe commonly used surgical instruments.
   - Know the basic operation and properties of carbon dioxide and diode lasers and develop a basic knowledge of laser safety protocol.
   - State advantages of surgical stapling and list common surgical stapling devices.
3. Discuss vascular sealing devices and list commonly used instruments and equipment for ophthalmic, orthopedic, arthroscopic, and laparoscopic procedures.
4. Do the following regarding surgical instrument packs, instrument care, and the use of surgical drapes and gowns.
   - List surgical instruments and supplies routinely included in general and emergency surgical packs for small and large animals.
   - Describe procedures for cleaning, packing, and sterilizing instruments.
   - Describe procedures for folding and packing cloth surgical drapes and gowns.
5. Do the following regarding the processes of sterilization and disinfection as part of aseptic technique:
   - Differentiate between sterilization and disinfection.
   - List and describe physical and chemical methods of sterilization and methods of quality control of sterilization methods.
   - Know the appropriate sterilization processes for sensitive equipment.
   - State safe storage times and conditions for sterile packs.
   - List and describe common antiseptic and disinfectant compounds.
   - Describe requirements for preparation of the operating room and maintenance of operating room sterility.
6. Describe preparation requirements for both small animal and equine patients, including skin preparation, patient positioning, and draping.
7. Describe preparation requirements for the surgical team and explain the procedures that may be used for hand scrubbing before surgery, the procedure for donning surgical attire, and the procedures for opening sterile items.

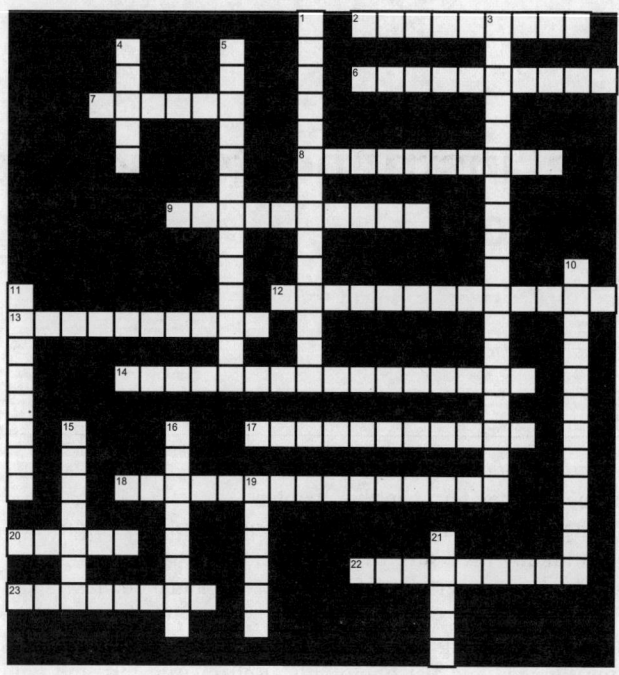

Across

2 One of the two self-retaining retractors commonly used to retract muscle during orthopedic and neurologic surgical procedures

6 A group of surgical instruments named _____ forceps are used to crush blood vessels and tissues in order to stop the source of bleeding

7 The common name for the frequently used disinfectant, sodium hypochlorite

8 The general name for instruments, the primary function of which is to improve visualization in the surgical field during soft-tissue and orthopedic procedures

9 Partially or fully threaded bone screws that comprise wider threads designed to increase gripping in soft bone

12 An antiseptic agent that has effective antimicrobial properties as well as a rapid onset and long-lasting residual activity

13 The type of cleaning unit designed to remove debris that is tightly bound to instruments and clean areas on the instruments that cannot be reached by scrub brushes

14 Large hemostatic forceps with longitudinal grooves in the jaws and cross-grooves at the tip

17 The type of cloth drape that comes premade with an opening in the center for easy placement over the predetermined incision site

18 The jaws of needle holders that are of high quality often contain replaceable _____ _____ inserts that help grip needles and prevent wear (2 words)

20 Another name for emergency sterilization

22 The smooth, stainless steel bone pins that can range in diameter from 1/16 to 1/4 inch

23 The iodine solution for skin that is not commonly used in veterinary medicine, and is comprised of 50% alcohol and 2% iodine

Down

1 A disinfectant solution that is used for cold sterilization. Can cause chemical synovitis and chondrocyte damage if not rinsed off

3 A cannula-type instrument into which the obturator is placed for arthroscopic procedures (2 words)

4 One of the two self-retaining retractors commonly used to retract muscle during orthopedic and neurologic surgical procedures

5 The chemical gas that is capable of killing all microorganisms (2 words)

10 The process that allows one to create and maintain a desired level of abdominal distention during laparoscopic procedures

11 Instruments designed with small cup-like formations on one or both ends used to scrape dense tissues like cartilage or bone

15 The retractor that comprises one single blade and a handle; used to lever tissues out of the line of view

16 The hand-held instrument characterized by sharp tips that appear cupped; used for cutting small pieces of dense tissues like cartilage, bone, or fibrous tissues

19 The sharp pointed instrument inserted inside an arthroscope sleeve

21 Surgical wire with T-shaped handles used in orthopedic procedures for cutting bone in a saw-like motion

EXERCISE 31.2 DEFINITIONS: KEY TERMS

Instructions: Define each term in your own words.

1. Coherent light:_____

_____

2. Latent thermal damage:_____

_____

3. Collateral thermal damage:_____

_____

4. External fixation:_____

_____

5. Asepsis:_____

_____

6. Aseptic technique:_____

_____

7. Exogenous route:_____

_____

8. Endogenous route:_____

_____

9. Sterilization:_____

_____

10. Filtration:_____

_____

11. Disinfectant:_____

_____

12. Antisepsis:_____

_____

13. Antiseptic agents:_____

_____

14. Cold trays:_____

_____

15. Quarter drapes: _____

_____

16. Towel clamps: _____

_____

EXERCISE 31.3 MATCHING: SURGICAL INSTRUMENTS

Instructions: Match each definition in column A with its corresponding word in column B by writing the appropriate letter in the space provided.

Column A

1. _____ Heavy-duty operating scissors commonly used for cutting dense tissues

2. _____ Instruments used to grasp needles and pass suture material through tissues in addition to aiding with suture tying

3. _____ Thumb forceps with delicate intermeshing teeth, which make them good for grasping delicate tissues atraumatically

4. _____ The needle holder that is equipped with scissors built into the instrument

5. _____ Thumb forceps that are relatively atraumatic with multiple sets of delicate teeth and long narrow jaws that are often used for vascular surgeries

6. _____ A traumatic type of thumb forceps with a broad curved surface that is good for handling needles

7. _____ The classification of instruments with a locking mechanism that are used to clamp tissues

8. _____ The self-retaining retractor that facilitates retraction of the ribs for surgical site exposure within the thoracic cavity

9. _____ Traumatic tissue forceps that are used to securely grasp tissues but that leave the tissues crushed, used only on tissues that are to be removed during the procedure

10. _____ The hemostatic forceps designed with large transverse grooves used to clamp bundles of tissues and large vessels

11. _____ Thumb forceps with jaws composed of large interdigitating teeth that are primarily used for fascia or skin

12. _____ One of the two types of hemostatic forceps that are similar in design to Halsted mosquito forceps; contain grooves associated with only the distal-most aspect of the jaws

13. _____ Intestinal tissue forceps designed with atraumatic flexible jaws, which allows for safe clamping of viable portions of the bowel in addition to other delicate tissues

14. _____ Hemostatic forceps that are relatively small in size and designed to occlude small vessels

15. _____ The general type of forceps used for tissue manipulation that is designed with a spring action; used by compressing the two metal handles together to make the jaws meet

16. _____ Hemostatic forceps that are similar to the Rochester-Pean but have interdigitating teeth at the tips used for grasping tissues; commonly utilized in orthopedic or large animal surgery

17. _____ The tissue forceps that are similar to Allis tissue forceps but are considerably less traumatic for tissues as a result of their smoother grasping surface and less stiff design

Column B

A. Kirschner wire

B. Rochester-Ochsner

C. Allis

D. Adson

E. Babcock

F. Halsted mosquito

G. Jamshidi

H. DeBakey

I. Kelly

J. Russian

K. Rochester-Carmalt

L. Mayo dissecting scissors

M. Rochester-Pean

N. Conical

O. Olsen-Hegar

P. Army-Navy

Q. Needle holders

R. Malleable

S. Finochietto

T. Rat-tooth

U. Kerrison

V. Doyen

W. Trephine

X. Tissue forceps

Y. Thumb forceps

18. _____ Hemostatic forceps that are large in size with longitudinal grooves and cross-grooves at the tip of the jaws, which aid in traction for crushing and clamping across vessels; commonly used in spay procedures

19. _____ A hand-held surgical retractor that is designed with smooth blades and used to retract skin, fat, or muscles

20. _____ A specific type of rongeur, with a gun-shaped appearance, used for spinal surgeries

21. _____ A T-shaped, stainless steel, reusable instrument that has a cutting cylindrical blade, similar to the appearance of a general biopsy punch

22. _____ The type of bone pin that is similar to an intramedullary pin but is smaller in size and may be used to pin small fragments of bone

23. _____ The type of needle that shares similarities with a trephine but is often disposable, making it only good for a single use

24. _____ An atraumatic hand-held surgical retractor composed of specialized metal that allows the retractor to be bent into a desired shape, making it especially useful for retracting thoracic and abdominal organs

25. _____ The type of obturator used to penetrate the synovial membrane of the joint capsule to allow further advancement of the arthroscope sleeve into the joint space; provides a reduced risk of causing articular cartilage damage

EXERCISE 31.4 PHOTO QUIZ #1: SURGICAL INSTRUMENT PARTS

Instructions: Name each surgical instrument part (indicated by the arrows).

Part Names

A. _____

B. _____

C. _____

D. _____

E. _____

F. _____

EXERCISE 31.5 PHOTO QUIZ #2: SURGICAL INSTRUMENTS

Instructions: Write the name of each general class of surgical instruments pictured. Then respond to each of the follow-up queries.

General Classes of Surgical Instruments

Suction tips
Scissors
Self-retaining retractors
Thumb forceps
Scalpel handles and blades

Tissue forceps
Hemostatic forceps
Needle holders
Hand-held retractors

1.

1. General class of instruments:_____

Name each instrument and then indicate how you can differentiate each by its size and jaw pattern.

Name: **Criteria used to differentiate:**

1a. _____   _____

1b. _____   _____

Name: **Criteria used to differentiate:**

1c. _____   _____

1d. _____   _____

1e. _____   _____

1f. _____   _____

2.

2. General class of instruments:_____

Name each instrument and then indicate whether it is primarily used to cut wire suture, delicate tissue, bandage material, suture, or fascia and other dense tissue, or if it is used for general-purpose cutting.

Name: **Primary use:**

2a. _____   _____

2b. _____   _____

2c. _____   _____

2d. _____   _____

2e. _____   _____

2f. _____   _____

3.

3. General class of instruments: _____

Name each instrument and then indicate whether it is primarily used to expose the abdominal cavity, expose the thoracic cavity, or retract muscle for orthopedic and neurologic surgeries.

Name: **Primary use:**

3a. _____   _____

3b. _____   _____

3c. _____   _____

3d. _____   _____

4. General class of instruments:_____

Name each instrument and then indicate whether it is primarily used to hold tissue and needles, skin and fascia, delicate tissue, vessels, needles only (because of tissue trauma), or wound dressing.

Name: **Primary use:**

4a. _____   _____

4b. _____   _____

4c. _____   _____

4d. _____   _____

4e. _____   _____

4f. _____   _____

5. General class of instruments:_____

Indicate the number of each blade.

5a._____ 5b. _____ 5c. _____ 5d. _____

5e. _____ 5f. _____ 5g. _____

Indicate the number of the scalpel handle on the bottom: _____

Which blades will fit on this handle? _____

Indicate the number of the scalpel handle on the top: _____

Which blades will fit on this handle? _____

6. General class of instruments:_____

Name each instrument and then indicate whether it is primarily used to suction fluid from a body cavity or a joint or for general-purpose suctioning.

Name: **Primary use:**

6a. _____   _____

6b. _____   _____

6c. _____   _____

7. General class of instruments:_____

Name each instrument and then indicate whether it is primarily used to hold tissue that will be removed, bowel and other delicate tissues, tissue that will not be removed, or surgical drapes.

Name: **Primary use:**

7a. _____   _____

7b. _____   _____

7c. _____   _____

7d. _____   _____

8.

8. General class of instruments: _____

Name each instrument and then indicate whether it is primarily used to retract skin, fat and muscle, abdominal and thoracic organs, the horn of the uterus, or tissues during orthopedic surgery.

Name: **Primary use:**

8a. _____   _____

8b. _____   _____

8c. _____   _____

8d. _____   _____

8e. _____   _____

9. General class of instruments: _____

What is the specific name of each instrument?

Name:

9a. _____

9b. _____

What is the difference between these two instruments?

_____

Examine this sterile field, identify the labeled instruments and supplies according to general type, and describe the primary purpose for each. (For instance, the needle holders on the upper left [A] are used to handle suture needles and material while suturing tissue.) Item H will be covered in Chapter 32 and may be left blank for this exercise.

A. _____

Primary purpose:_____

B. _____

Primary purpose:_____

C. _____

Primary purpose:_____

D. _____

Primary purpose:_____

E. _____

Primary purpose:_____

F. _____

   Primary purpose: _____

G. _____

   Primary purpose: _____

H. _____

   Primary purpose: _____

I. _____

   Primary purpose: _____

J. _____

   Primary purpose: _____

EXERCISE 31.7 TRUE OR FALSE: COMPREHENSIVE

Instructions: Read the following statements and write "T" for true or "F" for false in the blanks provided. If a statement is false, correct the statement to make it true.

1. _____ It is necessary to shave between the patient and the ground plate when using electrocautery technology in order to prevent the occurrence of burns.

2. _____ The use of a ground plate is required for bipolar electrosurgery.

3. _____ The wavelength and frequency of light emitted by a laser are uniform.

4. _____ When using a laser, muscle tissue is more likely to cause scatter radiation than bone.

5. _____ CO_2 laser beams are produced from a liquid medium.

6. _____ CO_2 lasers emit a "free" laser beam.

7. _____ The diode laser and YAG laser have similar wavelengths.

8. _____ The beam of the YAG or diode laser is transmitted by fibers.

9. _____ MPE is the acronym for minimum permissible exposure to laser radiation.

10. _____ The majority of lasers used in the medical field are class IV and are capable of causing damage to the skin and eyes.

11. _____ Certain laser types can penetrate through clear glass.

12. _____ Lasers generate a potentially toxic substance called "plume" when used on tissues.

13. _____ Brown-Adson thumb forceps are not commonly used in the veterinary field.

14. _____ Waterless hand antiseptics have many advantages over traditional hand-scrubbing and are an acceptable substitute for surgical hand-scrubbing.

15. _____ Kelly forceps are characterized by transverse grooves that extend along the entire length of the jaw, whereas the jaws of Crile forceps only contain grooves on the distal aspect.

16. _____ Another name for the "spay hook" is the Snook ovariohysterectomy hook.

17. _____ Most bone-holding forceps are self-retaining.

18. _____ Chisels and osteotomes are produced from a hard metal and therefore can be used to cut other materials besides bone.

19. _____ The threads of bone pins are located only on the end of the pin.

20. _____ External fixators are used to hold bone pins in position and can be made of metal or acrylic material.

21. _____ Bone screws should never be used in conjunction with a bone plate or interlocking nail.

22. _____ Large bone screws commonly have a slotted head.

23. _____ Arthroscopes are used to examine joint structures of large and small animals.

24. _____ Triangulation is a technique used primarily in arthroscopic operations.

25. _____ Once a fibrous joint capsule has been penetrated by a sharp trocar, the trocar is replaced with the arthroscope.

26. _____ Gas insufflation with the use of CO_2 or nitrous oxide is an acceptable method of joint distention.

27. _____ Pressurized bag systems are used to deliver fluid into the joint.

28. _____ Laparoscopy may be performed on horses with the use of local anesthetics and sedatives.

29. _____ Nitrous oxide gas is used to insufflate the abdomen when performing laparoscopy.

30. _____ Stainless steel surgical instruments with a polished finish are preferred over those with a satin finish.

31. _____ Only surgical instruments made from the same material should be ultrasonically cleaned at the same time.

32. _____ Oil is used to lubricate and maintain the proper function of surgical instruments.

33. _____ Cloth drapes and gowns are designed for repeated use.

34. _____ Radiation is a safe alternative for sterilizing certain materials that would otherwise be damaged by other methods of sterilization.

35. _____ As compared with dry heat, wet heat requires a greater period of time to achieve sterilization and is also more difficult to control.

36. _____ Wet heat sterilization with boiling water at ambient pressures is a reliable method to achieve sterilization.

37. _____ After the sterilization process is finished, the pack should be allowed to self-cool prior to handling by fully opening the autoclave door for at least 20 minutes.

38. _____ It is common among veterinary practices to use a combination of autoclave tape on the outside of a surgical pack as well as a chemical indicator strip in the center of the pack to assure proper sterilization was achieved.

39. _____ Liquid chemicals should not be used for instrument sterilization.

40. _____ Ethylene oxide is a toxic, colorless, and explosive gas used for instrument sterilization.

41. _____ Ethylene oxide gas is capable of penetrating through paper and plastic packaging materials.

42. _____ Proper placement of surgical packs and materials in the sterilization chamber is extremely important in order for effective sterilization to take place with the use of ethylene oxide gas.

43. _____ Disinfectants are capable of killing vegetative bacteria as well as effective at destroying spores.

44. _____ Iodine compounds are antimicrobial agents that are extremely effective against bacterial spores.

45. _____ Aqueous iodine solutions contain a lower level of free iodine than iodophors, resulting in less bactericidal activity.

46. _____ By diluting iodophor stock solutions, the bactericidal activity will increase, and the cytotoxicity will decrease.

47. _____ Povidone-iodine is commonly used in the veterinary field as a surgical scrub and is effective in reducing bacteria.

48. _____ The residual bactericidal effect of povidone-iodine is greatly reduced by the presence of organic matter.

49. _____ Chlorhexidine is an antiseptic agent that provides effective antimicrobial activity without causing significant skin irritation or complications, as seen with povidone-iodine solutions.

50. _____ Methyl alcohol is more effective than ethyl and isopropyl alcohol when used as a disinfectant.

51. _____ Glutaraldehyde is an effective antimicrobial agent that can be used on living tissues.

52. _____ Arthroscope and laparoscope components (light cable and camera) should be cleaned only by gas or cold sterilization.

53. _____ A thorough weekly cleaning of operating equipment should be performed on the same day each week.

54. _____ The final sterile scrub should be performed on the patient just before entering the operating room.

55. _____ One-step prep skin preparation solutions may be used in place of traditional scrubs for preparing surgery sites, as they have comparable antimicrobial killing capabilities.

56. _____ Feline castration surgical prep involves shaving the scrotum.

57. _____ Lateral recumbency is the most desirable position for most abdominal surgeries.

58. _____ The sleeves, the front of the gown, and the neckline are considered to be sterile on a scrubbed-in person.

59. _____ Scrubbed-in assistants are responsible for opening all sterile items for the surgeons.

Instructions: Circle the one correct answer to each of the following questions.

1. The laser energy applied to tissue is measured in
   a. volts.
   b. watts.
   c. joules.
   d. amperes.

2. Which of the following laser types is not commonly used in the veterinary field?
   a. CO2
   b. Nd:YAG
   c. Argon
   d. Diode

3. Elements of a safety protocol for laser use in the veterinary practice should include all except which of the following?
   a. A fire extinguisher should be readily available for the surgeon at all times to protect against the possibility of flash fires in the surgical field.
   b. Flammable anesthetic agents, such as pressurized oxygen, should never come in contact with the laser beam.
   c. The patient's eyes should be shielded from the beam.
   d. Shielded endotracheal tubes should be used if laser penetration of the trachea or upper respiratory tract is possible.

4. Which of the following is most susceptible to damage from laser injury?
   a. Thyroid glands
   b. Eyes
   c. Reproductive organs
   d. Hands

5. The surgical scissors most commonly utilized for soft-tissue dissection are
   a. Metzenbaum scissors.
   b. Mayo dissecting scissors.
   c. iris scissors.
   d. operating scissors.

6. The type of surgical instrument sometimes used to secure surgical drapes and instrument cords (such as those used for cautery) is
   a. Allis tissue forceps.
   b. Babcock forceps.
   c. Doyen forceps.
   d. Russian thumb forceps.

7. Tissue forceps are used for
   a. cutting and clamping tissues.
   b. occluding and grasping vessels.
   c. crushing and cutting tissues.
   d. clamping and holding tissues.

8. Which of the hemostatic forceps listed are most commonly used for large animal surgery or orthopedic procedures?
   a. Rochester-Ochsner forceps
   b. Rochester-Pean forceps
   c. Crile forceps
   d. Kelly forceps

9. The Poole suction tip is primarily used in the
   a. abdominal cavity.
   b. sinuses.
   c. joints.
   d. Both A and B

10. Which of the following is not a recognized material used for orthopedic implants?
    a. Cobalt-chromium alloys
    b. Titanium
    c. Stainless steel alloy
    d. Aluminum alloys

11. The most commonly used arthroscope for canine arthroscopy is
    a. 4-mm outer diameter, and a 25-degree angled lens.
    b. 4-mm outer diameter, and a 32-degree angled lens.
    c. 5-mm outer diameter, and a 10-degree angled lens.
    d. 2.7-mm outer diameter, and a 30-degree angled lens.

12. The inner pressure of an insufflated abdominal cavity should not exceed
    a. 10 to 15 mm Hg.
    b. 15 to 20 mm Hg.
    c. 20 to 25 mm Hg.
    d. 25 to 32 mm Hg.

13. Which of the following is not classified as an exogenous source of contamination?
    a. Air
    b. Surgical instruments
    c. Patient skin
    d. Oral cavity bacteria

14. Which of the following is NOT a type of surgical stapler?
    a. EEA
    b. TAV
    c. TA
    d. Skin stapler

15. Which of the following is not classified as a general type of physical sterilization?
    a. Filtration
    b. Radiation
    c. Heat
    d. Ethylene oxide

16. Which of the following statements is true regarding radiation sterilization?
    a. Materials that are easily damaged should not be sterilized by radiation.
    b. Radiation destroys microorganisms.
    c. Radiation produces high temperatures during the sterilization process.
    d. Radiation is not used for sterilization of medical supplies.

17. The most common sterilization method is
    a. wet heat.
    b. filtration.
    c. radiation.
    d. hydrogen peroxide gas plasma.

18. Which of the following products is most effectively sterilized by dry heat?
    a. Rubber
    b. Fabrics
    c. Metals
    d. Oils

19. In which type of surgical pack would you be most likely to find Senn retractors?
    a. Spay/neuter
    b. Soft tissue/general
    c. Orthopedic
    d. Emergency

20. Which of the following products is most effectively sterilized by moist heat?
    a. Powders
    b. Petroleum products
    c. Oils
    d. Rubber

21. The adequate amount of spacing between each pack in an autoclave chamber to ensure proper steam penetration is
    a. 2.5 to 7.5 cm.
    b. 3.5 to 8.5 cm.
    c. 5.0 to 10 cm.
    d. 7.5 to 12 cm.

22. The recommended exposure time and temperature for flash-sterilization is
    a. 2 minutes at 250° F.
    b. 3 minutes at 131° C.
    c. 4 minutes at 270° F.
    d. 5 minutes at 131° F.

23. To prevent rapid cooling of packs after a sterilization cycle has finished, the autoclave door should be slightly cracked open for a minimum of
    a. 5 minutes.
    b. 10 minutes.
    c. 15 minutes.
    d. 20 minutes.

24. Fusible pellet glass indicators provide evidence that a(n)
    a. pressure of 27 psi was reached.
    b. adequate level of steam saturation was achieved.
    c. time of 15 minutes passed.
    d. temperature of 118° c was reached.

25. Which of the following statements is false in regard to culture test indicators?
    a. They use spores of a particular strain of bacteria.
    b. They yield rapid results.
    c. They are the only type of indicator that provides evidence that microorganisms were destroyed.
    d. They do not indicate if proper steam penetration has been achieved.

26. Which of the following events would render a sterile surgical pack contaminated?
    a. The pack was stored in an open cabinet.
    b. The pack was stored in an upside-down position.
    c. The outside of the pack came in contact with a nonsterile instrument.
    d. The pack was dropped but the tape sealing the pack remained intact.

27. The general operating temperature for ethylene oxide is between
    a. 21° C and 140° C.
    b. 15° C and 60° C.
    c. 21° C and 60° C.
    d. 21° F and 70° F.

28. The minimum humidity requirement for effective sterilization to occur by the use of ethylene oxide is
    a. 20%.
    b. 25%.
    c. 32%.
    d. 35%.

29. Which of the following statements is not true of hydrogen peroxide gas plasma sterilization?
   a. Gas plasma is capable of inactivating mycobacteria and bacterial spores.
   b. Gas plasma is capable of inactivating viruses and fungi.
   c. Gas plasma is considered to be safer for the environment when compared with ethylene oxide.
   d. Gas plasma sterilization is considered to be a more hazardous form of chemical sterilization when compared with ethylene oxide.

30. The residual bactericidal activity of povidone-iodine when left on the skin is
   a. 2 to 4 hours.
   b. 4 to 6 hours.
   c. 6 to 8 hours.
   d. 8 to 10 hours.

31. Skin irritation or acute dermatitis related to the use of povidone-iodine iodophors in veterinary practice can affect up to
   a. 10% of canine patients.
   b. 25% of canine patients.
   c. 50% of canine patients.
   d. 75% of canine patients.

32. Which is not a sterilization indicator used with autoclave sterilization?
   a. Chemical sterilization indicators
   b. Infrared thermometer indicators
   c. Melting pellet glass
   d. Culture tests

33. The required exposure time when soaking instruments to achieve cold sterilization should exceed
   a. 32 minutes.
   b. 1 hour.
   c. 2 hours.
   d. 3 hours.

34. For which of the following procedures is it not acceptable to use cold-sterilized instruments?
   a. Dental surgery
   b. Superficial laceration
   c. Debridement
   d. Lumpectomy

35. The factor most consistently observed to influence the incidence of wound contamination and subsequent infection is
   a. the type of surgery performed.
   b. the degree of pre-surgical contamination of the wound.
   c. whether the patient was properly fasted prior to surgery.
   d. the length of time the patient is under general anesthesia.

36. The general recommendation for initial skin preparation of a surgical site consists of scrubbing and rinsing
   a. 2–3 times.
   b. 3–5 times.
   c. 4–7 times.
   d. 5–8 times.

37. Which of the following statements is not true regarding the surgical hand scrub?
   a. The two basic methods include "counted brush strokes" and "timed."
   b. The "counted brush stroke" method is more commonly used.
   c. Ten to 25 brush strokes are performed on all surfaces prior to rinsing.
   d. After completion of the scrub, the hands are rinsed in water so that the water flows from the fingers to the elbow.

38. Which of the following is not acceptable for scrubbed-in personnel?
   a. Resting gloved hands on a sterile drape
   b. Clasping gloved hands in front of the body between shoulders and waist
   c. Crossing arms at chest height
   d. Touching the gown within the sterile zone while wearing gloves

39. Which of the following is a false statement regarding towel clamps?
   a. The Roeder towel clamp has a metal ball stop on the jaws.
   b. The Backhaus towel clamp prevents deep tissue penetration.
   c. Towel clamps are designed to secure drapes to the patient.
   d. Towel clamps have tips that join together like tongs.

Instructions: Fill in each of the spaces provided with the missing word or words that complete the sentence.

1. Lasers emit energized light produced from a crystal, a _____, or a _____.

2. A laser's _____ within the light spectrum determines the effect it will have on tissue.

3. The result of laser-tissue interaction is dependent on the tissue's _____ and _____.

4. In addition to the expected effect of a laser on the surgery site, lasers also cause thermal tissue damage that is classified either as _____ or _____.

5. The two most commonly used needle holders in the veterinary field are _____ and _____.

6. Adson thumb forceps are commonly used for the dissection of delicate _____ tissue and _____.

7. _____ and _____ hemostatic forceps share similarities in appearance but differ in their jaw tooth pattern, which covers the entire jaw in one and only the distal aspect of the jaw in the other.

8. The _____ is a specialized surgical instrument designed to act as a hand-held retractor that is used to grasp uterine horns during ovariohysterectomy procedures.

9. The suction tip designed for general purpose use is referred to as a _____ tip.

10. The periosteal elevator most commonly utilized in small animal orthopedics is known as the _____ elevator.

11. The type of bone-holding forceps equipped with a ratcheted handle for secure bone clamping is known as the _____ bone-holding forceps.

12. Two surgical devices made from soft metals that are used for bone cutting are the _____ and _____.

13. The points of bone pins come in varieties, like the _____, trocar, and _____ trocar.

14. The most commonly used sizes of stainless steel cerclage wire for small animal surgery are _____ gauge, _____ gauge, and _____ gauge.

15. The two basic types of bone screws are the _____ and the _____.

16. When using a laparoscope, the abdominal cavity is accessed through the _____ in horses or through the _____ _____ in both dogs and horses.

17. The use of a sharp _____ and a cannula is needed to penetrate subcutaneous tissues and the lining of the peritoneum in order to create a portal for a laparoscope.

18. The most commonly used gas for insufflation is _____ because it is noncombustible, making it relatively safe.

19. The box lock of instruments should remain in the _____ position when going through the ultrasonic cleaner.

20. Instruments with a(n) _____ finish are less resistant to discoloration and spotting caused by cleaning.

21. After instruments are cleaned, they should be rinsed thoroughly with _____ water and allowed to completely dry prior to autoclaving to prevent _____ formation.

22. _____ and _____ heat are the two general types of heat sterilization.

23. The two primary methods of sterilization used by manufacturers for packaging and the production of certain surgical supplies are _____ and _____.

24. Downward displacement or _____ displacement sterilizers use steam introduced into the top of the autoclave chamber to push air to the bottom.

25. Rapid and even penetration of steam by use of a _____ sterilizer is achieved by a vacuum pump that evacuates air before steam is allowed to enter the chamber.

26. Ethylene oxide and _____ are the two most commonly used agents for gas sterilization.

27. Ethylene oxide sterilization is slowly being overtaken by _____ sterilization because it is safer for personnel and the environment.

28. _____ indicators are used to show that hydrogen peroxide was present in gas plasma sterilization, whereas _____ indicators are used to test for sterility.

29. The quaternary ammonium compound most commonly used as a disinfectant is _____ chloride.

30. The two most commonly used aldehydes in veterinary medicine are _____ and _____.

31. The _____ skin preparation is performed in the patient preparation room to remove gross contamination.

32. _____ recumbency means the animal is placed on its back.

33. _____ recumbency means the animal is laying on either the right or left side of the body.

34. _____ recumbency means the animal is lying on its belly.

35. The two methods for donning surgical gloves are _____ gloving and

_____ gloving.

EXERCISE 31.10 CASE STUDY: INSTRUMENT CLEANING AND PACKING

Signalment: Mary, a 1-year-old female domestic shorthair tabby
Chief complaint: Mary is being admitted to the hospital for a routine spay.
Minimum database: Mary's database is normal, including physical examination findings and basic lab work. There is no history of previous medical problems.
Disposition of the case: Mary's surgery went well with no complications. Now you are responsible for cleaning, maintaining, repacking, and sterilizing the instruments used for this case. Your goals are to ensure efficient operation of the surgery suite, prevent instrument damage, and ultimately prepare the instruments in such a way that makes them safe for use on the next surgical case.
Please answer the following questions related to this case.

1. Describe the protocol that should be followed to prevent instrument corrosion.

   _____

   _____

   _____

2. Explain the process of cleaning instruments, listing each step in the proper order. Include information regarding both hand cleaning and ultrasonic cleaning, including the agents and equipment used.

   _____

   _____

   _____

   _____

   _____

   _____

3. How should instruments be rinsed, dried, and lubricated?

   _____

   _____

   _____

4. Instruments should always be inspected before repacking them. During this inspection, what will you look for?

_____

_____

_____

5. What are the principles of packing the instruments in preparation for sterilization? What instruments would be in a typical pack?

_____

_____

_____

_____

6. Explain the principles of using an autoclave to sterilize the pack, including preparation, loading the autoclave, maintenance, and ensuring safety.

_____

_____

_____

_____

_____

_____

Find the words listed below. The words may be located horizontally, vertically, or diagonally, and may be reversed.

```
G E S T E I N M A N N P I N U H A D A O A S
R B A A N I A O A R T H R O S C O P E L I Y
H S R N I O S O E L E C L Q L E N T C A C E
E B N Q D P S S R O N G E U R S H O L P D L
L R O R I O L T E R S D E A I Y H O E A C N
E D R N X P R P E O P G H T L O H H E R S T
E I O P E R I O S T E A L E L E V A T O R B
R S E G H C Q G E A C N N R T T Y C S S E L
O I O C R C U L S N R E L N S D A G S C I I
R N L C O O A T R U O F L A B T L E S O R P
R F L N L D I I T X F I T R A U I T E P H C
N E I I H I U I I I G O T Y T A L Y L E O L
S C R A C U I D F O N A V A S O P I N A C D
N T D F E I E I I N I G R M L O R O I C A S
A A R R L I H C E A D A F M O U L E A C E Y
G N I N I A T E R F L E S O O S G A T O P O
E T A S R O H P O D O I G N R G S N S R P H
Y L L O I I O T E T H R F I I C A E A D O A
A R L E T I H H F O E O O U R A E O N I E F
E N A T R N Y O L F N O E M P U R P S O R S
L C H H N D E T I R O L H C O P Y H S N O T
L E O N E L L Y N O B S R U D H I D P P C B
```

SelfRetaining
Phenols
Balfour
Hypochlorite
PeriostealElevator
Alcohol
BonecuttingForceps
QuaternaryAmmonium
BoneholdingForceps
HallAirDrill
SteinmannPin
Arthroscope
Triangulation
Rongeurs
Laparoscope
StainlessSteel
Accordion
Glutaraldehyde
EthyleneOxide
Disinfectant
Iodophors
Chlorhexidine

32 Surgical Assistance and Suture Material

LEARNING OBJECTIVES

When you have completed this chapter, you will be able to:
1. Pronounce, define, and spell all key terms in this chapter.
2. Describe the role of the veterinary technician in surgical assistance for large and small animal patients.
3. Explain preoperative preparation as it applies to the small animal surgical patient, including review of clipping and surgical scrub techniques with respect to patient positioning, and discuss considerations for operating room sterility and instrument table organization.
4. Discuss intraoperative duties of the surgical assistant, including surgical lighting, instruments, hemostasis, suture cutting, lavage and suction, camera manipulation, tissue manipulation, retraction, and organ positioning.
5. Describe the most common temporary and permanent forms of surgical implants and their uses.
6. Discuss the considerations involved in choosing a type of suture material and list and describe commonly used suture materials and needles and their application.
7. Describe the role of the surgical assistant in the postoperative management of patients.
8. Discuss surgical assisting in equine patients, including draping techniques, instrument setup, tissue handling, and common types of suture materials.

EXERCISE 32.1 MATCHING #1: TERMS AND DEFINITIONS

Instructions: Match each term in column A with its corresponding definition in column B by writing the appropriate letter in the space provided.

Column A	Column B
1. _____ Fenestrated	A. Does not allow water to penetrate
2. _____ Impervious	B. Surgical incision into the abdominal wall
3. _____ Ingesta	C. Relating to surgery on the skeleton
4. _____ Laparotomy	D. Having a window or one created in a surgical drape
5. _____ Orthopedic	E. "Squeezed on," as with a suture needle onto suture
6. _____ Swaged	F. Food material in the intestinal tract

EXERCISE 32.2 MATCHING #2: CHARACTERISTICS OF SUTURE MATERIAL

Instructions: Match each characteristic of suture material in column A with its corresponding classification in column B by writing the appropriate letter in the space provided. (Note that responses may be used more than once.)

Column A

1. _____ Passes more easily through tissue

2. _____ Better knot security

3. _____ Greater capillary action

4. _____ More susceptible to bacterial colonization

5. _____ Made of a single strand

Column B

A. Monofilament

B. Multifilament

EXERCISE 32.3 MATCHING #3: TRADE AND GENERIC NAMES OF SUTURE MATERIAL

Instructions: Match each trade name in column A with its corresponding generic name in column B by writing the appropriate letter in the space provided.

Column A

1. _____ Vicryl

2. _____ Dexon

3. _____ Monocryl

4. _____ PDS

5. _____ Maxon

6. _____ Nylon

7. _____ Prolene

8. _____ Novafil

9. _____ Mersilene

Column B

A. Polydioxanone

B. Polybutester

C. Polyglyconate

D. Polyglactin 910

E. Polypropylene

F. Polyester

G. Poliglecaprone 25

H. Polyamide

I. Polyglycolic acid

EXERCISE 32.4 MATCHING #4: CLASSIFICATION OF SUTURE MATERIAL

Instructions: Match each suture material in column A with its corresponding classification in column B by writing the appropriate letter in the space provided. (Note that responses may be used more than once.)

Column A

1. _____ Polyglyconate

2. _____ Stainless steel

3. _____ Polybutester

4. _____ Silk

5. _____ Polypropylene

6. _____ Polydioxanone

7. _____ Polyglycolic acid

8. _____ Poliglecaprone 25

9. _____ Polyglactin 910

10. _____ Polyamide

11. _____ Polyester

Column B

A. Monofilament, absorbable

B. Monofilament, nonabsorbable

C. Multifilament, absorbable

D. Multifilament, nonabsorbable

E. Monofilament or multifilament, absorbable

F. Monofilament or multifilament, nonabsorbable

394

Instructions: Respond to the queries associated with each photo in the spaces provided.

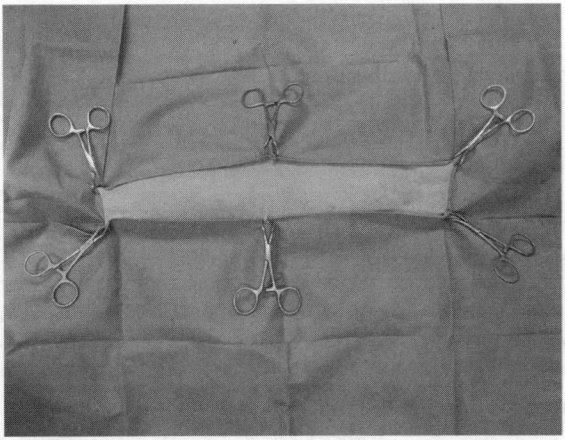

1a. Identify the instruments in this image.

_____

1b. What principles must be followed when placing these clamps?

_____

_____

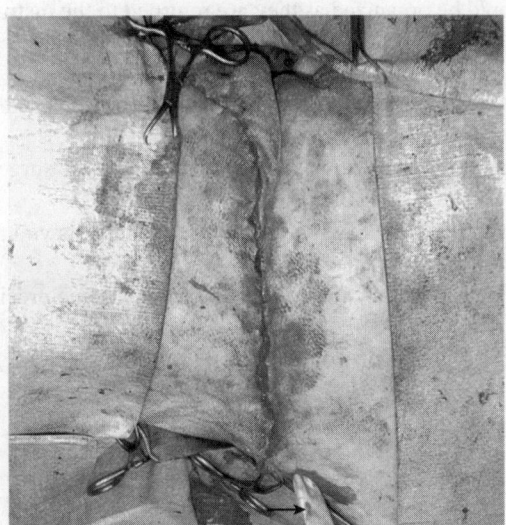

2a. Identify the type of drain used in this image.

_____

2b. What is the purpose of this drain in this case?

_____

2c. Is this drain passive or active? What does this mean regarding the way that it works?

_____

_____

2d. What are some of the principles of caring for this drain?

_____

_____

EXERCISE 32.6 TRUE OR FALSE: COMPREHENSIVE

Instructions: Read the following statements and write "T" for true or "F" for false in the blanks provided. If a statement is false, correct the statement to make it true.

1. _____ The main purpose of drapes is to cover the hair, which is not sterile.

2. _____ Once a towel clamp is removed from the patient, it is considered contaminated and must be removed from the surgery site and instrument table.

3. _____ Sterile stockinettes can be used as an additional drape material to allow the surgeon and surgical assistant to maneuver a leg without continually touching the skin.

4. _____ When surgery is performed on an extremity, and the surgeon wishes to maintain mobility of the limb, it is often desirable for the limb to be prepped using the hanging-limb technique.

5. _____ Oral surgeries are considered sterile procedures.

6. _____ Generally, instruments should be organized as they are returned to the instrument table after use to help prevent delays in accessing them again.

7. _____ The handles used to adjust operating room lights should be placed before the patient is draped.

8. _____ Utilizing a surgical assistant to pass instruments is convenient for the surgeon but increases surgery time.

9. _____ Any portion of the scissors may be used for cutting sutures as long as you are not in the surgeon's way.

10. _____ Bipolar (as opposed to unipolar) electrocautery is used when extreme precision is necessary.

11. _____ Iso-osmotic fluids are used for lavage of wounds and surgical sites.

12. _____ Once prepped, the skin is considered sterile.

13. _____ The urinary bladder is located in the cranial part of the abdomen.

14. _____ USP 2-0 suture is smaller in diameter than USP 2 suture.

15. _____ Suture with high memory holds knots better than suture with low memory.

16. _____ Suture material classified as absorbable loses the majority of its breaking strength in 21 days.

17. _____ Catgut absorbs in an unpredictable fashion.

18. _____ Polypropylene suture has the greatest tensile strength of all suture materials.

19. _____ Swaged needles are more traumatic to tissue.

20. _____ Locations where taper needles are commonly used include the intestines, subcutaneous tissue, and fascia.

21. _____ Formation of a watertight seal is an advantage of continuous suture patterns.

22. _____ The surgical nurse is vital to decreasing surgery and anesthesia time in the large animal patient.

23. _____ Irrigation during bone drilling is helpful in removing debris but is not required.

24. _____ Self-retaining retractors are critical to adequate organ exposure in equine abdominal surgery.

25. _____ Blood loss in most surgical procedures of horses is not a major concern.

EXERCISE 32.7 MULTIPLE CHOICE: COMPREHENSIVE

Instructions: Circle the one correct answer to each of the following questions.

1. When placing quarter drapes, the drape should be placed
   a. a few cm from the incision and pulled closer to the incision if needed to adjust it.
   b. a few cm from the incision and pulled farther away from the incision if needed to adjust it.
   c. 5 to 10 cm from the incision and pulled closer to the incision if needed to adjust it.
   d. 5 to 10 cm from the incision and pulled farther away from the incision if needed to adjust it.

2. If a surgical glove becomes contaminated during surgery, it should be
   a. removed and replaced.
   b. covered.
   c. flushed with sterile saline.
   d. wiped clean.

3. Quarter drapes are held in place by
   a. Allis tissue forceps.
   b. Babcock forceps.
   c. Rochester forceps.
   d. Backhaus towel clamps.

4. When preparing for an abdominal exploration, the patient should be placed in
   a. right lateral recumbency.
   b. dorsal recumbency.
   c. sternal recumbency.
   d. left lateral recumbency.

5. The proper patient position for a right lateral intercostal thoracotomy is
   a. dorsal recumbency.
   b. left lateral recumbency.
   c. right lateral recumbency.
   d. sternal recumbency.

6. A break in aseptic technique is most likely to occur
   a. as the patient is being prepped.
   b. interoperatively.
   c. as the patient is being draped.
   d. during suturing and as the drapes are being removed.

7. Surgical instruments that are most commonly used should be placed in a location that the surgeon can easily access. These instruments most commonly include
   a. retractors, scalpel, and hemostats.
   b. hemostats, needle holders, and retractors.
   c. scalpel, tissue forceps, and scissors.
   d. scissors, needle holders, and thumb forceps.

8. The portions of the surgery gown that are considered sterile are
   a. front from waist to shoulders.
   b. front and sides from waist to shoulders.
   c. front and sides from midchest to waist.
   d. front from midchest to waist.

9. Scalpel blades are placed on the scalpel handle using
   a. Halstead mosquito forceps.
   b. Allis tissue forceps.
   c. fingers.
   d. a needle holder.

10. The suction tip that is best for suctioning large volumes of fluid out of body cavities is called the
    a. Yankauer tip.
    b. Hohmann tip.
    c. Poole tip.
    d. Frazier tip.

11. Which organ can be lifted out of the abdomen during an exploratory laparotomy, because it is very mobile?
    a. Liver
    b. Spleen
    c. Kidney
    d. Stomach

12. A dog's left kidney can be best viewed by retracting the
    a. duodenum ventrally and to the left.
    b. descending colon and spleen to the right.
    c. ascending colon ventrally and caudally.
    d. spleen cranially.

13. Which retractors are the most appropriate choice for retracting lungs when performing a thoracotomy?
    a. Gelpi
    b. Army-Navy
    c. Malleable
    d. Senn

14. Which of the following tissues heals more slowly and therefore requires the use of nonabsorbable suture?
    a. Tendon
    b. Stomach
    c. Bladder
    d. Uterus

15. Which of the following sutures is available with an antibacterial coating?
    a. Silk
    b. Polydioxanone
    c. Catgut
    d. Polyglactin 910

16. Which suture has the best handling characteristics but stimulates inflammation?
    a. Catgut
    b. Polyglycolic acid
    c. Silk
    d. Polydioxanone

17. The most commonly used curved needles are
    a. 1/4-circle and 5/8-circle.
    b. 3/8-circle and 1/2-circle.
    c. 5/8-circle and 1/2-circle.
    d. 3/8-circle and 1/4-circle.

18. A cutting needle would be the most appropriate choice for
    a. skin.
    b. intestine.
    c. fascia.
    d. bladder wall.

19. The suture needle point recommended for suturing organs like the liver and kidney is
    a. cutting.
    b. reverse-cutting.
    c. taper.
    d. blunt.

20. The closure of the equine abdominal wall usually requires
    a. USP 4-0 or 5-0 suture.
    b. USP 2-0 or 3-0 suture.
    c. USP 0 or 1 suture.
    d. USP 2 or 3 suture.

EXERCISE 32.8 CASE STUDY: SUTURE NEEDLES

You are working at a busy multiple-doctor practice as the head surgery technician. A new veterinary assistant has come to talk to you because she is confused about the different suture needles. When the doctor asked her to get one earlier in the day, she had no idea what to do. She asks you to give her some information about needles so she will have a better understanding of them and can get the proper one when asked. Explain the structure and function of suture needles, including the general shapes they come in, the different types of points, and the methods of suture attachment. In each case, discuss the circumstances under which each type is used.

a. Shapes: _____

_____

_____

_____

_____

_____

b. Needle points: _____

_____

_____

_____

_____

_____

c. Suture attachment: _____

_____

_____

_____

_____

_____

33 Small Animal Surgical Nursing

LEARNING OBJECTIVES

When you have completed this chapter, you will be able to:
1. Pronounce, spell, and define all key terms in the chapter.
2. Regarding surgical preparation and animal positioning:
    - Describe the perioperative responsibilities of the veterinary technician.
    - Describe indications and use of prophylactic antibiotics.
    - Describe signs of blood loss in the postoperative patient.
    - Discuss concerns related to hypothermia in perioperative patients and be able to manage it.
    - Evaluate surgical incisions for complications and be able to remove skin sutures or staples.
3. Understand restraint of the anesthetized patient for surgical procedures.
4. Differentiate between elective and nonelective surgeries.
5. List and describe perioperative considerations for commonly listed surgical procedures.
6. List considerations related to client education for discharged surgical patients.

Across

1 The term used to describe low blood pressure
5 Male cats with urologic syndrome may experience urethral _____
6 A dog should be placed in _____ recumbency for a simple orchidectomy procedure
7 The name of the hernia found more commonly in female dogs
8 A common symptom of cats with urologic syndrome
11 A specific type of collar used to prevent animals from licking and/or chewing at an affected area
13 A term that means surgical removal of the testicles
14 The term cesarean delivery was derived from the name of _____, who was thought to be the first person to be born by this surgical technique
18 A specific type of hernia in which omentum and intraabdominal fat protrudes through a defect in the abdominal wall
19 A syndrome associated with a loss of stamina in working breeds that is a complication of ovariohysterectomy
21 A surgical procedure performed in male dogs with penile scar tissue to establish normal urine flow (2 words)
22 The name of the hernia where a classic visual sign is a "tucked-up" abdomen
26 Cesarean delivery is usually performed on animals experiencing _____
27 The most critical anesthetic period for an animal with a diaphragmatic hernia
28 _____ radiographs should be taken to confirm the diagnosis of a diaphragmatic hernia.
29 During an ovariohysterectomy procedure, before closing the abdominal wall, the _____ stump must be visualized to check for hemorrhage

Down

2 A surgical procedure performed in male cats that experience urethral obstruction secondary to feline urologic syndrome (2 words)
3 The removal of the scrotum at the same time as removing the testicles is called scrotal _____
4 Some animals experiencing urologic syndrome may need lifesaving measures to protect their heart if this electrolyte value is too high
9 A term used to describe general bleeding
10 The surgical treatment recommended for an animal with a pyometra
12 The term used to describe narrowing of the opening of the urethra because of excessive formation of scar tissue
15 A complication of an umbilical hernia in which there is a loss of intestinal blood supply
16 A term used to describe bloody urine
17 A term used for intestinal entrapment
20 A surgical procedure performed to remove bladder stones
23 The drug used to increase uterine muscular contractions
24 An alternative name for bladder stones
25 The medical term for an internal organ

Chapter **33** **Small Animal Surgical Nursing**

EXERCISE 33.2 DEFINITIONS: KEY TERMS

Instructions: Define each term in your own words.

1. Abdominocentesis: _____

_____

2. Capillary refill time: _____

_____

3. Anastomosis: _____

_____

4. Arthrodesis: _____

_____

5. Enterotomy: _____

_____

6. Onychectomy: _____

_____

7. Strangulation: _____

_____

8. Thoracocentesis: _____

_____

9. Urethrostomy: _____

_____

EXERCISE 33.3 MATCHING: TERMS AND DEFINITIONS

Instructions: Match each term in column A with its corresponding definition in column B by writing the appropriate letter in the space provided.

Column A

1. _____ Evisceration

2. _____ Gastrotomy

3. _____ Intussusception

4. _____ Ileus

5. _____ Osteochondrosis

6. _____ Ostectomy

7. _____ Celiotomy

8. _____ Orchidectomy

9. _____ Dehiscence

Column B

A. The telescoping of one portion of an animal's bowel into another

B. The surgical removal of part of a bone

C. The surgical removal of an animal's testicles

D. Surgical incision into the abdominal cavity

E. The uncontrolled exposure of abdominal organs through a surgical incision as a result of trauma or dehiscence

F. Temporary loss of intestinal motility

G. A surgical incision made into the stomach

H. Abnormally thickened portion of the articular cartilage

I. Separation of the sutured layers of an incision

EXERCISE 33.4 TRUE OR FALSE: COMPREHENSIVE

Instructions: Read the following statements and write "T" for true or "F" for false in the blanks provided. If a statement is false, correct the statement to make it true.

1. _____ Water should be offered to animals before food postoperatively.

2. _____ It is best to vaccinate a puppy or kitten the day of surgery rather than before.

3. _____ Prophylactic antibiotics should be given to all animals undergoing surgery.

4. _____ To achieve therapeutic drug levels in a surgical wound, antibiotics should be administered no less than 20 minutes prior to the first incision.

5. _____ It is not unusual for a patient's PCV and TP to drop to 10% as a result of anesthesia and surgery.

6. _____ The size of the surgical incision can affect the patient's body temperature during a surgical procedure.

7. _____ Heat lamps are a safe alternative to heating blankets to maintain adequate body temperature in an anesthetized patient.

8. _____ For small dogs and cats, it is acceptable to use a warm water bath postoperatively to raise their body temperature quickly.

9. _____ During an anesthetic procedure, an increased heart rate is a direct indicator of pain, which should be managed by increasing the anesthetic levels.

10. _____ It is best to assess how much pain an animal is in postoperatively prior to administering pain medication.

11. _____ Topical antibiotic ointments can delay the healing process when applied directly to incision sites.

12. _____ Noxious-tasting agents should be placed directly on an incision to prevent licking and chewing.

13. _____ Tail docking is most commonly performed for aesthetic reasons to conform to breed standards.

14. _____ Gastrointestinal surgery often involves glove changes and new packs during surgery.

15. _____ Ideally, dewclaws should be removed during the first week of the animal's life.

16. _____ The medical term for surgical removal of the claw and its associated distal phalanx is onychectomy.

17. _____ Gastric dilation-volvulus is a condition commonly seen in toy dog breeds.

18. _____ Spaying a dog or cat during estrus does not affect the potential risks of the surgical procedure.

19. _____ Remaining ovarian tissue left from a spay procedure may result in recurrent heat cycles and stump pyometra.

20. _____ Animals that have been spayed may have an increase in body weight after the surgery.

21. _____ In preparation for canine castration, the scrotum is normally shaved and draped into the surgical field.

22. _____ Alcohol should not be used when preparing the scrotum for castration in male cats.

23. _____ Shaving scrotal hairs is an acceptable alternative to plucking scrotal hairs when prepping for feline castration.

EXERCISE 33.5 MULTIPLE CHOICE: COMPREHENSIVE

Instructions: Circle the one correct answer to each of the following questions.

1. The surgical procedure that is most likely to require the veterinary technician to act as a surgical assistant is a(n)
   a. orthopedic procedure.
   b. hernia repair.
   c. feline ovariohysterectomy.
   d. laceration or abscess repair.

2. At what body temperature is it safe to stop using heat sources to warm the patient postoperatively?
   a. 103° F
   b. 102° F
   c. 101° F
   d. 100° F

3. Which of the following procedures would be considered least painful?
   a. Fracture repair
   b. Amputation
   c. Declaw
   d. Mass removal

4. What is the earliest that it is safe to remove sutures after a surgical procedure?
   a. 6 to 8 days
   b. 10 to 14 days
   c. 20 to 24 days
   d. 25 to 30 days

5. Which surgery would be considered a nonelective procedure?
   a. Declaw
   b. Splenectomy
   c. Castration
   d. Ovariohysterectomy

6. What is the ideal age to perform tail docking on puppies?
   a. 2 to 3 days
   b. 3 to 5 days
   c. 6 to 10 days
   d. 10 to 12 days

7. What are three known techniques used for feline claw removal?
   a. Rescoe nail trimmers, #12 scalpel blade, CO2 laser
   b. Surgical scissors, #15 scalpel blade, CO2 laser
   c. #12 scalpel blade, surgical scissors, Rescoe nail trimmers
   d. Rescoe nail trimmers, #15 scalpel blade, CO_2 laser

8. How many hours post onychectomy should the postoperative bandages be removed?
   a. 12 hours
   b. 24 hours
   c. 6 hours
   d. 8 hours

9. What is not a typical early complication of an onychectomy procedure?
   a. Loose bandage
   b. Removal of the bandage by the patient
   c. Skin sloughing
   d. Hemorrhage

10. What is the proper name for a surgical incision into the abdominal cavity?
   a. Celiotomy
   b. Gastrotomy
   c. Pyometra
   d. Orchidectomy

11. The most common approach to the abdominal cavity is
   a. ventral midline.
   b. paramedian.
   c. paracostal.
   d. flank.

12. What is the standard clipping for ventral midline celiotomy surgery?
   a. 2 cm cranial to xiphoid to 2 cm caudal to the pubis and to the nipples laterally
   b. 2 cm cranial to umbilicus to 2 cm caudal to pubis, and 2 to 4 cm lateral to the nipples
   c. 2 cm cranial to xiphoid to 2 cm caudal to pubis, and 2 to 4 cm lateral to the nipples
   d. 2 cm cranial to umbilicus to 2 cm caudal to pubis and to the nipples laterally

13. What is the proper term to describe an incision made into the stomach?
   a. Enterotomy
   b. Cystotomy
   c. Perineal urethrostomy
   d. Gastrotomy

14. What color should a normal gastrointestinal tract be when viewed in an open abdominal surgery?
   a. Pale tan
   b. Brown
   c. Gray
   d. Pink

15. A devitalized intestinal track can be recognized by
   a. bleeding of the cut surface.
   b. decreased motility.
   c. red discoloration.
   d. lack of fluorescein dye uptake.

16. Which of the following is not a classic clinical sign of gastric dilatation-volvulus?
   a. Vomiting
   b. Retching
   c. Increased appetite
   d. Distention of stomach

17. Which radiographic view of the abdomen is most beneficial when evaluating stomach rotation or bloat on a dog?
   a. Left lateral
   b. Right lateral
   c. VD
   d. DV

18. Which of the following is not a good indication for castrating a dog or cat?
   a. Decreasing population growth
   b. Treatment of perineal hernias
   c. Reducing exercise requirements
   d. Prevention of reproductive system tumors

19. Which of the following is removed during a spay?
   a. Broad ligament and the ovaries
   b. Ovaries and uterus
   c. Suspensory ligament and uterine horn
   d. Oviducts and ovaries

20. A spay hook is a surgical instrument that is specifically used to
   a. exteriorize the uterine horns.
   b. elevate the ovaries to the level of the incision.
   c. immobilize the uterine vessels.
   d. ligate the uterine body.

21. When performing a spay after parturition, it should be done when the puppies or kittens are weaned and lactation ceases at approximately
   a. 2 to 4 weeks later.
   b. 4 to 6 weeks later.
   c. 6 to 8 weeks later.
   d. 8 to 10 weeks later.

22. A condition of the uterus involving endometrial hyperplasia, increased uterine secretions, and accumulation of fluid in the uterus with secondary infection is known as
   a. pyometra.
   b. uterine prolapse.
   c. mucometra.
   d. hydrometra.

23. Which is not a major indication for feline castration?
   a. Prevent fighting
   b. Decrease urine odor
   c. Prevent roaming
   d. Decrease vocalization

24. What is the most common indication for cystotomy in small animals?
   a. Remove tumors
   b. Correct congenital defects
   c. Remove cystic calculi
   d. Repair traumatic rupture in the bladder

25. The name for a hernia in which abdominal contents protrude into the thoracic cavity is
    a. umbilical hernia.
    b. diaphragmatic hernia.
    c. inguinal hernia.
    d. abdominal hernia.

26. Approximately what percentage of mammary tumors in cats are malignant?
    a. 10% to 15%
    b. 25% to 50%
    c. 50% to 60%
    d. 80% to 90%

27. The most common neurologic disorder involving the spine in dogs is
    a. atlantoaxial subluxation.
    b. spinal trauma.
    c. lumbosacral stenosis.
    d. intervertebral disc rupture.

28. What are the first three steps that should always be performed when encountering an animal with a long bone fracture?
    a. (1) Stabilize the animal, (2) check for open wounds associated with the fracture, and (3) immobilize the fracture.
    b. (1) Administer pain medication, (2) assess the fracture, and (3) immobilize the fracture.
    c. (1) Anesthetize the animal for emergency surgery, (2) administer pain medication, and (3) immobilize the fracture.
    d. (1) Manipulate the bones back into place, (2) administer pain medication, and (3) immobilize the fracture.

29. After long bone or joint surgery, what level of activity is most appropriate for optimal recovery?
    a. Leash walking
    b. Playing with other dogs
    c. Cage confinement
    d. Off-leash activities

EXERCISE 33.6 FILL-IN-THE-BLANK: COMPREHENSIVE

Instructions: Fill in each of the spaces provided with the missing word or words that complete the sentence.

1. Evisceration is the uncontrolled exposure of organs through a surgical incision because of _____ of the wound.

2. Ileus is the term used to describe the temporary loss of _____ motility.

3. _____ is an infection along tissue planes.

4. The _____ is the required time it takes for blood to refill small capillary beds of mucus membranes after digital blanching has occurred.

5. _____ is the term used to describe a localized area of fluctuant swelling that is not usually painful or warm to the touch

6. Onychectomy is the removal of the claw and the associated _____ phalanx.

7. Celiotomy (laparotomy) is a surgical incision into the _____ cavity.

8. Vomiting, retching, and severe distention of the stomach are classic signs of _____.

9. Animals suffering from GVD are usually in _____, and if left untreated, will die as a result of cardiovascular collapse.

10. A gastropexy is performed on the _____ ventrolateral aspect of the body wall near the last rib.

11. The primary indication for ovariohysterectomy is the prevention of _____ and the subsequent production of unwanted puppies and kittens.

12. Ovariohysterectomy performed before the animal's first estrus cycle will greatly decrease the risk of _____ neoplasia in dogs.

13. Another name for false pregnancy is _____.

14. There is not an optimal age for canine castration, but it is often performed around _____ months of age.

15. _____ is enlargement of the uterus with serous fluid.

16. The accumulation of sterile mucoid fluid within the uterus is known as _____.

17. Basic discharge instructions on a postoperative patient would include _____ administration, _____ monitoring, _____ restriction, and contact information in the event of a problem.

18. _____ delivery is when an incision is made into the abdominal cavity and then into the uterus to deliver a neonate.

19. Cesarean delivery is usually performed on animals that are experiencing _____.

20. _____ is the incision into the urinary bladder to expose the interior contents or lumen of the urinary bladder.

21. Perineal urethrostomy in male cats is often recommended to manage multiple episodes of _____ associated with feline urologic syndrome.

EXERCISE 33.7 CASE STUDY #1: DELIVERY OF PUPPIES BY CESAREAN SECTION

A 3-year-old pregnant female Mastiff is scheduled for a planned Cesarean section tomorrow at the practice where you were recently hired. You are going to be a part of a small team that will receive and care for the newborn puppies. Wanting to provide competent care, you study your notes the night before to be sure you are prepared to assist. Also, because time is of the essence when reviving puppies delivered by Cesarean, you want to prepare the necessary equipment well beforehand.

1. In addition to the equipment necessary to clamp and tie off the umbilical cords, what other equipment do you need to have ready?

_____

_____

_____

2. What exactly will you do when you are handed the first neonate?

_____

_____

_____

_____

_____

_____

_____

_____

EXERCISE 33.8 CASE STUDY #2: MONITORING FOR POSTOPERATIVE BLEEDING

You have just completed an ovariohysterectomy on a 1-year-old female bearded collie mix named Mandy. This patient was in heat at the time of the surgery, and there was more bleeding than usual during the procedure. Although the surgery went well, the doctor has asked you to monitor this patient for intra-abdominal hemorrhage postoperatively. Answer the following questions regarding the management of this case.

1. What changes in this patient's vital signs and general physical findings would alert you to this serious postoperative complication?

_____

_____

_____

_____

_____

2. What general diagnostic tests could be performed to help determine if intra-abdominal bleeding was occurring?

_____

_____

_____

_____

_____

3. If signs of hemorrhage were observed, what general types of treatment strategies could be used for Mandy?

_____

_____

_____

_____

_____

_____

_____

_____

4. Mandy recovered uneventfully and was ready for discharge the following day. Discuss in detail the appearance of a normal postoperative incision between the time of surgery and suture removal. Then, discuss the signs that an incision is not healing normally.

   a. Appearance of a normal incision postoperatively:

   _____

   _____

   _____

   _____

   _____

   b. Signs that an incision is not healing normally:

   _____

   _____

   _____

   _____

   _____

   _____

_____

_____

_____

_____

_____

_____

_____

5. When Mandy's incision is healed, the sutures or staples will need to be removed.

a. Typically, how many days after surgery are sutures or staples removed?

_____

b. Describe the procedure that will be used to remove her sutures or staples.

_____

_____

_____

_____

_____

_____

Find the words listed below. The words may be located horizontally, vertically, or diagonally and may be reversed.

```
A E O E U Y P Z E T E E I R E G R A T U
I S A O T M R L N H V L A A M O R E S L
M E E N R O M D E E U D V N P S A L Y C
E A R C Z T T S O M I E G A S C L I B E
O P L S N C A L P A C I G L H T L S G A
A C T I V E T E L T S E I G A E O S E E
G M E C N R C T A O R N U E U X C E M O
C C T I T T I S S M E O Z S A D N A A O
C Y A N O S I S I A R I M I A T A E E E
Y R A M M A M N A H S T E C I L H E N P
D A Y V S G A L T A E T E S G S T M Y S
A I A A A L B E T U M D M F T M E D M R
R T E S L A K S Q R A A I O Y C B M E V
S G R A T I A I Y X E P O R T S A G R C
M H S I R T N I E O I E Y M L I Z R S I
I I N T E R V E R T E B R A L D I S C O
E L S M U A B G L A A S S L T O L U G I
L N D O Q P A S S I V E O I G V E E I A
A Z T V R E M D A A R S I N T C A B O O
E U L L E A R R D R A A O G O M R R L A
```

Seroma
GDV
Hematoma
Nose
Dehiscence
Mammary
Drain
Neoplasia
ElizabethanCollar
Lumpectomy
Active
Metastasize
Passive
Analgesics
Strikethrough
IntervertebralDisc
Formalin
Tourniquet
Radial
Germinal
Laser
Cyanosis
Ileus
LineaAlba
Gastropexy
PartialGastrectomy

Chapter **33** **Small Animal Surgical Nursing**

Large Animal Surgical Nursing

LEARNING OBJECTIVES

When you have completed this chapter, you will be able to:
1. Pronounce, spell, and define all key terms in this chapter.
2. Describe the preoperative preparation needed for equine patients, as well as the responsibilities of the veterinary technician before, during, and after equine surgery, including postoperative monitoring, medication administration, bandage care, and grooming.
3. List the surgical procedures commonly performed in equine patients and describe indications and preoperative, intraoperative, and postoperative considerations for common surgical procedures in equine patients.
4. List the surgical procedures commonly performed in bovine patients and describe indications and preoperative, intraoperative, and postoperative considerations for common surgical procedures in bovine patients.
5. Discuss the surgical procedures of young stock, including dehorning, castration, and umbilical hernias and infections.
6. Do the following related to small ruminants:
   - Discuss selected conditions of small ruminants related to the urinary and ophthalmic systems.
   - Describe the surgical procedures commonly performed in small ruminants, including indications and preoperative, intraoperative, and postoperative considerations for common surgical procedures in small ruminants.

EXERCISE 34.1 DEFINITIONS: KEY TERMS

Instructions: Define each term in your own words.

1. Colpotomy:_____

_____

2. Laparotomy:_____

_____

3. Rumenotomy:_____

_____

4. Urachus:_____

_____

EXERCISE 34.2 TRUE OR FALSE: COMPREHENSIVE

Instructions: Read the following statements and write "T" for true or "F" for false in the blanks provided. If a statement is false, correct the statement to make it true.

1. _____ A "preference card" is a system that details the instruments, supplies, and equipment a specific surgeon typically requests for procedures, alleviating the need for a preoperative planning discussion between the veterinary technician and the surgeon.

2. _____ A tourniquet bandage is wrapped around the limb in a spiral fashion, moving from proximal to distal to a point below the surgery site.

3. _____ When performing lower limb surgery on a horse, a tourniquet may be used to assist with hemostasis. To prevent any potentially serious side effects, a tourniquet should be applied for a maximum period of 2 hours.

4. _____ To help prevent myositis during general anesthesia in the equine patient, the down forelimb should be pulled forward to minimize the pressure on the triceps and radial nerve.

5. _____ Shoes are generally removed from an equine patient prior to surgery to prevent them from falling off and contaminating the surgery site.

6. _____ Urethral obstruction is most commonly seen in show or pet goats and lambs who are being fed a high-grain, low-roughage diet.

7. _____ Arthrotomy is preferred to arthroscopy for joint surgery in equine patients because of its lower morbidity and mortality rates.

8. _____ Tendons are poorly vascularized and heal very slowly.

9. _____ Secondary sinusitis in horses is related to upper respiratory infections caused by *Streptococcus*.

10. _____ Equine castration requires extensive surgical facilities and specialized equipment.

11. _____ Lacerations are the most common type of open wound in horses.

12. _____ The best way to repair major fractures of long bones in horses is with screws and bone plates.

13. _____ Behavior and mentation are most accurately observed when the food animal is in its natural environment with minimal human disturbance.

14. _____ Laminitis, a serious, often life-threatening disease in the horse, is defined as inflammation of the lamina in the spine.

15. _____ Complete dehorning in adult goats should be avoided as it has been shown to cause depressed behavior following horn removal.

16. _____ The left recurrent laryngeal nerve is involved in about 90% of cases of laryngeal hemiplegia.

17. _____ Removing a dairy cow's tail is referred to as "tail-jacking."

18. _____ Prolapse of the vagina usually involves the entire vagina and cervix through the vulva.

19. _____ Exteriorizing the cow's uterus during a C-section should be avoided unless it is impossible.

20. _____ When placing a jugular catheter in the bovine patient, it is advisable to make a stab incision in the skin to prevent burring of the catheter.

414

Chapter **34** **Large Animal Surgical Nursing**

21. _____ Extra-label use refers to the use of a new animal drug in a food-producing animal in a manner that is not in accordance with the drug labeling.

22. _____ Puncture wounds generally cause little damage to an animal.

23. _____ Open castration is the most common castration method used in calves and small ruminants.

24. _____ Most oral lacerations in the bovine patient require surgical intervention, daily mouth lavage, and systemic antibiotics.

25. _____ The majority of flank laparotomies in the bovine patient are performed while the patient is standing, using local anesthetic techniques.

26. _____ The majority of lameness in cattle is caused by foot problems originating in the claws.

27. _____ Claw amputation is the best treatment option to treat interdigital hyperplasia.

28. _____ The Liptak test can be used to diagnose TRP.

29. _____ Many food animal surgeries are performed in the field and are considered "clean" surgeries.

30. _____ Sinus trephination, also called face flap surgery, involves the creation of a bone flap into the affected sinus, allowing for better access.

31. _____ Chondritis is a condition most commonly affecting young racehorses.

32. _____ Scrotal hernias are seen exclusively in stallions.

33. _____ When in stocks, a horse undergoing a rectal procedure does not pose a safety risk.

34. _____ When drug information specific to a species is not on the bottle or package insert, it can be found on the Food Animal Residue Avoidance Databank (FARAD).

35. _____ Preputial prolapse is commonly seen in pigs.

36. _____ Lacerations are of greater concern with equine patients than their food-animal counterparts.

37. _____ Teat lacerations are most common in dairy cows and goats.

38. _____ Perineal lacerations are rare in all species.

39. _____ Tusk trimming on the pig can be done without causing pain or infection due to the lack of a pulp cavity above the gingival margin.

EXERCISE 34.3 MULTIPLE CHOICE: COMPREHENSIVE

Instructions: Circle the one correct answer to each of the following questions.

1. The leading cause of death in horses is
   a. laminitis.
   b. dystocia.
   c. colic.
   d. long bone fracture.

2. The use of elastrator bands to perform castration of calves has been associated with the development of
   a. self-mutilation.
   b. seromas.
   c. infection.
   d. incomplete sloughing.

3. Labor in the mare is completed quickly, usually in
   a. 20 to 35 minutes.
   b. 5 to 10 minutes.
   c. 45 to 60 minutes.
   d. 15 to 20 minutes.

4. _____ is/are likely the most common cause of acute lameness encountered in equine practice.
   a. Subsolar abscesses
   b. Seedy toes
   c. Laminitis
   d. Bowed tendon

5. The most common surgical approach to the equine abdominal cavity is through a
   a. lateral flank incision.
   b. ventral midline incision.
   c. paramedian incision.
   d. paracostal incision.

6. Which is the most common type of hernia seen in equine veterinary practice?
   a. Umbilical
   b. Inguinal
   c. Incisional
   d. Hiatal

7. Improvement in weak flexor tendons in foals can be encouraged by
   a. the use of bandages.
   b. applying a cast for 3 to 5 days.
   c. providing a firm surface to stand on.
   d. extensive periods of controlled exercise.

8. Which is not typically used during equine arthroscopy?
   a. Trocars
   b. CO_2 insufflation
   c. Cannula
   d. VAPR system

9. The Caslick's procedure is typically performed when
   a. more than 6 cm of the vulva lies ventral to the pelvis.
   b. more than 4 cm of the vulva lies dorsal to the pelvis.
   c. more than 4 cm of the vulva lies ventral to the pelvis.
   d. when the vulva and anus are on the same plane.

10. Mares with granulosa cell tumors often display
   a. aggressive behavior.
   b. dog-sitting stance.
   c. lameness.
   d. depression.

11. Inguinal hernias are most commonly seen in
   a. stallions.
   b. mares.
   c. foals.
   d. geldings.

12. Laminitis should be suspected in a horse displaying a(n) _____ stance.
   a. over at the knees
   b. knock-kneed
   c. cow-stretching
   d. dog-sitting

13. Prior to general anesthesia, feed should be withheld from an adult food-animal patient for
   a. 6 to 12 hours.
   b. 12 to 24 hours.
   c. 18 to 36 hours.
   d. 36 to 48 hours.

14. Manifestations of pain in the colic patient do not include
   a. vomiting.
   b. lying down.
   c. sweating.
   d. rolling.

15. Horses should typically receive preoperative medications such as antibiotics and anti-inflammatories _____ prior to induction.
   a. 1 to 2 days
   b. 3 to 4 hours
   c. 1 to 2 hours
   d. 15 to 30 minutes

16. Which regional analgesic technique involves the injection of lidocaine behind the last rib and just below the transverse process of the lumbar vertebrae?
   a. Line block
   b. Inverted L block
   c. Distal paravertebral block
   d. Proximal paravertebral block

17. To ensure that the entire surgical team is thoroughly prepared and working from the same information, a surgical checklist, time-out, or call-out should be performed right before
   a. the first surgical incision.
   b. the presurgical scrub.
   c. the placement of the final suture.
   d. the induction of the patient.

18. Abdominal fluid obtained via abdominocentesis is graded according to all except which factor?
    a. Gross appearance
    b. Cell count
    c. pH
    d. Total protein concentration

19. What bovine disease may lead to peritonitis, liver or reticular abscesses, pericarditis, or vagal indigestion?
    a. Traumatic reticuloperitonitis
    b. Abomasal displacement
    c. Osteomyelitis
    d. Abomasal volvulus

20. A rumenotomy is performed by entering the patient's abdomen from an incision made in the
    a. right flank.
    b. left flank.
    c. ventral midline.
    d. dorsal midline.

21. For a patient with traumatic reticuloperitonitis, in which the foreign body remains embedded in the reticulum wall despite the use of a rumen magnet, surgery is performed by entering the patient's abdomen from an incision made in the
    a. right flank.
    b. left flank.
    c. ventral midline.
    d. dorsal midline.

22. Abomasal displacements are most likely to occur in the first _____ weeks after parturition.
    a. 6
    b. 8
    c. 12
    d. 16

23. In a bovine patient with foot problems, which claws are most likely involved because they are the weight-bearing claws?
    a. Front lateral and hind medial
    b. Front medial and hind medial
    c. Front lateral and hind lateral
    d. Front medial and hind lateral

24. _____ is the ideal means of assessment of the internal umbilical structures in the foal.
    a. Radiography
    b. Manual palpation
    c. The use of forceps
    d. Ultrasonography

25. Postsurgical care for equine ovariectomy patients is largely dependent on
    a. the age of the mare.
    b. the type of approach used.
    c. the condition of the ovaries.
    d. the breed of horse.

26. Failure to deliver a foal within _____ of onset of second-stage labor is associated with dramatically increased foal mortality.
    a. half an hour
    b. an hour
    c. two hours
    d. three hours

27. Cattle with a pendulous sheath, a large preputial orifice, and a relaxed preputial membrane and penis are especially prone to
    a. obstructive urolithiasis.
    b. preputial prolapse.
    c. paraphimosis.
    d. phimosis.

28. The best time to dehorn a calf is between
    a. 8 to 12 weeks of age.
    b. 12 to 16 weeks of age.
    c. 5 to 7 weeks of age.
    d. 4 to 6 weeks of age.

29. Initial management of a horse with a fracture begins with
    a. radiography.
    b. administration of a sedative.
    c. stabilization.
    d. aseptic preparation of the skin.

30. The most widely used bone plate in equine surgery is the
    a. LCP.
    b. DCP.
    c. LC-DCP.
    d. DLP.

Instructions: Fill in each of the spaces with the missing word or words that complete the sentence.

1. In general, a significant economic drive underlies veterinary care in the food animal industry, so _____ will likely be a major consideration in decisions to treat the patient.

2. _____ allow practitioners to perform a greater number of surgical and diagnostic procedures and make an excellent addition to food animal practices.

3. A food animal that is undergoing surgery with general anesthesia or is at risk of significant blood loss during surgery should have preoperative blood work to include, at a minimum, values for _____ and _____.

4. Preoperative fasting for food animals should include withholding water for _____.

5. If an animal is to be recumbent during surgery, appropriate _____ must be used.

6. The _____ refers to the time before marketing or slaughter during which antibiotics, analgesics, or anesthetics cannot be used in an animal.

7. Typically, in mature cattle but also in calves and small ruminants older than six months of age, the _____ will be exposed when the horns are removed.

8. It is important to know the patient's vaccination history prior to dehorning, specifically _____ immunity.

9. _____, _____, and _____ from castrated males is more consistently of higher quality and palatability than their intact male counterparts.

10. Castration in commercial swine should be performed _____ after birth.

11. The _____ breed of dairy calves is most susceptible to umbilical hernias.

12. Performing a laparotomy on a standing animal facilitates _____ exploration and manipulation.

13. Hereford and Brahman breeds are especially sensitive to the sedative _____ and require only very small doses.

14. After successful rumenotomy, healthy rumen contents need to be replaced in the animal by performing a(n) _____.

15. "Hardware disease" is a common name for _____.

16. Conservative treatment of abomasal displacement involves _____ the patient to encourage the abomasum to flip back into place.

17. Livestock kept in _____ tend to see a higher incidence of lameness.

18. Vaginal prolapse can be classified according to _____ and severity of the condition.

19. The surgery used to remove scar tissue and shorten a bull's prepuce is commonly referred to as
_____.

20. Urolithiasis refers to the formation of "stones," or concretions of mucus, protein, and_____
in the urinary tract of male small ruminants.

EXERCISE 34.5 FILL-IN-THE-BLANK #2: SURGICAL NURSING OF HORSES

1. A(n) _____ used in a circular motion will loosen mud, dirt, or dander worked into the
equine patient's coat.

2. Preoperative blood work on a horse should minimally include a(n) _____ and
_____ determination.

3. Presurgical clipping should be performed with a number _____ blade against the grain
of the hair in a(n) _____ fashion with straight edges.

4. Care should be used to avoid clipping hair on the horse's _____ and
_____; those areas should only be clipped when absolutely necessary.

5. When gas anesthesia is to be used, the horse's _____ should be thoroughly rinsed
_____ immediately before induction.

6. Upon opening surgical packs, instruments, and supplies, both the OR technician and the scrubbed surgical team
should visually and verbally confirm that all internal process indicators show adequate changes to denote the
_____ of the instruments.

7. Postoperatively, changes in distal pulse palpation and hoof and coronary band temperature are early indications of
_____ and should be communicated immediately.

8. Most, but not all, of the causes of colic involve the _____ system, and the treatment may
or may not be surgery.

9. When using a nasogastric tube for gastric decompression, net _____ should always be
measured and recorded.

10. The composition of abdominal fluid, retrieved via _____, is determined by the condition
of the organs that are bathed by this fluid.

11. If monopolar cautery might be used, the OR technician should ensure that a(n) _____ is
in place before beginning the surgical site prep.

12. Hernias which admit _____ or less should be allowed time to resolve on their own.

13. Castrated males, or _____, are generally preferred by the average horse owner.

14. Mares should be monitored closely for the first 24 hours following ovariectomy, especially for signs of
_____ suggestive of internal blood loss.

15. The Caslick's procedure must be _____ on mares when foaling is imminent and sometimes before the act of breeding.

16. _____ should be used if the foal is dead and the malposition cannot be corrected.

17. _____ is defined as any deviation from the normal gait or posture and can be due to pain, mechanical function, or neurologic disease.

18. The loss of structural integrity in a fracture can be classified as either _____ or _____.

19. In arthroscopy, a sterile _____ is used to distend the joint.

20. Two types of tendon problems occur in young horses: _____ and _____.

21. _____ of the carpus is the most common limb deformity in growing foals.

22. Supportive therapy for laminitis includes controlling pain and inflammation with NSAIDs and analgesics and promoting blood flow with _____ drugs.

23. A foot with a subsolar abscess should be soaked in povidone iodine (Betadine) and magnesium sulfate (Epsom salt), and a(n) _____ dressing applied to encourage drainage.

24. In the horse, conformational factors, including long-sloping pasterns and low _____, can contribute to a horse's predisposition to tendon injuries.

25. Horses referred to as "roarers" are likely suffering from _____.

26. A reduction in the laryngeal luminal diameter is a hallmark of _____.

27. A horse has _____ pairs of sinuses.

28. Lacerations in which tissues have been torn away are called _____.

29. _____ and _____are the primary causes of clinical signs of colic in foals.

30. Clinical signs of a diseased umbilicus include _____ with the navel area exhibiting swelling, heat, and drainage.

31. Most horses are castrated at _____ months to allow for physical development before behavioral changes and management challenges occur.

32. The _____ procedure is a very common surgery performed in mares with pneumovagina.

33. The rotation of the uterus on its long axis is termed _____.

34. _____ is a severe and life-threatening disease process that causes reduced blood flow to a horse's foot and subsequent breakdown of the attachments of the hoof.

35. Subtotal spinus _____ is an effective method of surgical treatment for impinged dorsal spinus processes or "kissing spines."

36. Fistulous withers involves the _____ overlying the first thoracic vertebral spines and first presents as swelling on one or both sides of the poll.

37. Both fistulous withers and poll evil are often, but not always, associated with infection of the bacteria _____, which is more common to cattle.

38. The action of a horse setting his front teeth on a horizontal object such as the edge of a stall, bucket, or fence post, arching his neck, pulling back, and swallowing huge gulps of air, often accompanied by a grunting sound, is called _____.

39. _____ is the removal of the eyeball globe along with the adjacent connective, muscular, and glandular tissue.

40. The upper respiratory disease that affects a horse's upper airway and results in paralysis of the arytenoid cartilage is _____.

41. A condition of enlarged mucosal folds surrounding the epiglottis and narrowing the airways is called _____.

42. Entropion, commonly occurring as a birth defect, presents as a neonate's eyelid _____ _____.

35 Veterinary Dentistry

LEARNING OBJECTIVES

When you have completed this chapter, you will be able to:
1. Pronounce, spell, and define all key terms in this chapter.
2. Explain terminology used in veterinary dentistry to designate location and direction; describe the modified Triadan system for numbering teeth; and describe normal occlusion in dogs and cats, common malocclusions, and orthodontic treatment in small animals.
3. Discuss aspects of the complete medical history as they relate to veterinary dentistry and describe aspects of extraoral and intraoral examinations in dogs and cats.
4. Describe equipment and supplies used for dental radiography and understand the different angles used in dental radiography.
5. Differentiate between the stages of periodontal disease seen in dogs and cats, including gingivitis, and periodontitis, and state the goal of periodontal debridement.
6. Describe equipment and procedures for professional dental cleaning with power and hand scalers and explain methods for sharpening dental instruments.
7. Discuss the rationale and procedures for polishing teeth.
8. Compare and contrast regional nerve blocks for oral surgery for dogs and cats.
9. Explain the grading system for periodontal disease and the importance of home care in veterinary dentistry.
10. Discuss indications for restorative dentistry, endodontics, and exodontics.
11. Describe common dental conditions and pathology seen in small animals.
12. List and describe equine dental clinical practices and common problems and treatments.

Across

2 The tip of the tooth root
4 The study and treatment of the inside of the tooth and periapical tissues
7 The condition in which the mandible is abnormally short in relation to the maxilla
10 The area between the roots of a multirooted tooth
11 Tooth decay that results from demineralization of hard tooth structures by acid-producing oral bacteria
12 Term for mammals that have two sets of teeth (primary and deciduous)
15 The term used to indicate an upper jaw that is wider than the lower jaw (normal in most species)
18 Having a wide skull and a short maxilla
19 Light brown or yellow, raised, mineralized deposit adherent to the tooth and root surfaces
20 Anatomic term describing the attachment structures of the teeth.
21 Tooth structure that consists of nerves, blood vessels, lymphatics, and connective tissue
23 Tooth type that has a large reserve crown and root structure that allows for continued growth over an animal's lifetime
24 Diffuse inflammation of the entire oral cavity
25 Hard layer covering the surface of the root of a tooth

Down

1 Having a narrow skull and long maxilla
3 The extraction of diseased teeth
5 Gap between teeth seen normally in many species
6 Tooth type in which the crown is relatively small compared with the size of the well-developed roots
8 Inflammation of the gingiva
9 Thin layer covering the crown that is the hardest tooth substance
13 The most commonly used system of numbering teeth. (2 words)
14 Misalignment of the teeth or jaws
16 Having a well-proportioned skull width and maxillary length
17 Inflammation of the gingiva and other supporting tooth structures
22 A white-tan film that collects on teeth and is composed of bacteria, exfoliated cells, food debris, and saliva

EXERCISE 35.2 MATCHING #1: DENTAL MORPHOLOGY

Instructions: Match each definition in column A with its corresponding term in column B by writing the appropriate letter in the space provided.

Column A

1. _____ The most rostral teeth in cats and dogs; used for gnawing and grooming

2. _____ Having two sets of teeth

3. _____ The type of teeth seen in horses, rodents, and lagomorphs

4. _____ Large teeth found caudally to premolars

5. _____ Primary or "baby" teeth

6. _____ Spatial relationship of teeth within the mouth

7. _____ Adjective used to describe the largest shearing tooth of the upper and lower jaws in carnivores

8. _____ Smooth convex bulge located on the palatal side of the gingival third of incisor teeth

9. _____ Teeth used for prehending and holding

10. _____ Describe the adjacent or near-adjacent surfaces of teeth

Column B

A. Diphyodont

B. Canine

C. Carnassial

D. Molars

E. Deciduous

F. Cingulum

G. Mesial, distal

H. Incisors

I. Hypsodont

J. Occlusion

EXERCISE 35.3 MATCHING #2: TRIADAN NUMBERING SYSTEM

Instructions: Using the numeric Triadan system for tooth identification saves time when performing detailed dental charting. Match each canine or feline tooth listed with its corresponding Triadan number by writing the appropriate number in the space provided. (Refer to Figures 35.3 and 35.4 in the textbook for these numbers.) Not all teeth are present in a normal adult cat. Write "not present" if the tooth listed is not present in a normal adult cat.

1. _____ Canine left maxillary second incisor tooth

2. _____ Feline right mandibular third premolar tooth

3. _____ Canine left maxillary second molar tooth

4. _____ Canine right maxillary canine tooth

5. _____ Feline left mandibular second premolar tooth

6. _____ Feline right mandibular third incisor tooth

7. _____ Canine right maxillary fourth premolar tooth

8. _____ Feline right maxillary first premolar tooth

9. _____ Canine right mandibular third molar tooth

10. _____ Feline left mandibular fourth premolar tooth

11. _____ Canine deciduous right maxillary first incisor tooth

12. _____ Feline deciduous left mandibular canine tooth

EXERCISE 35.4 MATCHING #3: CLINICAL STAGES OF PERIODONTAL DISEASE

Instructions: Match each clinical description in column A with its corresponding grade of periodontal disease in column B by writing the appropriate letter in the space provided. (Note that responses may be used more than once.)

Column A

1. _____ Root debridement, gingival curettage, and periodontal surgery are often required

2. _____ Inflammatory changes are confined to the gingiva (gingivitis)

3. _____ Root debridement or subgingival curettage *may* be required

4. _____ Periodontitis where 50% or more of the attachment structures of the tooth have been lost

5. _____ Early form of periodontitis

6. _____ This grade is easily reversible with a routine dental cleaning

7. _____ Periodontitis where 25% to 50% of attachment structures of the tooth have been lost

8. _____ Early attachment loss is present

9. _____ Fair to guarded prognosis to save affected teeth

10. _____ Frequently, affected teeth cannot be saved

Column B

A. Grade I periodontal disease

B. Grade II periodontal disease

C. Grade III periodontal disease

D. Grade IV periodontal disease

EXERCISE 35.5 MATCHING #4: HOME DENTAL CARE BRUSHING TECHNIQUES

Instructions: Match each description in column A with its corresponding brushing technique in column B by writing the appropriate letter in the space provided. (Note that responses may be used more than once.)

Column A

1. _____ Toothbrush bristles are placed along the gingival margin and the sulcus

2. _____ A gentle sweeping motion of toothbrush bristles is directed apical to coronal

3. _____ Toothbrush bristles do not enter the sulcus

4. _____ The bristles are directed at a 45-degree angle toward the marginal gingiva

5. _____ Toothbrush bristles are placed apical to the gingival margin

6. _____ Toothbrush bristles enter the gingival sulcus

7. _____ A mesial to distal motion of brushing is employed

8. _____ Sometimes used in areas of periodontal surgery

Column B

A. Bass brushing technique

B. Modified Stillman brushing technique

EXERCISE 35.6 MATCHING #5: LOCAL ANESTHETIC AGENTS

Instructions: Match each characteristic in column A with its corresponding local anesthetic agent in column B by writing the appropriate letter in the space provided. (Note that responses may be used more than once.)

Column A

1. _____ Onset of effect in 6 to 10 minutes

2. _____ Onset of effect in 2 to 5 minutes

3. _____ Duration of action 0.5 to 2 hours

4. _____ Duration of action 4 to 8 hours

5. _____ Most commonly used local anesthetic in veterinary dentistry

Column B

A. Bupivacaine 0.5%

B. Lidocaine 2%

EXERCISE 35.7 MATCHING #6: DENTAL NERVE BLOCKS

Instructions: Match each description in column A with its corresponding dental nerve block in column B by writing the appropriate letter in the space provided. (Note that responses may be used more than once.)

Column A

1. _____ For this block, the needle is inserted perpendicular to the soft palate just caudal to the molar approximately ½ cm deep in cats and 1 cm deep in dogs.

2. _____ The foramen for this block is located dorsal to the roots of the maxillary third premolar.

3. _____ This block affects the sensation of the soft tissue and bone of the entire ipsilateral mandible.

4. _____ This block may cause numbness of the tongue and, therefore, self-inflicted trauma.

5. _____ The foramen for this block is located below the mesial root of the mandibular second premolar.

6. _____ The foramen for this block is located caudal and ventral to the mandibular third molar in the dog and the mandibular first molar in the cat.

7. _____ This block requires a needle that is bent 1 cm from the tip.

8. _____ This block is placed just caudal to the dog's maxillary second molar or the cat's maxillary first molar.

9. _____ This block helps prevent sensation to the ipsilateral mandible rostral to the labial frenulum.

10. _____ Lidocaine may be the preferred local anesthetic for this block.

11. _____ This block causes a loss of sensation rostral only to the third premolar on the ipsilateral maxilla.

12. _____ This block prevents sensation of the entire maxillary quadrant on the buccal and palatal sides of the teeth.

13. _____ This block has an intraoral and extraoral approach described.

Column B

A. Infraorbital nerve block

B. Middle mental nerve block

C. Inferior alveolar nerve block

D. Maxillary nerve block

Instructions: Answer the questions for each picture.

1. Identify this type of occlusion.

   _____

2. Identify this lesion in the dog.

   _____

3. Identify this lesion in the cat that is lateral to the palatoglossal folds (see arrows).

_____

4. Identify these instruments and their uses.

_____

_____

_____

_____

_____

_____

_____

_____

5. Identify this method of holding a dental instrument.

_____

6. Identify this instrument and describe its proper use.

_____

_____

_____

_____

_____

_____

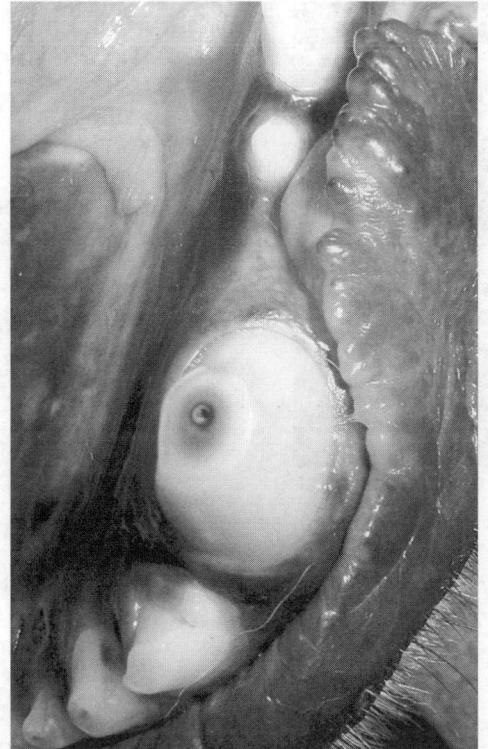

7. Identify this lesion. What instrument is used to confirm the diagnosis?

_____

_____

8. Based on this picture, what is the measurement of the gingival sulcus of this patient?

_____ mm

9. What accumulation is indicated by the asterisk in this picture? What subsequent formation is indicated by the arrows?

_____

_____

A   B

10. Which instrument (A or B) is better used for scaling the rostral portion of the mouth?

_____

_____

_____

11. Which patient is older: A or B? How do you know this from looking at the radiographs?

_____

_____

_____

12. Identify this malocclusion by class.

_____

13. Identify this malocclusion by class.

_____

14. Identify the two malocclusions present in this patient.

a. _____

b. _____

15. Describe this therapy and the most likely reason for its use.

    a. Therapy:_____

    b. Reason for its use:_____

16. Identify these instruments, their use, and the species in which they are used.

    a. Instruments:_____

    b. What they are used for:_____

    c. Species:_____

Instructions: Read the following statements and write "T" for true or "F" for false in the blanks provided. If a statement is false, correct the statement to make it true.

1. _____ Each dental or oral surgical procedure should begin with a comprehensive extraoral and intraoral examination.

2. _____ Alveolar mucosa refers to the mucosa that begins at the mucocutaneous junction and lines the cheeks and lips.

3. _____ When performing an intraoral examination, missing teeth should be documented on the dental chart by placing an "X" through the missing tooth.

4. _____ The normal gingival sulcus depth is 0 to 3 mm in dogs and 0 to 1 mm in cats.

5. _____ Probing depths greater than normal should be documented on the dental chart as pockets.

6. _____ Abrasion refers to the normal wear associated with a patient's tooth-to-tooth contact over time with normal mastication.

7. _____ During the periodontal examination of multirooted teeth, a bifurcation should be assessed from the buccal and lingual-palatal surfaces.

8. _____ Many dental X-ray units have an internally set level of kilovoltage and milliamperes, and only exposure time may be changed for a darker or lighter technique.

9. _____ Intraoral packaged film is the standard of the industry, used since the 1920s.

10. _____ To ensure good diagnostic quality, the dental sensor may be held in the patient's mouth, provided the handler wears appropriate protective gear.

11. _____ Direct-method computed digital radiography involves using an electronic intraoral sensor, a computer, and an X-ray machine to capture an image and convert it to a digital format of pixels.

12. _____ The epithelial attachment to the tooth crown forms the bottom of the gingival sulcus.

13. _____ Early in plaque formation, the bacterial population consists mainly of endotoxin-producing Gram-positive anaerobic rods and spirochetes.

14. _____ When performing a dental cleaning, the most important patient safety precaution is to intubate the patient and check to ensure that the endotracheal tube cuff is fully inflated.

15. _____ Standard-size universal and broad-tip ultrasonic scalers are designed to provide better access to subgingival pockets and furcation areas.

16. _____ The ultrasonic scaler tip should be directed at a 90-degree angle toward the tooth surface to avoid damaging the enamel.

17. _____ A curette with a straight shank in relation to the long axis of the handle is best suited for use on rostral teeth.

18. _____ If the face of a curette is offset at an angle of 60 to 70 degrees, as in Gracey curettes, the instrument is considered to be area-specific, and only one of the cutting edges may be adapted to the tooth.

19. _____ Sickle scalers are used to scale the crowns of teeth. Their sharp tip can cause lacerations if the instrument is used subgingivally.

20. ____ When sharpening hand instruments, the angle between the stone and the face should be no greater than 85 degrees.

21. ____ Sharpening stones typically used for dental instruments include Arkansas, India, ceramic, and a synthetic composition that differs in coarseness and the type of lubricant required to reduce heat friction.

22. ____ No restorative material is as strong as the original tooth structure.

23. ____ Indications for restorative dentistry include teeth with dental caries, fractured teeth, and endodontically treated teeth.

24. ____ As an animal ages, the pulp chamber and root canal become narrower as a result of the continued production of secondary dentin.

25. ____ Given radiation risks, dental radiographs are not strictly necessary when performing endodontic treatments.

26. ____ Exodontics involves relatively risk-free and straightforward procedures.

27. ____ Complicated tooth fractures can lead to the formation of a periapical abscess, facial swelling, and draining tracts.

28. ____ Complicated tooth fractures should be monitored for a period of time before endodontic or exodontic therapy is performed.

29. ____ Tooth root abscesses in the horse occur as a result of exposure of the pulp to the oral environment or death of the tooth.

30. ____ Horses do not get dental caries.

EXERCISE 35.10 MULTIPLE CHOICE: COMPREHENSIVE

Instructions: Circle the one correct answer to each of the following questions.

1. The radicular hypsodont type of dental morphology is found in which species?
   a. Rabbits
   b. Horses
   c. Cats
   d. Pigs

2. The "cheek teeth" in canines and felines are the
   a. canines and incisors.
   b. incisors and molars.
   c. premolars and canines.
   d. premolars and molars.

3. How many permanent teeth are there in the normal adult canine dentition?
   a. 32
   b. 36
   c. 42
   d. 44

4. At what age would a cat be expected to have all of its permanent teeth erupted?
   a. 6 months
   b. 8 months
   c. 10 months
   d. 12 months

5. Which clinical symptoms of oral disease may manifest later in the disease process?
   a. Rubbing the face along furniture
   b. Anorexia
   c. Dropping food
   d. Pawing at the mouth

6. The only easily palpable major salivary gland of the dog and cat is the
   a. sublingual.
   b. parotid.
   c. zygomatic.
   d. mandibular.

7. Which tissue would not be considered part of the periodontium?
   a. Alveolar bone
   b. Gingival connective tissue
   c. Dentin
   d. Cementum

8. The instrument used to measure gingival sulcus depth is a periodontal
   a. explorer.
   b. curette.
   c. probe.
   d. scaler.

9. When performing dental radiographs, which technique is most useful for obtaining images of the mandibular teeth caudal to the mandibular 4th premolar?
   a. Bisecting angle technique
   b. Occlusal technique
   c. Paralleling technique
   d. Cone-cutting technique

10. Which anatomic structure would be the most radiopaque on a dental radiograph?
    a. Cementum
    b Enamel
    c. Dentin
    d. Lamina dura

11. Once plaque has formed on a tooth, how long does it take to mineralize if left undisturbed?
    a. 1 day
    b. 3 days
    c. 7 days
    d. 2 weeks

12. For operator safety, what is the appropriate protective equipment that should be worn during a dental cleaning procedure?
    a. Scrub top, mask, gloves
    b. Cap, eye protection, gloves
    c. Mask, eye protection, gloves, gown
    d. Gown, eye protection, gloves

13. Intrinsic staining of the teeth that is often seen on the occlusal surface of maxillary molars in dogs would not be caused by
    a. trauma.
    b. tetracycline antibiotics during tooth development.
    c. food pigments.
    d. developmental defects.

14. According to the Mobility Scoring Index, how would a patient's tooth be classified if mobility were increased in any direction other than axial over a distance of more than 0.5 mm and up to 1.0 mm?
    a. Stage 0 (M0)
    b. Stage 1 (M1)
    c. Stage 2 (M2)
    d. Stage 3 (M3)

15. Which form of local anesthetic delivery is most commonly used in veterinary dentistry?
    a. Splash block
    b. Local infiltration
    c. Regional anesthesia
    d. Both B and C

16. Which of the following is an example of regional anesthesia?
    a. Placing bupivacaine in an open wound to provide topical anesthesia
    b. Placing lidocaine at the foramen of the infraorbital nerve
    c. Placing bupivacaine into the periodontal ligament of the left maxillary fourth premolar
    d. Placing lidocaine into the periodontal ligament of the right mandibular first molar

17. Which of the following is not a reason that bupivacaine 0.5% is commonly used in veterinary dentistry?
    a. Long duration of action
    b. Intraoperative pain management
    c. Postoperative pain relief
    d. Beneficial synergistic effect with lidocaine

18. What is the maximum safe dose for bupivacaine, 0.5% for the dog?
    a. 1 mg/kg
    b. 1.5 mg/kg
    c. 2 mg/kg
    d. 3 mg/kg

19. What is the maximum safe dose for bupivacaine, 0.5% for the cat?
    a. 1 mg/kg
    b. 1.5 mg/kg
    c. 2 mg/kg
    d. 3 mg/kg

20. Which grade of periodontal disease often requires tooth extraction?
    a. I
    b. II
    c. III
    d. IV

21. What is the minimum depth of a periodontal pocket where doxycycline can be placed?
    a. 3 mm
    b. 4 mm
    c. 6 mm
    d. 7 mm

22. What is not a reason why doxycycline gel is the drug of choice for the treatment of periodontal pockets?
    a. It has a good antimicrobial spectrum against periodontal pathogens.
    b. It has anti-inflammatory effects.
    c. It has a space-occupying effect, which prevents food and debris from filling the pocket.
    d. It has never been indicated in allergic reactions in cats or dogs.

23. What is recommended as an antibacterial oral rinse when treating periodontal disease?
    a. 0.12% chlorhexidine
    b. 1.2% chlorhexidine
    c. 0.2% chlorhexidine
    d. 2% chlorhexidine

24. Attempts to save teeth with advanced periodontal surgery should not be performed unless the client is able to
    a. apply a 2% chlorhexidine rinse.
    b. consent to doxycycline gel therapy.
    c. perform daily tooth brushing.
    d. provide a soft-food diet for the rest of the patient's life.

25. Why is human toothpaste not used for tooth brushing in veterinary patients?
    a. They cause gingival ulceration.
    b. The mint flavoring is toxic.
    c. They can cause stomach upset if swallowed.
    d. Both B and C

26. Which type of diet is best to help control plaque?
    a. A diet that has been manufactured and tested to reduce plaque accumulation.
    b. Any diet of hard foods is appropriate.
    c. Soft diets are best in order to avoid gingival trauma from hard abrasive foods.
    d. All veterinary diets now provide plaque control.

27. Which organization has been established to recognize products that have been shown to meet predetermined standards of plaque and calculus retardation?
    a. The Veterinary Oral Health Council (VOHC)
    b. The American Veterinary Medical Association (AVMA)
    c. The American Veterinary Dental College (AVDC)
    d. The Food and Drug Administration (FDA)

28. How do mechanical cleansing diets help prevent plaque and tartar accumulation?
    a. Long fibers oriented in one direction within a large kibble are designed to scrape the side of the teeth as the teeth penetrate the kibble.
    b. Crisscrossed fibers oriented in a large kibble are designed to scrape the side of the teeth as the teeth penetrate the kibble.
    c. Small particles of digestible vegetable carbohydrate are placed in the large kibble designed to scrape the side of the teeth as the teeth penetrate the kibble.
    d. Microscopic particles of inert silica are placed in the large kibble designed to scrape the side of the teeth as the teeth penetrate the kibble.

29. What is the function of hexametaphosphate (HMP) in a chemical cleansing diet that helps prevent plaque and tartar accumulation?
    a. HMP decreases the production of saliva, which contains the minerals associated with tartar accumulation.
    b. HMP sequesters calcium in plaque fluids effectively preventing the mineralization of plaque.
    c. HMP binds with magnesium in order to decrease mineral deposition in plaque.
    d. HMP generates a thermal response in the oral cavity, effectively killing plaque-forming organisms.

30. Which of the following chew toys has no potential for harmful effects when used to help prevent plaque and tartar accumulation?
    a. Rawhide chews
    b. Cow hooves
    c. Hard nylon bones
    d. All of the choices listed above have some potentially harmful effects.

31. Which of the following is not an indication for restorative dentistry?
    a. Dental caries
    b. Fractured teeth
    c. Stained occlusal surfaces
    d. Endodontically treated teeth

32. Which is not a factor when considering treatment options for teeth with endodontic disease?
    a. Age
    b. Gender
    c. Duration of endodontic disease
    d. Tooth anatomy

33. On which teeth of the dog are crowns more commonly placed?
    a. Canines and mandibular first molars
    b. Maxillary fourth premolars and mandibular first molars
    c. Canines and maxillary fourth premolars
    d. Canines and maxillary first molars

439

34. What is the minimum age at which conventional root canal therapy is usually performed on dogs and cats?
    a. 6 months of age
    b. 12 months of age
    c. 15 months of age
    d. 18 months of age

35. What does the term CUPS refer to?
    a. Chronic ulcerative papillary sepsis
    b. Chronic ulcerative paradental stomatitis
    c. Caustic ulcerative papillary stomatitis
    d. Canine upper premolar syndrome

36. Which of the following is not an indication for exodontics?
    a. A grave prognosis for saving a tooth
    b. Owner financial constraints that preclude the use of salvage techniques
    c. Multiple anesthetic episodes are contraindicated
    d. Aggressive biting behavior

37. What is recommended as a lavage solution once exodontia is performed?
    a. Sodium hypochlorite
    b. Isotonic saline
    c. 0.12% chlorhexidine solution
    d. Both B and C

38. What is the suture type and pattern recommended to close an exodontic area?
    a. 4.0 or 5.0 absorbable braided in a simple interrupted pattern
    b. 4.0 or 5.0 absorbable monofilament in a simple interrupted pattern
    c. 4.0 or 5.0 nonabsorbable monofilament in a simple continuous pattern
    d. 4.0 or 5.0 nonabsorbable braided in a simple continuous pattern

39. In what location are feline resorptive lesions usually seen clinically?
    a. Cervical (neck) region
    b. Apex of the root
    c. Occlusal surface of the crown
    d. All locations are equally seen

40. What is the treatment of choice for cats with tooth resorption?
    a. Deep root planing followed by fluoride gel
    b. Root canal followed by crown restoration with glass ionomer
    c. Exodontics
    d. Nothing, because cats rarely have clinical signs with tooth resorption

41. Which of the following is not an example of a class I malocclusion?
    a. The mandible is relatively shorter than the maxilla.
    b. The mandibular canines are lingually displaced.
    c. The maxillary incisors are positioned lingual to the mandibular incisors.
    d. A maxillary premolar is positioned lingual to the opposing mandibular premolar.

42. Mandibular brachygnathism (mandibular distoclusion) belongs to which class of malocclusion?
    a. I
    b. II
    c. III
    d. IV

43. Mandibular prognathism (mandibular mesioclusion) belongs to which class of malocclusion?
    a. I
    b. II
    c. III
    d. IV

44. Dolichocephalic skull types are typical of
    a. Persian cats.
    b. Labrador retrievers.
    c. greyhounds.
    d. boxers.

45. Which of the following is not true for dental impressions?
    a. Dental impressions are important in the treatment plan for orthodontic disease.
    b. Alginate is the material used to fill the dental impression tray.
    c. Dental stone is used to fill the impression to create a positive image of the mouth.
    d. Dental impressions should be taken during every annual veterinary visit.

46. Which dog breed is more likely to experience persistent deciduous teeth?
    a. Cavalier King Charles Spaniel
    b. Border collie
    c. Doberman pinscher
    d. Yorkshire terrier

47. Discolored teeth in the dog are commonly a result of which disease or condition?
    a. Canine distemper
    b. Pulpitis (pulp necrosis)
    c. Periodontal disease
    d. Class IV malocclusion

48. Stomatitis, seen most commonly as lymphocytic-plasmacytic stomatitis in cats, has what cause?
    a. Immune-mediated
    b. Uremia
    c. Viral disease
    d. Foreign-body reaction

49. What therapy resovles stomatitis in approximately 80% of cases in cats?
    a. Doxycycline at 2 mg/kg for 14 days
    b. Dental cleanings every 3 months
    c. Full mouth or nearly full mouth extractions
    d. Crown restorations

50. What is the cause of masticatory myositis?
    a. Viral infection of the muscle of mastication
    b. Antibody formation toward a specific component of myosin found only in the muscles of mastication
    c. A caustic reaction to a 2% chlorhexidine oral rinse
    d. Periapical abscess formation from an untreated, complicated fracture of the maxillary fourth premolar

51. What is the definitive method of diagnosis for masticatory myositis?
    a. Serum and muscle tissue analysis
    b. Viral isolation with electron microscopy
    c. History of inappropriate use of chlorhexidine with cytology of oral mucosa
    d. Internal oral examination and dental radiography of the maxillary fourth premolar

52. What is the usual treatment of choice for masticatory myositis?
    a. Saline rinses of the oral cavity twice daily for 2 weeks
    b. Acyclovir orally once daily for 1 month
    c. Endodontic or exodontic treatment of the maxillary fourth premolar fracture
    d. An immunosuppressive dose of steroids tapered to a maintenance dose

53. What is one of the most common types of jaw fracture in the dog and cat?
    a. Temporomandibular disarticulation
    b. Ramus fracture
    c. Symphyseal separation of the mandible
    d. Fracture of the angle of the mandible

54. Attrition refers to wear
    a. due to chewing inappropriately.
    b. from teeth contacting teeth.
    c. from chewing at hair.
    d. from chewing on metal.

55. What is the purpose of the varied grooves and ridges on the occlusal surfaces of the premolars and molars in the horse?
    a. Determination of age
    b. Grinding of food
    c. Defense against predators
    d. Prehension of food

56. In which teeth is cemental hypoplasia known to occur in horses?
    a. All teeth
    b. Premolars
    c. Incisors
    d. First molars

57. What is the most accurate method of determining a horse's age based on its dentition?
    a. Gracey groove
    b. Dental star
    c. Eruption times
    d. Galvayne groove

58. What is the term used to describe the process of mechanically adjusting the occlusal surface of horse teeth by removing raised areas?
    a. Floating
    b. Bishoping
    c. Curettage
    d. Sailing

59. What is not one of the clinical signs associated with a wry nose in the horse?
    a. Difficulty suckling
    b. Difficulty prehending food
    c. Severe dyspnea
    d. Head shaking, rubbing, and tilting

60. What is the mechanism by which horses' teeth are kept clean?
    a. Daily brushing
    b. Placement of HMP in drinking water
    c. Normal mastication of abrasive substances
    d. All of the above

EXERCISE 35.11 FILL-IN-THE-BLANK: COMPREHENSIVE

Instructions: Fill in each of the spaces provided with the missing word or words that complete the sentence.

1. Because of the variation in severity of disease at the time of treatment, the term dental prophylaxis is largely being replaced with the term _____.

2. Members of the _____ are technicians who have completed a credentialing process and passed a specialty examination to verify an advanced level of dental knowledge.

3. The root apices of _____ teeth are open for a limited time during tooth eruption and development and therefore do not continually grow or erupt.

4. Another term meaning aradicular hypsodont is _____.

5. The adjective _____ is used to describe the maxillary fourth premolar and mandibular first molar of dogs and cats, which play a significant role in shearing food during mastication.

6. A history of sneezing after drinking water may indicate the presence of a(n) _____, which is a common problem in small-breed dogs with advanced periodontal disease.

7. An important component of the extraoral examination is a technique called _____, which involves gently pushing on the closed eyelids with your thumbs to assess the ability of the globes to move caudally in the orbit.

8. The _____ is a raised structure located on the midline behind the maxillary incisors of dogs and cats.

9. The rostral two-thirds of the hard palate is covered by palatal mucosa that has hard ridges, called _____, ranging from 8 to 10 in number.

10. Radiographic evaluation of areas that have missing teeth is imperative because _____ can develop as a result of an unerupted tooth.

11. Dental instruments are held with a(n) _____, in which the first three fingers are in a triangular position on the instrument, and the ring finger is used as a rest on an adjacent oral structure.

12. The _____ is a cribriform plate of bone lining the tooth socket and appears radiographically as a white line adjacent to the periodontal space.

13. The term _____ more truly describes the periodontal health of a tooth because it accounts for both pocket depth and gingival recession.

14. _____ occurs when the dental X-ray beam misses portions of the sensor, plate, or film, resulting in areas without image.

15. Inaccurate vertical angulation of the x-ray beam causes the resultant image to appear shortened, which is termed _____, or lengthened, which is termed _____.

16. The _____ is composed of strong fibers that connect the tooth to alveolar bone.

17. A normal anatomic structure called the _____ is located apical to the mandibular second premolar in dogs and can be misinterpreted as periapical pathology when superimposed over a tooth root.

18. The term _____ refers to the use of nonsurgical instrumentation to remove hard and soft deposits from all tooth surfaces, along with the disruption of nonadherent bacteria within the gingival sulcus.

19. In today's veterinary practices, _____ are the instruments primarily used for routine debridement and advanced periodontal therapy.

20. The portion of an ultrasonic scaler handpiece that converts electrical energy into mechanical energy is called the _____.

21. In general, dental hand instruments consist of three parts: (1) the _____, (2) the _____, and (3) the _____.

22. Designed for subgingival scaling and root planing, a(n) _____ has two cutting edges and can be adapted for all surfaces of the teeth.

23. Three benefits of nerve blocks in veterinary dentistry are _____ analgesia, _____ analgesia, and a decreased concentration of _____ agents.

24. One should aspirate prior to injecting local analgesic when performing a dental nerve block to ensure that the needle is not in a(n) _____ _____.

25. A(n) _____ -gauge needle is most commonly used for dental nerve blocks.

26. _____ materials are those that do not induce new bone but act as a scaffold to allow existing bone cells to fill the defect.

27. _____ materials are those that will induce new bone growth by stimulating osteoblast precursors to form.

28. The three basic categories of home dental care intended to reduce oral bacteria are _____, _____, and use of _____.

29. Of the three basic categories of home dental care listed previously, _____ provides the most thorough method of plaque control for pets.

30. _____ is the facial morphology in which the upper jaw is wider than the lower jaw.

31. A(n) _____ refers to wound irrigation directly into an open incision, providing topical anesthesia.

32. _____ refers to the infiltration of local anesthetic along planned incision lines or into the periodontal ligament of a tooth of interest.

33. The _____ toothbrushing technique is sometimes used in areas of periodontal surgery to minimize plaque accumulation while preventing trauma to the reattaching gingival tissue.

34. During endodontic therapy, _____ is defined as filling the canal with material that will seal it from the periapical area.

35. When sharpening hand instruments, the angle between the stone and the face should be approximately _____ degrees.

36. The veterinary technician's role in oral surgery is to have the proper equipment ready, place the regional _____, take pre- and post-surgical _____, retract tissue, and assist in hemostasis.

37. When significant periodontal disease exists, an iatrogenic jaw fracture more easily occurs when extracting the _____ mandibular molar and the mandibular _____ in cats and small-breed dogs.

38. When performing exodontia, the handle of the dental elevator should rest securely in the palm of the hand, and the _____ is placed at the tip of the dental elevator to prevent inadvertent advancement of the tip into deeper structures.

39. _____ extraction is a type of tooth extraction that uses dental elevators placed in the periodontal space on the mesial or distal surface of the crown to fatigue the periodontal ligament.

40. _____ extraction is a type of tooth extraction in which a gingival flap is created, and then a window is created in the buccal bone over the tooth to be extracted.

41. The most commonly used numbering system for dentition is the _____.

42. The _____ is the animal species that is most commonly affected with tooth resorption.

43. There are _____ classes of malocclusion.

44. Class _____ malocclusion is the most common type receiving orthodontic correction in pets.

45. _____ is a nonspecific term for a form of unilateral maxillary-mandibular asymmetry.

46. _____ is the term used to describe the extraction of persistent deciduous or adult teeth that are problematic because of malocclusion.

47. Mandibular permanent canines erupt _____ in relationship to the persistent deciduous teeth, whereas maxillary permanent canines erupt _____ in relationship to the persistent deciduous teeth.

48. The best time to remove persistent deciduous teeth is before they cause _____ of their permanent counterparts.

49. The three typical types of dental trauma in dogs and cats are _____, a(n) _____ tooth fracture (in which there is no pulp exposure), and a(n) _____ tooth fracture (in which there is pulp exposure).

50. The most common oral tumor in the cat is _____.

51. The most common benign oral tumor in the dog is a(n) _____.

52. The four common malignant oral tumors in the dog are malignant _____, _____, _____, and _____.

53. A(n) _____ muzzle may be the treatment of choice in young animals with jaw fractures.

54. "Wolf teeth" is a term used to describe the permanent _____ in the horse and are more commonly seen in the _____ arcade.

55. The premolars and molars in the horse are collectively known as _____.

56. A common term for mandibular brachygnathism in horses is _____.

57. Sinusitis and chronic unilateral nasal discharge related to dental disease in the horse usually affect the maxillary fourth _____; the first, second, and third _____ teeth; and the _____ sinus.

58. Extraoral exodontia is usually performed on the _____ teeth in the horse.

59. _____ is the term for deviation of the incisive bone, maxilla, and nasal septum laterally from the midline in the foal.

EXERCISE 35.12 CASE STUDY: PROFESSIONAL DENTAL CLEANING

You have just been hired as a veterinary technician in a small animal practice that emphasizes quality dental care. On your first day on the job, you are directed to the dental suite and asked to perform a professional dental cleaning on a 9-year-old, neutered male Toy Poodle. Wanting to make a good impression by providing excellent care to your patient, you mentally review the procedure. Respond to each of the following queries about professional dental cleaning.

1. Power scaling instruments use a water-cooled vibrating tip to remove hard and soft deposits from the teeth and periodontal pockets.

   a. Explain how the vibrations of power scalers are measured.

   _____

   _____

   b. Briefly describe the two types of power scalers and how each operates.

   i. _____

   _____

   _____

   ii. _____

   _____

   _____

   c. Explain the disadvantages of using a sonic scaler.

   _____

   _____

2. The ultrasonic scaling unit contains an electronic generator inside a plastic housing connected to a foot pedal by a cable. The handpiece is also connected to a water supply by tubing to provide a water stream from the ultrasonic scaler tip.

a. List the benefits of the water stream that comes from the ultrasonic scaler tip.

_____

_____

_____

_____

_____

b. Identify the patient and human safety precautions that should be taken to reduce the amount of aerosolized bacteria caused by the ultrasonic scaler's water mist.

_____

_____

_____

_____

c. How should the patient's eyes be protected during ultrasonic scaling?

_____

_____

d. Why is it important to intubate the patient and ensure that the endotracheal cuff is fully inflated prior to ultrasonic scaling?

_____

_____

3. The magnetostrictive scaler is the most common type of power scaler used in human and veterinary dentistry. Describe how the tip of a magnetostrictive scaler functions and how the tip should be properly used on tooth surfaces.

_____

_____

_____

_____

_____

_____

4. The power and water knobs of magnetostrictive units must be properly adjusted prior to the periodontal debridement procedure.

a. What does the power knob do?

_____

_____

_____

b. When should the high-power versus low-power setting be used?

_____

_____

_____

c. Why is it necessary to have adequate water flow through the ultrasonic scaler handpiece?

_____

_____

_____

5. Describe the proper technique required for removing dental calculus using a supragingival hand scaler.

_____

_____

_____

_____

_____

6. Angulation refers to the relationship of the face of a hand scaling instrument to the tooth. Explain proper curette angulation and the technique for removal of dental deposits from the gingival sulcus.

_____

_____

_____

_____

_____

_____

7. Polishing is the final but critical step performed on a dental patient as part of routine cleaning or advanced periodontal therapy.

a. Explain the rationale for dental polishing.

_____

_____

_____

b. Describe proper polishing technique when using a motor-driven handpiece and rubber cup, including desired polishing paste, cup pressure, speed setting, and polishing time per tooth surface.

_____

_____

_____

_____

_____

_____

_____

_____

c. After polishing, what is the final step that should be performed to finish the complete dental cleaning procedure?

_____

_____

_____

36 Geriatric and Hospice Care: Supporting the Aged and Dying Patient

When you have completed this chapter, you will be able to:

1. Pronounce, define, and spell all key terms in the chapter.
2. Discuss the aging process and explain when dogs and cats are geriatric.
3. Identify and explain changes seen in various body systems as dogs and cats age.
4. Identify cognitive impairment and how it might influence geriatric pet behavior.
5. Discuss the management of quality of life as pets age.
6. Discuss what is involved in a geriatric wellness program.
7. Explain hospice and palliative care, including pain management and physical rehabilitation for the geriatric patient.
8. Explain the nursing care of the geriatric patient, including hydration, assisted nutrition, bladder and fecal hygiene, and mobility assistance.
9. Discuss companion animal death and dying.
10. Explain the changing nutritional needs of aging pets.
11. Discuss components of hospice nursing care for geriatric dogs and cats, including identifying the appropriate time to discuss euthanasia with a pet's owner.
12. Discuss components of the physical examination of a geriatric horse.
13. List and describe disorders commonly seen in geriatric horses, including oral/nasal, vision, cardiac, respiratory, gastrointestinal, kidney, skin, neurologic, and orthopedic problems.
14. Identify and explain the chronic conditions that most commonly affect geriatric horses, such as pituitary pars intermedia dysfunction (PPID), equine odontoclastic tooth resorption and hypercementosis (EOTRH), heaves, laminitis, dental problems, sinusitis, equine recurrent uveitis (ERU), and neurologic and musculoskeletal defects.
15. Discuss geriatric horses' management, nutrition, and nursing care, including end-of-life issues.

EXERCISE 36.1 DEFINITIONS: TERMS AND DEFINITIONS

Instructions: Define each term in your own words.

1. Laminitis:_____

   _____

2. Geriatric:_____

   _____

3. Hirsutism:_____

   _____

4. Hospice:_____

   _____

5. Incontinence:_____

_____

6. Senescence:_____

_____

7. Wave mouth:_____

_____

8. Sarcopenia:_____

9. Frailty:_____

10. Cachexia:_____

EXERCISE 36.2 MATCHING: EQUINE RECURRENT UVEITIS (ERU)

Instructions: Match the term in column A with its corresponding description in column B by writing the appropriate letter in the space provided.

Column A

1. _____ Corneal edema

2. _____ Hyphema

3. _____ Fungal ulcers

4. _____ Enucleation

5. _____ Hypopyon

6. _____ Neovascularization

7. _____ Subpalpebral lavage system

8. _____ Anterior uveitis

Column B

A. Removal of an eye

B. Cellular debris in the eye

C. Blood vessel growth on the cornea

D. Bluish-white tint to the cornea

E. A difficult-to-treat condition requiring medications several times a day

F. Inflammation in the front chamber of the eye

G. A device placed for ease of treatment of ERU

H. Hemorrhage in the eye

EXERCISE 36.3 TRUE OR FALSE: COMPREHENSIVE

Instructions: Read the following statements and write "T" for true or "F" for false in the blanks provided. If a statement is false, correct the statement to make it true.

1. _____ Cognitive dysfunction is a neurodegenerative disorder seen in senior dogs and cats characterized by rapid cognitive decline over a short period.

2. _____ The speed with which the aging process occurs in animals varies according to the size and breed.

3. _____ Aging is considered a disease process.

4. _____ The client's capacity to care for their pet is an important consideration in developing the treatment plan, since it relies on their active involvement.

5. _____ It is imperative that both euthanasia and natural (unassisted) death not be discussed too soon after the caregiver/hospice-provider relationship has been established.

6. _____ Mouth size is a significant risk factor for periodontal disease in dogs.

7. _____ It is recommended that dogs and cats in the last 25% of their predicted life span have routine healthcare visits, including a minimum laboratory database, every 6 months.

8. _____ It is notoriously difficult to maintain weight and body condition in older horses.

9. _____ The most common initial sign of EOTRH reported by horse owners is lengthening teeth with sharp areas.

10. _____ When managing pain in the geriatric patient, a preemptive, multimodal approach should be implemented.

11. _____ Older patients often have subclinical diseases that affect their nutritional status and health.

12. _____ Two common neurologic diseases of older cats are degenerative myelopathy (DM) and intervertebral disc disease (IVDD).

13. _____ Chronic renal failure is common in aging cats, with up to 75% of cats >12 years of age affected.

14. _____ Heaves in horses is often related to a dust or mold allergy.

15. _____ In a horse with heaves, wheezes will be heard on both sides of the chest, especially during inhalation.

16. _____ In an aged horse, laminitis usually develops as a secondary condition to a pre-existing problem.

17. _____ Eye pain and swelling in an aged horse requires treatment but is usually not serious.

18. _____ Geriatric horses often develop degenerative joint disease in the coxofemoral joints, stifles, and lumbar vertebrae.

19. _____ Decreased skin elasticity and brittle claws have been noted in apparently healthy older cats.

20. _____ Small, medium, and large dogs are classified as senior at 9 years of age.

21. _____ A giant-breed dog ages more rapidly than a small-breed dog or a cat.

22. _____ In general, a dog needs more energy from food as it ages.

23. _____ Palliative care is specialized medical care for animals with serious illnesses.

24. _____ A 14-lb, 6-year-old dog is the equivalent age of a 52-year-old human.

25. _____ Aortic saddle thrombus is believed to cause moderate pain in animals.

26. _____ Owner education is a critical role of the veterinary technician or nurse working with horses at risk of laminitis.

27. _____ Rehabilitation is often capable of halting the loss of muscle mass that occurs in geriatric patients, but it cannot reverse it.

28. _____Castrated dogs live longer on average than those that are not castrated.

29. _____Mix breed dogs have a shorter life expectancy than purebred dogs.

30. _____Clinical Metrology Instruments for dogs and cats help clients identify pain and functional limitations.

31. Testing for PPID is different for early, moderate, and advanced stages.

451

Instructions: Circle the one correct answer to each of the following questions.

1. The most common central nervous system tumor in older pets is
   a. lymphosarcoma.
   b. glioma.
   c. oligodendroglioma.
   d. meningioma.

2. A Great Dane that is 8 years of age is considered to be a
   a. young adult.
   b. mature adult.
   c. senior.
   d. geriatric.

3. Which of the following is not a change you would expect to see in an aging patient?
   a. Decreased skin elasticity
   b. Decreased ability to combat infection
   c. Decreased cardiac output
   d. Decreased calculus accumulation

4. Which of the following is not a change you would expect to see in an aging patient?
   a. Decreased percentage of body fat
   b. Urinary incontinence
   c. Loss of muscle mass
   d. Thickened footpads in dogs

5. Which of the following is not a core competency of the veterinary hospice nurse role?
   a. Medical caregiver
   b. Educator
   c. Mediator
   d. Advocate

6. Medical conditions appropriate for hospice or palliative care include all of the following except
   a. terminal diagnosis.
   b. progressive, undiagnosed disease.
   c. acute disability.
   d. terminal geriatric status.

7. The "A" in the acronym DISHA stands for
   a. avoiding interactions.
   b. alertness diminished.
   c. altered mental status.
   d. activity changes.

8. Cachexia is characterized by all of the following except
   a. weakness.
   b. anorexia.
   c. weight gain.
   d. perceived poor quality of life.

9. The geriatric wellness exam should include all of the following except
   a. a hearing test.
   b. abdominal and rectal palpation.
   c. a full orthopedic examination.
   d. assessment of the cardiopulmonary system.

10. The most important goal of palliative care and hospice is to help patients achieve
    a. longevity.
    b. good quality of life.
    c. improved renal functioning.
    d. the restoration of health.

11. A geriatric horse with a long, wavy hair coat that does not shed completely in the spring is likely to have
    a. hypothyroidism.
    b. laminitis.
    c. PPID.
    d. heaves.

12. The most common abnormal heart rhythm in geriatric horses is
    a. ventricular tachycardia.
    b. first-degree AV heart block.
    c. sinus arrhythmia.
    d. atrial fibrillation.

13. The development of hypertrophied external abdominal oblique muscles as a result of increased effort on exhalation is typically seen in horses with
    a. recurrent airway obstruction.
    b. sinusitis.
    c. chronic heaves.
    d. laryngeal paralysis.

14. Pituitary pars intermedia dysfunction (PPID) was formerly known as
    a. recurrent airway obstruction.
    b. equine recurrent uveitis.
    c. equine Cushing disease.
    d. hirsutism.

15. The reluctance of a horse to touch its nose to its shoulder is generally indicative of pain affecting the
    a. nose.
    b. neck.
    c. jaw.
    d. shoulder.

16. The signs of PPID in horses include hirsutism, abnormal sweating, polyuria, polydipsia, and
    a. weight loss.
    b. laminitis.
    c. muscle hypertrophy.
    d. hyperactivity.

17. An important aspect of treatment for horses with heaves is
    a. minimizing contact with allergens.
    b. bronchoalveolar lavage.
    c. ultrasound of the thoracic cavity.
    d. regular use of an inhaler.

18. Which type of feeding tube does not require anesthesia for placement?
    a. Esophageal
    b. Jejunostomy
    c. Nasoesophageal
    d. Gastrostomy

19. Which of the following is typically not an underlying cause of acute or chronic weight loss in the geriatric horse?
    a. Tooth loss
    b. Inability of the GI tract to absorb nutrients
    c. Neoplasia
    d. ERU

20. A geriatric horse that lives in a barn with poor air circulation, has a history of allergic reactions, and exhibits tachypnea and dyspnea may be exhibiting signs of
    a. laminitis.
    b. heaves.
    c. sinusitis.
    d. DJD.

21. Pretreatment with a(n) _____ is recommended in horses with a history of vaccine reactions.
    a. steroid
    b. bronchodilator
    c. NSAID
    d. antibiotic

22. All of the following are considered rehabilitative therapies except
    a. laser therapy.
    b. acupuncture.
    c. pulsed electromagnetic field therapy.
    d. subpalpebral lavage.

EXERCISE 36.5 FILL-IN-THE BLANK: COMPREHENSIVE

Instructions: Fill in each of the spaces provided with the missing word or words that complete the sentence.

1. Many veterinarians recommend that healthy geriatric small animals (those over _____ years of age) should be examined _____ time(s) a year.

2. Physiologic changes that occur in dogs and cats as they age are categorized as changes in _____, _____, and _____.

3. Considerations for equine euthanasia are often multifactorial but are usually related to failures in either the _____ system or the _____ system.

4. When the healthcare team, working in collaboration with the pet owner, successfully addresses the patient's physical, social, and _____ needs, they are best able to maximize comfort and minimize suffering.

5. Recumbent patients require soft bedding, impeccable hygiene, and _____ to avoid complications such as bed sores, muscle stiffness, and atelectasis.

6. In emaciated or geriatric patients, when compatible history and physical examination findings are present, it is reasonable to assume 7% _____ and treat accordingly.

7. The position for bladder expression may vary from patient to patient. For instance, the bladder can usually be expressed when a patient is in _____ recumbency or when it is _____.

8. Aged horses are generally considered to be those older than _____ years.

9. A systolic murmur auscultated on the left side of the equine thorax suggests a common valvular disease of the geriatric horse known as _____.

10. Common tumors in horses include squamous cell carcinomas, which often develop on the _____, and melanomas, which often develop around the _____ area.

11. PPID in horses causes a collection of clinical signs resulting from chronic high blood _____ levels.

12. PPID in horses is treated with the dopamine agonist _____.

13. To maintain health and keep the horse comfortable, a geriatric horse should have its hooves trimmed every _____ weeks and dental floating every _____ months.

14. Dogs that weigh _____ more than their ideal body weight are generally classified as overweight, while those that weigh _____ more than their ideal body weight are classified as obese.

15. The most common behavioral changes in old cats are grouped under the acronym _____, which stands for _____.

16. Animals fully change bone content every _____ years.

EXERCISE 36.6 SHORT ANSWER: COMPREHENSIVE

Instructions: Provide a short answer to each of the following questions in the space provided.

1. Discuss ways to improve access to food and water for elderly dogs and cats.

_____

_____

_____

_____

_____

_____

_____

_____

2. Discuss ways to increase comfort in sleeping areas for elderly dogs and cats.

_____

_____

_____

_____

_____

_____

_____

_____

3. Discuss ways to help animals with severe cognitive dysfunction or anxiety function optimally within their environments.

_____

_____

_____

_____

_____

_____

_____

_____

_____

4. What are the three categories of the major physical and functional changes associated with aging in animals? Give examples of each.

a. _____

   _____

   _____

   _____

   _____

b. _____

   _____

   _____

   _____

   _____

c. _____

   _____

   _____

   _____

5. Discuss the importance of and activities associated with bladder and fecal hygiene maintenance in pets approaching the end of life.

   _____

   _____

   _____

   _____

   _____

   _____

6. Aging horses can develop one of a number of chronic diseases. For each chronic disease of the aged equine patient under Disease Condition, indicate the part of the body it affects and several common clinical signs associated with the condition, focusing on those that occur most frequently.

Disease Condition	Part of the Body Affected by This Condition	Clinical Signs of This Condition
PPID		
Heaves		
Acute laminitis		
Wave mouth		
Chronic sinusitis		
Equine recurrent uveitis		
Neurologic deficits		

7. Due to inadequate caloric intake, geriatric horses with poor body condition may require dietary changes or supplementation. What specific dietary changes can be employed to maintain body weight in these patients?

_____

_____

_____

_____

_____

_____

_____

8. Discuss how the World Health Organization's definition of Quality of Life is applied to animals.

_____

_____

_____

9. Detail the ten steps to make a geriatric health care program successful.

37 The Human-Animal Bond and Euthanasia

LEARNING OBJECTIVES

When you have completed this chapter, you will be able to:
1. Pronounce, define, and spell each of the key terms in this chapter.
2. Discuss aspects of the human–animal bond.
3. List and describe the elements of grief and the role of veterinary professionals in grief counseling.
4. Do the following regarding euthanasia:
   - Discuss the impact of euthanasia and client grief on members of the veterinary health care team.
   - Discuss the legal and ethical issues related to euthanasia.
   - Discuss the role of the veterinary health care team in counseling owners facing the death of their pet and factors that owners need to consider when making decisions regarding euthanasia, natural death, and aftercare.
   - Describe the considerations in training staff and preparing for unexpected events during euthanasia.
   - List the signs and symptoms of staff burnout.
   - List and describe the common methods of euthanasia in large and small animals.
   - Discuss the special considerations related to euthanasia of large animals.

EXERCISE 37.1 MATCHING: TERMS AND DEFINITIONS

Instructions: Match each term in column A with its corresponding definition in column B by writing the appropriate letter in the space provided.

Column A

1. _____ Paradigm
2. _____ Partnering
3. _____ Normalizing
4. _____ Dysthanasia
5. _____ Euthanasia
6. _____ Compassion fatigue
7. _____ Natural death
8. _____ Empathy

Column B

A. A death that happens without euthanasia

B. A healthy approach to help grieving client understand that what they are feeling is acceptable

C. The ability to identify with the emotions and feelings of others

D. Method of intentionally ending a life to relieve suffering

E. A philosophical or theoretical framework that underlies and guides a school of thought

F. A death in which the patient suffers

G. The gradual loss of the ability to respond with empathy due to the frequency and number of demands for such responses

H. Establishing a profound connection with a grieving client

EXERCISE 37.2 DEFINITIONS: KEY TERMS

Instructions: Define each term in your own words.

1. Bond-centered care:_____

_____

2. Anticipatory grief:_____

_____

3. Complicated grief: _____

_____

4. Disenfranchised grief: _____

_____

5. Mourning: _____

_____

6. Burnout: _____

_____

EXERCISE 37.3 TRUE OR FALSE: COMPREHENSIVE

Instructions: Read the following statements and write "T" for true or "F" for false in the blanks provided. If a statement is false, correct the statement to make it true.

1. _____ People often view their pets as family members, children, or companions.

2. _____ The human brain makes no distinction between the loss of a pet and the loss of a human family member.

3. _____ There is currently no formal education for veterinary technicians who wish to specialize in the counseling of grieving clients.

4. _____ Euthanasia is one of the most commonly performed procedures in veterinary medicine.

5. _____ The dominant paradigm in veterinary medicine addresses the emotions surrounding end-of-life care.

6. _____ Veterinary professionals usually receive extensive training on how to counsel grieving clients in professional or technical school as a part of the regular curriculum.

7. _____ Counseling clients during a pet's end-of-life is the job of the veterinarian and is beyond the scope of practice for the veterinary technician or nurse.

8. _____ It is not appropriate to discuss memorialization with the client until death is near.

9. _____ Anthropomorphism is increasingly accepted and even encouraged.

10. _____ Some clients become angry with the veterinary staff in response to loss.

11. _____ The veterinary assistant should not place the intravenous catheter for euthanasia in front of the patient.

12. _____ After death, clients may be permitted to wash the body, take paw imprints, trim hair, or perform other tasks of memorialization.

13. _____ If the client requests euthanasia, the veterinarian must comply.

14. _____ In certain cases, it is clear that euthanasia is the humane thing to do.

15. ____ Sodium pentobarbital may be injected directly into the heart of a cat and small dog.

16. ____ Clients who bury pets on their property risk contaminating the soil and groundwater with euthanasia drugs.

17. ____ Other pets living with the dying or deceased patient will have behavioral changes in the time period leading up to and after death.

EXERCISE 37.4 MULTIPLE CHOICE: COMPREHENSIVE

Instructions: Circle the one correct answer to each of the following questions.

1. Which is an open-ended question?
   a. "Did you adopt her as a puppy?"
   b. "How old is she?"
   c. "What questions do you have about hospice care?"
   d. "Is she in pain?"

2. Which statement made by the veterinary technician is inappropriate?
   a. "Have you thought about what you want to do with his remains?"
   b. "I've been in your shoes before."
   c. "What is most important to you as time grows short?"
   d. "What is your understanding of your pet's condition and prognosis?"

3. A client comes into your practice to euthanize her pet. During the process, she says, "If only I had fed her a better quality food, maybe this would not be happening." This statement best characterizes which stage of the grief process?
   a. Denial
   b. Sadness
   c. Guilt
   d. Relief

4. How can veterinary technicians help a client decide whether or not to euthanize?
   a. Veterinary technicians can explain what they would do if it were their pet.
   b. Veterinary technicians can relate what other clients have done in similar situations.
   c. Veterinary technicians can help the client draw "lines in the sand."
   d. Veterinary technicians can provide a quality of life score.

5. The emotions most deeply felt by grieving clients are
   a. sadness and loneliness.
   b. guilt and sadness.
   c. loneliness and helplessness.
   d. helplessness and sadness.

6. In general, the best way to assist clients who are grieving is to
   a. refer them to a mental health professional.
   b. remind them of the happier times with the pet.
   c. suggest adopting a new pet.
   d. assure them that their feelings are normal.

7. Which is a role of the veterinary technician in end-of-life care?
   a. Recommending when to euthanize
   b. Recommending a natural death
   c. Advocating for quality end-of-life care
   d. Discouraging euthanasia for convenience

8. A reliable measure of the most pet's quality of life is
   a. how much or how often the pet eats.
   b. whether the pet enjoys eating.
   c. how the pet appears physically.
   d. how much the pet weighs.

9. What is an appropriate response to a client who wants to have her dog put down because he is not housetrained?
   a. "That is unethical, and not a good reason to end his life."
   b. "Have you considered rehoming him?"
   c. "Performing convenience euthanasia is illegal in all fifty states."
   d. "You are the world's expert on your pet."

10. Technicians who work for shelters or in research facilities where part of the job is depopulation are specifically susceptible to
    a. denial.
    b. disorganization.
    c. rationalization.
    d. compassion fatigue.

11. The first action of a lethal dose of a barbiturate is to
    a. stop the heart.
    b. restrict respirations.
    c. paralyze the patient.
    d. depress the neurons in the brain stem.

12. _____ is the most common injectable drug for inducing euthanasia.
   a. Intrathecal lidocaine
   b. Magnesium chloride
   c. Potassium chloride
   d. Sodium pentobarbital

13. What kind of drug is dexmedetomidine?
   a. Sedative
   b. Narcotic
   c. Amphetamine
   d. Analgesic

14. If sodium pentobarbital is given in a one-step protocol, which routes must be used?
   a. IV or oral
   b. Intrathecal or intrarenal
   c. IM or subcutaneous
   d. Intrahepatic or intracardiac

15. Why is safety a concern during the euthanasia procedure for a horse?
   a. The patient often thrashes during the administration of anesthesia.
   b. The patient must be reduced to recumbency.
   c. A horse in pain behaves unpredictably.
   d. The patient may resist because it senses its owner's sadness.

16. Which sign is present in the hours before death?
   a. Fluid buildup
   b. Strabismus
   c. Cool extremities
   d. Weight gain

17. The purpose of acepromazine is
   a. Sedation
   b. Analgesia
   c. Tranquilization
   d. Anesthesia

EXERCISE 37.5 FILL-IN-THE-BLANK: COMPREHENSIVE

Instructions: Fill in each of the spaces provided with the missing word or words that complete the sentence.

1. _____ is the term for stretched limbs and a backward arched head.

2. Ultimately, every technician is responsible for his or her own _____, the first line of defense against the emotional hazards of the work.

3. Seen most often in large animals, a patient euthanized without drugs (i.e. by physical methods) may simply be left for

   _____ and for the natural decomposition process to return the body to simpler forms of matter that will support new plant and animal life.

4. The respiratory struggling of an animal in the minutes before it passes is called _____ breathing.

5. _____ is the decomposition of the remains in an alkaline solution of potassium hydroxide and sodium hydroxide in water.

EXERCISE 37.6 MATCHING: PRE-SEDATION, ANESTHESIA, AND EUTHANASIA DRUGS

Instructions: Match each drug in column A with its corresponding purpose in column B by writing the appropriate letters in the space provided. Note that a given drug may have more than one function.

Column A

1. _____ Diazepam

2. _____ Ketamine

3. _____ Xylazine

4. _____ Nalbuphine

5. _____ Hydromorphone

6. _____ Detomidine

7. _____ Pentobarbital

Column B

A. Sedation

B. Muscle relaxation

C. Anesthesia

D. Analgesia

E. Euthanasia

EXERCISE 37.7 CASE STUDY #1: HELPING CLIENTS THROUGH THE GRIEVING PROCESS

Mrs. Andreas came into your clinic today with her 12-year-old female Golden Retriever, Goldie. Goldie had not been feeling well for about a week, and Mrs. Andreas noticed a few large lumps under her jaw. A physical examination revealed generalized enlargement of the peripheral lymph nodes. A complete diagnostic workup was done, including a needle biopsy of the right submandibular lymph node. The tests revealed lymphoma (cancer of the lymph nodes). While the doctor was explaining the disease and the prognosis, Mrs. Andreas looked away and seemed preoccupied with other thoughts. The doctor then tried to discuss treatment options, but Mrs. Andreas cut him off and said she had to leave or Goldie would be late for an appointment at the groomer.

1. Describe an approach you might take to help Mrs. Andreas understand her feelings.

_____

2. What type of grief is Mrs. Andreas experiencing in the days after receiving Goldie's diagnosis?

_____

3. What are some constructive steps you could take to help Mrs. Andreas come to terms with the diagnosis?

_____

_____

_____

_____

_____

_____

4. What can you do to help Mrs. Andreas decide whether it is time to euthanize Goldie?

_____

_____

_____

_____

_____